MATHEMATICAL METHODS
IN
MEDICINE

PART I: STATISTICAL AND ANALYTICAL TECHNIQUES

HANDBOOK OF APPLICABLE MATHEMATICS

Chief Editor: Walter Ledermann

Editorial Board: Robert F. Churchhouse
Harvey Cohn
Peter Hilton
Emlyn Lloyd
Steven Vajda

Assistant Editor: Carol van der Ploeg

GUIDEBOOKS

1: MATHEMATICAL METHODS IN SOCIAL SCIENCE
David J. Bartholomew, *London School of Economics and Political Science*

2: MATHEMATICAL METHODS IN MANAGEMENT
Geoffrey Gregory, *Loughborough University of Technology*

3: MATHEMATICAL METHODS IN MEDICINE
Part I Statistical and Analytical Techniques
Edited by David Ingram, *The Medical College of St. Bartholomew's Hospital*
Ralph Bloch, *McMaster University, Ontario*

4: MATHEMATICAL METHODS IN MEDICINE
Part II Applications in Clinical Specialities
Edited by David Ingram and Ralph Bloch

5: MATHEMATICAL METHODS IN ENGINEERING
Edited by Glyn A. O. Davies, *Imperial College*

6: MATHEMATICAL METHODS IN ECONOMICS
Edited by Frederick van der Ploeg, *London School of Economics and Political Science*

CORE VOLUMES

Volume I: ALGEBRA
Edited by Walter Ledermann, *University of Sussex* and Steven Vajda, *University of Sussex*

Volume II: PROBABILITY
Emlyn Lloyd, *University of Lancaster*

Volume III: NUMERICAL METHODS
Edited by Robert F. Churchhouse, *University College, Cardiff*

Volume IV: ANALYSIS
Edited by Walter Ledermann, *University of Sussex* and Steven Vajda, *University of Sussex*

Volume V: COMBINATORICS AND GEOMETRY (PARTS A AND B)
Edited by Walter Ledermann, *University of Sussex* and Steven Vajda, *University of Sussex*

Volume VI: STATISTICS (PARTS A AND B)
Edited by Emlyn Lloyd, *University of Lancaster*

MATHEMATICAL METHODS
IN
MEDICINE

PART I: STATISTICAL AND ANALYTICAL TECHNIQUES

Edited by

D. INGRAM

Department of Medicine
The Medical College of St Bartholomew's Hospital,
London

R. F. BLOCH

Department of Medicine
McMaster University Medical Centre, Hamilton,
Ontario

A Wiley–Interscience Publication

JOHN WILEY AND SONS

Chichester · New York · Brisbane · Toronto · Singapore

Library of Congress Cataloging in Publication Data:

Ingram, D.
    Mathematical methods in medicine.

    'A Wiley–Interscience publication.'
    Guidebook 3–4 to Handbook of applicable mathematics.
    Includes bibliographical references.
    Contents: pt. 1. Statistical and analytical
techniques.
    1. Medicine—Mathematics. I. Bloch, R. F.
II. Handbook of applicable mathematics. III. Title.
[DNLM: 1. Statistical and analytical techniques.
2. Mathematics. 3. Medicine. QT 35 M4265]
R853.M3153   1984   510'.24616   83-17044

ISBN 0 471 90045 1 (pt. 1)

British Library Cataloguing in Publication Data:

Ingram, D.
    Mathematical methods in medicine.—(Handbook
    of applicable mathematics)
    Pt.1: Statistical and analytical techniques
    1. Medicine—Mathematics
    I. Title   II. Bloch, R. F.   III. Series
    510'.246   R853.M3

    ISBN 0 471 90045 1

Photosetting by Thomson Press (India) Limited, New Delhi
Printed by Page Bros. (Norwich) Ltd.

CONTENTS

Editorial Note xiii

Preface xv

Contributors to the Guidebook xix

Introduction: Mathematics for Medicine 1

1   Medical Statistics: Basic Concepts and Methods 9
    1.1   Introduction 9
        1.1.1   Variation in biology and medicine 10
        1.1.2   The idea of a variable 11
        1.1.3   Descriptive statistics (1): central tendency or location   12
        1.1.4   Descriptive statistics (2): scatter 13
    1.2   Distributions in theory and practice 15
        1.2.1   Distributions, populations and samples 15
        1.2.2   Discrete distributions, independence 16
        1.2.3   Distribution of a continuous variable 18
        1.2.4   The Normal distribution 20
        1.2.5   The χ^2, t and F distributions 21
        1.2.6   Random and non-random samples, randomization   22
        1.2.7   Robustness and 'Normality' 23
        1.2.8   Likelihood and sufficiency 25
        1.2.9   Transformations 26
    1.3   Introduction to statistical inference 27
        1.3.1   Estimation (point estimation) 28
        1.3.2   Hypothesis testing 30
        1.3.3   Type I and type II errors, power 32
        1.3.4   Interpretation of statistical significance 34
        1.3.5   One-sample t test, degrees of freedom 34
        1.3.6   Two-sample t test 36
        1.3.7   Paired t test 38
        1.3.8   Simple non-parametric methods 38
        1.3.9   The chi-squared test on observed counts 40
        1.3.10   Chi-squared on 'contingency tables' 41
        1.3.11   Confidence limits (interval estimation) 43
        1.3.12   Analysis of proportions 45

1.3.13   Simple linear regression   47
1.3.14   Residuals   50
1.3.15   Correlation   52
1.3.16   Different approaches to statistical inference   . . .   53
1.4   Design of medical investigations   55
1.4.1   Asking the right questions   56
1.4.2   The use of controls   57
1.4.3   Deciding sample size for *t* tests and other tests   . .   59
1.4.4   Crossover trials   61
1.4.5   Sequential methods   63
Summary of formulae   64

2   **Medical Statistics: Advanced Techniques and Computation**   . . .   69
2.1   Building statistical models in more complex situations. . .   69
2.1.1   Analysis of variance (ANOVA)   69
2.1.2   Two-way ANOVA and other options.   73
2.1.3   Interpretation of ANOVA for more complicated
        designs   76
2.1.4   Dangers of non-orthogonal ANOVA, missing values   79
2.1.5   Multiple linear regression   81
2.1.6   Analysis of covariance (ANCOVA)   86
2.1.7   Further analysis of proportions and rates   88
2.1.8   Further details on categorical data   91
2.2   Multivariate analysis   94
2.2.1   Introduction to multivariate analysis   94
2.2.2   Principal components analysis   95
2.2.3   Discriminant analysis   98
2.2.4   Other multivariate techniques   99
2.3   Survival analysis   101
2.4   Computation   103
2.4.1   Statistical calculation   104
2.4.2   Computer programs.   105
2.4.3   Uses and abuses of computers   108
References   110

3   **Formal Approaches to the Analysis of Clinical Decisions**   119
3.1   Introduction   119
3.1.1   A place for mathematics   119
3.1.2   The clinical decision problem   120
3.1.3   Diagnosis   122
3.1.4   Further introductory reading   124
3.2   Decision theory   124
3.2.1   A prescription for clinical decision-making   124

3.2.2 Some illustrative examples 129
3.2.3 Assessment of utility 134
3.3 Mathematical methods for diagnosis 136
3.3.1 Principles of discriminant analysis 136
3.3.2 Predictive procedures 141
3.3.3 Bayes' independence model 143
3.3.4 Other methods for modelling feature likelihoods . . 146
3.3.5 Logistic discrimination 148
3.3.6 Use of artificial intelligence 149
3.4 Other related topics 150
3.4.1 Developing a diagnostic rule 150
3.4.2 Measuring observer error 152
3.4.3 Measuring the performance of diagnostic systems . 154
References 156

4 Statistical Methods in Human Genetics and Immunology 161
4.1 Introduction to population genetics 161
4.2 The Hardy–Weinberg theorem 162
4.2.1 Application of the Hardy–Weinberg theorem: estimates of gene frequency 163
4.2.2 Detecting departures from Hardy–Weinberg equilibrium 166
4.2.3 Some effects of inbreeding on the genotypic distribution 169
4.2.4 Some effects of selection and mutation on the genotypic distribution 171
4.3 Comparisons of populations: genetic distance, relative risk and linkage disequilibrium 176
4.3.1 The comparison of genotypic distributions in samples 177
4.3.2 Measures of genetic distance 179
4.3.3 Testing for linkage disequilibrium and the estimation of relevant parameters 184
4.3.4 Studies of the distribution of genetic markers in individuals with diseases 189
4.4 Introduction to genetic studies of human disorders 193
4.5 Estimation of parameters and testing of some simple genetic hypotheses 194
4.5.1 Estimating the probability of ascertainment . . . 194
4.5.2 Testing the hypothesis of a single gene with full penetrance using information about the immediate families of affected individuals 196
4.5.3 Estimation of parameters assuming polygenic transmission 200

4.6   Testing more complex genetic hypotheses   205
       4.6.1   Methods for testing a more general major gene
                hypothesis for qualitative traits   205
       4.6.2   Methods for testing a major gene hypothesis for
                quantitative traits   207
       4.6.3   Linkage studies   209
       A short glossary of terms   214
       References   216

5   **Biological Signal Processing**   225
     5.1   Introduction   225
     5.2   Event and boundary detection   229
            5.2.1   Bayes' theorem for a two-class detector   230
            5.2.2   Detection of small P-waves   232
            5.2.3   Onsets and end-points of waves   235
            5.2.4   Dichrotic notches in arterial pressure waves . . .   238
     5.3   Patterns from signals   240
            5.3.1   Frequency spectrum   240
            5.3.2   Covariance matrix   241
            5.3.3   Typification   241
            5.3.4   Practical implementation   241
     5.4   Data reduction and segmentation   243
            5.4.1   Segmentation of the electrocardiogram   243
            5.4.2   Segmentation for reduction of foetal heart rate
                     patterns   244
            5.4.3   Segmentation of electroencephalograms   244
     5.5   Systems for signal processing   245
            5.5.1   Function laboratories   246
            5.5.2   Computer-assisted intensive care   251
     5.6   Concluding remarks   254
     Appendix 5.A A summary of mathematical definitions and tech-
                  niques encountered in signal processing   255
            5.A.1   Statistical moments   255
            5.A.2   Signals and noise   256
            5.A.3   Transformations   267
     References   270

6   **Mathematical Aspects of Laboratory Medicine**   273
     6.1   Introduction   273
            6.1.1   The role of the clinical laboratory   273
            6.1.2   The place of mathematics in the clinical laboratory   274
     6.2   Definitions   274
            6.2.1   Precision, bias and accuracy   275

6.2.2   Error 275
6.2.3   Assay and assay run 275
6.2.4   Quality control 275
6.2.5   Normal and reference ranges 276
6.3   Laboratory logistics 276
6.4   Variation in biological samples 278
6.4.1   Sampling and the combination of errors 278
6.4.2   Biological rhythms 279
6.4.3   Dynamic tests 280
6.5   Analytical techniques and result derivation 283
6.5.1   The standard curve 283
6.5.2   Linear standard curves 284
6.5.3   Non-linear standard curves 284
6.5.4   Analysis of bio-assay data 285
6.5.5   Validity of curve-fitting 286
6.5.6   Uncertainty of position of the standard curve . . . 288
6.5.7   Assay bias 288
6.5.8   Inherent variation 289
6.5.9   Imprecision and replicate analysis 290
6.5.10 Drift 291
6.5.11 Comparison of analytical methods 293
6.6   Result assessment and quality control 294
6.6.1   Internal quality control techniques 295
6.6.2   External quality assessment techniques 300
References   302

7   **Mathematical Aspects of Pharmacokinetics and Protein–Ligand Binding** 307
71.   Introduction 307
7.2   Compartmental analysis 308
7.2.1   Introduction 308
7.2.2   Rapid intravenous injection in a two-compartment open model 309
7.2.3   First-order absorption in a two-compartment open model 314
7.2.4   A general input and output model 317
7.2.5   Multiple dosing 320
7.2.6   Non-linear systems 321
7.3   Evaluation of pharmacokinetic parameters 323
7.3.1   Graphical technique 323
7.3.2   Numerical technique 324
7.3.3   Examination of the fitted model 325
7.4   Simulation pharmacokinetics 327

7.5   Availability and clearance   328
7.6   Introduction to ligand binding   330
7.7   Mathematical models   331
       7.7.1   The stoichiometric model   332
       7.7.2   The site-binding model.   333
       7.7.3   Applicability of the models   334
7.8   Analysis of binding data   337
       7.8.1   Graphical techniques   337
       7.8.2   Numerical techniques   343
       7.8.3   A strategem for the analysis of binding data . . .   346
7.9   Interpretation of binding coefficients   347
       7.9.1   The affinity profile   347
       7.9.2   Drug distribution   348
7.10   A worked example of drug–protein binding   349
7.11   Further applications   354
References   356

8   **Tracer Techniques and Nuclear Medicine**   361
8.1   Introduction   361
8.2   Radioactive decay   362
       8.2.1   Exponential decay   362
       8.2.2   Parent–daughter relationship   362
       8.2.3   Example—The ^{99m}Tc generator   363
8.3   Radioactive sample counting.   364
       8.3.1   Counting statistics   364
       8.3.2   Combination of counting measurements.   364
       8.3.3   Dual isotope counting   365
       8.3.4   Example—dual isotope vitamin B12 absorption test   367
8.4   Curve processing.   369
       8.4.1   Radioactive decay correction.   369
       8.4.2   Background corrections   370
       8.4.3   Linear least squares fit   370
       8.4.4   Least squares fit to an exponential curve   373
       8.4.5   Exponential stripping   374
       8.4.6   Curve-smoothing.   375
       8.4.7   Deconvolution.   377
       8.4.8   Principal components analysis   380
       8.4.9   Gamma fit   382
8.5   Compartmental analysis   383
       8.5.1   Closed single-compartment system   385
       8.5.2   Open single-compartment system   385
       8.5.3   Example—exchangeable sodium determination . .   387
       8.5.4   Open two-compartment mamillary system   389

8.5.5 Example—Effective renal plasma flow (ERPF) determination 391
8.6 Blood flow 393
 8.6.1 Mean transit time 393
 8.6.2 Cardiac output 395
 8.6.3 Example—blood volume and cardiac output measurement 397
 8.6.4 Organ blood flow 399
 8.6.5 Regional blood flow 401
References 403
Bibliography 404

9 Control Techniques in Drug Administration 405
9.1 Introduction 405
9.2 Post-operative control of blood pressure 410
9.3 Control of anaesthesia 413
 9.3.1 Drug-induced unconsciousness 413
 9.3.2 Drug-induced muscle relaxation 416
 9.3.3 Post-operative pain relief 417
9.4 Control of blood glucose levels 422
9.5 Concluding remarks 425
Glossary of terms 426
References 428

10 Linear Graphs: An Approach to the Solution of Systems of Linear Equations 431
10.1 Introduction 431
10.2 The Laplace transform 432
10.3 Linear graphs; notation and rules for graph reduction . . 432
10.4 Solution of a three-compartment model using a linear graph 435
References 442

Index 443

Editorial Note

Mathematical skills and concepts are increasingly being used in a great variety of activities. Applications of mathematics range from intricate research projects to practical problems in commerce and industry.

Yet many people who are engaged in this type of work have no academic training in mathematics and, perhaps at a late stage of their careers, have neither the inclination nor the time to embark upon a systematic study of mathematics.

To meet the needs of these users of mathematics we have produced a series of texts or *guidebooks* with uniform title. One of these is *Mathematical Methods in Medicine* (with similar books on Engineering, Economics and so on). The purpose of this volume is to describe how mathematics is used as a tool in Medicine and to illustrate it with examples from this field. The guidebooks do not, as a rule, contain expositions of mathematics *per se*. A reader who wishes to learn about a particular mathematical topic, or consolidate his knowledge, is invited to consult the *core volumes* of the *Handbook of Applicable Mathematics;* they bear the titles

- I   Algebra
- II Probability
- III Numerical Methods
- IV Analysis
- V   Combinatorics and Geometry (Parts A and B)
- VI Statistics (Parts A and B)

The core volumes are specifically designed to elaborate on the mathematical concepts presented in the guidebooks. The aim is to provide information readily, to help towards an understanding of mathematical ideas and to enable the reader to master techniques needed in applications. Thus the guidebooks are furnished with references to the core volumes. It is essential to have an efficient reference system at our disposal. This system is explained fully in the Introduction to each core volume; we repeat here the following points. The core volumes are denoted by the Roman numerals mentioned above. Each mathematical item belongs to one of the six categories, namely:

- (i)   Definitions
- (ii) Theorems, propositions, lemmas and corollaries
- (iii) Equations and other displayed formulae

   (iv)   Examples
   (v)   Figures
  (vi)   Tables

A typical item is designated by a Roman numeral followed by three Arabic numerals a, b, c, where a refers to the chapter, b to the section and c to the individual item enumerated consecutively in each category. For example, 'IV Theorem 6.2.3' is the third theorem of section 2 in Chapter 6 of the core volume IV. We refer to equation 6.2.3 of Volume IV as IV (6.2.3), and section 6.2 of Volume IV as IV §6.2.

We trust that these guidebooks will contribute to a deeper appreciation of the mathematical methods available for elucidating and solving problems in all the various disciplines covered by the series.

Preface

The scope of medical research and clinical practice has expanded extremely rapidly over the recent decades and, in the process, many new linkages have been forged between medicine and the so-called 'hard' sciences (physics, chemistry), the biological sciences and the social sciences. The importance of anatomy and physiology for a rational approach to clinical practice and research has been recognized for several hundred years. During the last one hundred years biochemistry and pharmacology have joined these in becoming recognized as basic medical sciences and are now taught in most medical schools. During the same time discoveries in the physical sciences and their application to medical problems have also helped to transform the techniques of diagnosis of disease and the planning and control of treatments. This rapid and pervasive pattern of development, while intellectually very exciting, has created many problems in medical education, in the creation of many new specialities within the wide-ranging health services and in the overall management of these expensive services.

The concepts and computations of mathematics are now essential tools in medical science, in the provision of many routine clinical services and for the rational practice of medicine. The universality of mathematics places it in a special position as a common language which can span many facets of medical practice. However, mathematics itself is not easy and the mathematics applicable to biological science is often peculiarly difficult. It is thus a language not much spoken in clinical medicine. It cannot be applied without medical knowledge and insight since all too often the path may lead down blind-alleys of complexity and practical irrelevance. However, one can perhaps equally argue that without a coherent mathematical framework a rational development of these many interacting components of health services will prove impossible.

The concepts of statistical data analysis are generally accepted as relevant to the basic training of doctors and medical research workers. However, because of other pressures on their time and energy, members of the medical professions are often unaware of other mathematical concepts and techniques and the ways they could be used. The mathematician, on the other hand, frequently lacks insight into the need for certain tools and the value of those already available. Progress can be achieved in several ways: (i) the biomedical practitioner can develop a greater awareness of modern mathematics and of ways of finding methods most suited to a given problem; (ii) the mathematician can become more familiar with those biomedical areas that use mathematical techniques and the, as yet, unfilled needs for mathematical tools in medicine; and (iii) both should attempt to develop a common language sufficient to communicate clearly the nature of the need and the specific features of mathematical tools which might be applied.

The series of six core volumes in the *Handbook of Applicable Mathematics* offers an encyclopaedic view of mathematical concepts and techniques written for the non-mathematician. Yet the gap between these volumes and the traditional study and practice of medicine and biomedicine is still too wide to be crossed in one leap. The two volumes of this Guidebook for mathematical methods in medicine are designed to offer some stepping-stones between the two banks and pathways from both banks towards meeting places. They have four principal objectives:

(a) They should lead the physician or other medical specialist from the familiar medical areas to more abstract but relevant mathematical concepts and tools and indicate appropriate more advanced references.
(b) They should give the mathematically oriented reader an overview of how familiar mathematical techniques are used in various medical fields.
(c) They should define common quantitative terminology in an effort to reduce the risk of misunderstanding due to semantic confusion.
(d) They should directly explain the scope of application of mathematical techniques to the medical or other non-mathematical reader.

We have, of course, found it impossible to simultaneously optimize all four objectives. Individual chapters vary in style and in the emphasis placed on these objectives. Inevitably, the inherent complexity of the subject matter varies considerably between different types of application and it would not be helpful to disguise this fact by attempting to achieve a uniform level of mathematical treatment in the presentation. Part I (this volume) is concerned with the application of statistical methods in medicine and with other general analytical techniques which impinge on many medical specialities. The chapters of Part II (the second volume) discuss applications of mathematics grouped by medical topics, and the discussion of mathematical models is a prominent feature.

Because medicine has become linked with so many basic sciences and the provision of medical care involves so many areas of human activity, it is quite clear that the scope of the Medical Guidebook could easily overlap with virtually every other conceivable Guidebook in the series. We have thus tried to focus our attention on topics arising fairly immediately from consideration of the practice of medicine and medical research. Thus, for example, some may find more of interest to them in a Guidebook on Management Science, operations research skills being widely used in Health Care planning and organization. Informed readers may well differ on the appropriateness of the material chosen. With such a wealth of potential material, we have had to be selective, but perhaps in the course of time it will be possible to revise and update the Guidebook and add new sections to fill in gaps and explain new developments. Because the field is so wide, extensive reference lists are included and we hope these will, in themselves, be of value to readers who wish to follow the material in greater depth and range.

Some texts on mathematics in medicine start with an introductory *tour d'horizon* of the panoply of mathematical tools. That is not the style of this Guidebook since the introduction to basic mathematics is covered in the core volumes of the *Handbook*. We have sought, rather, to introduce in general terms the advantages and pitfalls in adopting quantitative methods in different areas. In a subject like medicine, the developments in application of mathematical methods are often extremely difficult and slow moving. We hope that the chapters of this Guidebook will give a representative view of the state of the art.

We would like to dedicate the books to two outstanding supervisors, supporters and colleagues, Professor John Dickinson and Professor Moran Campbell. Without their own long-standing academic collaboration, recently as Professors of Medicine at The Medical College of St Bartholomew's Hospital and McMaster University Medical School, we would probably never have met and our own collaboration would not have developed. If this work is remotely as successful as their collaborative works on Clinical Physiology it will be due in no small measure to the quality of their guidance and support, although they carry no responsibility for its limitations. It has taken us some three years to assemble and shape the material and we are most grateful to our authors for their support and tolerance of a sometimes rather demanding editorial regime. Also, to the many people who have helped in the preparation, reading and commenting on manuscripts, and especially to Professors E. H. Lloyd and L. Saunders, we express our thanks. We are both very mindful of the strength of support from our families and particularly to Jennifer and Esther.

London　　　　　　　　　　　　　　　　　　　　　　　D. Ingram
Hamilton　　　　　　　　　　　　　　　　　　　　　　R. F. Bloch

Contributors to the Guidebook

R. F. *Bloch*, McMaster University, Hamilton, Ontario, Canada
E. R. *Carson*, The City University, London, England
G. S. *Challand*, Charing Cross Hospital, London, England
T. G. *Coleman*, University of Mississippi, Jackson, U.S.A.
D. G. *Cramp*, Royal Free Hospital Medical School, London, England
C. *Davis*, McMaster University, Hamilton, Ontario, Canada
A. T. *Elliott*, The Western Infirmary, Glasgow, Scotland
S. J. W. *Evans*, The London Hospital Medical College, London, England
R. *Fleming*, The School of Pharmacy, London, England
D. N. *Ghista*, McMaster University, Hamilton, Ontario, Canada
J. E. *Hall*, University of Mississippi, Jackson, U.S.A.
J. *Hewson*, McMaster University, Hamilton, Ontario, Canada
A. S. *Houston*, Royal Naval Hospital, Haslar.
D. *Ingram*, The Medical College of St Bartholomew's Hospital, London, England
R. *Lawson*, The Royal Infirmary, Manchester, England
D. *Linkens*, The University of Sheffield, England
J. *Mazumdar*, University of Adelaide, Australia
E. *McCutcheon*, University of South Carolina, Columbia, U.S.A.
P. W. *Macfarlane*, University of Glasgow, Scotland
R. *McGee*, McMaster University, Hamilton, Ontario
N. R. *Mendell*, State University of New York at Stonybrook, U.S.A.
M. F. *Petrini*, University of Mississippi, Jackson, U.S.A.
J. E. H. *Shaw*, The Medical College of St Bartholomew's Hospital, London, England
M. *Sherriff*, The Royal Dental Hospital, London, England
A. *Skene*, University of Nottingham, England
R. D. *Speller*, Middlesex Hospital Medical School, London, England
P. *Stein*, Henry Ford Hospital, Detroit, U.S.A.
A. *Todd-Pokropek*, University College, London, England
J. H. *van Bemmel*, Free University, Amsterdam, Holland
F. E. *Ward*, Duke University, North Carolina, U.S.A.
T. E. *Wheldon*, MRC Cyclotron Unit, Hammersmith Hospital, London, England
D. R. *White*, St Bartholomew's Hospital, London, England

Mathematical Methods in Medicine
Edited by D. Ingram & R. F. Bloch
© 1984 John Wiley & Sons Ltd.

Introduction—Mathematics for Medicine

The practice of medicine has developed and fared well over the centuries without recourse to mathematics. Doctors have prided themselves on their mastery of a discipline involving a subtle balance of scientific knowledge, technical skills and insight in human relationships. Where the mechanisms of disease are discussed, often only a qualitative exposition is attempted and is usually difficult to improve upon because of the large inherent variability of living organisms. It is often felt that the precise formulations of mathematics are not applicable in such a complex field. However, as medicine itself has evolved extremely rapidly in recent times, the scientific support called upon by the practising clinician has often become complex.

In medicine, more than in most fields, research and practice are closely related. Many diseases which doctors have to treat are understood only incompletely and are still the subject of considerable research effort. Many treatments have been arrived at empirically and are studied in an attempt to understand their mode of action. In medical science, in contrast to the 'hard' sciences, one is studying and treating a complex living organism and devising methods to assist it in remaining or becoming 'healthy'. In the technological sciences the aim, by contrast, is to investigate and understand basic properties of matter and then make use of them to design systems which will meet specified requirements. Medicine intervenes in the natural control mechanisms of the body to restore, or assist the body itself to restore, a normal state of function, as far as can be achieved.

The practice of medicine, aside from its essentially human content, which is manifest in all areas, now incorporates scientific and technological support at many levels: in the processes of investigation of disease; in the reaching of decisions concerning treatments; in the implementation of treatments; in the assessment of the effectiveness and value of these various activities; in fundamental research aimed at increasing knowledge and understanding through which medical practice can be improved. Let us consider some specific examples.

A major innovation of the past decade has been the development of computerized tomographic scanning equipment based on detection of the decay of injected radioisotopes, on the transmission of X-rays or, now, on radiofrequency nuclear magnetic resonance. In all cases, a section of the body is scanned and the measurements processed to create a pictorial reconstruction of

1

the section. The image contains information in terms of the distribution of the radioisotope, attenuation of X-rays by the tissues, or magnetic resonance phenomena within the section 'viewed'. Such techniques for visualizing organ structure and function have become integral to many modern techniques of diagnosis and treatment.

In the early care of patients who have had a kidney transplant, there is continuous surveillance for signs of graft rejection and gearing of immuno-suppressant drug treatment to early signs of trouble. A high quality of information regarding the onset of rejection episodes is a clinical priority.

In the treatment of many diseases, the drugs used are themselves harmful agents chosen to attack the disease process but often, as a side-effect, capable of upsetting or damaging normal function of the body. This is perhaps particularly true of chemotherapy for treatment of cancers. Similarly, many treatments seek to maintain levels of measured variables such as blood pressure or blood glucose concentration where the normal control mechanism has broken down (perhaps temporarily, as in the control of blood pressure in a patient under intensive care following open-heart surgery, or permanently, as in the case of control of blood sugar concentrations in a patient with severe diabetes). In all cases precise procedure is a clinical necessity.

Rigorous means for assessment of the efficacy of medical procedures are important where, as with any scientific endeavour, the perils of self-deception must always be guarded against. There are many reasons for wanting to investigate or treat a patient in a particular way and for organizing resources accordingly—not all necessarily based on medical issues. Objective methods for weighing evidence and publishing informative conclusions are essential to the rational practice and development of medicine.

In the areas covered by these examples, there is a clear, well-appreciated, case for application of mathematical concepts and techniques. However, these are tools to be used with knowledge and understanding if they are to help to clarify, improve and develop medical science and patient care.

There would probably be no disagreement with this claim that mathematics is an important unifying language of a large number of diagnostic and therapeutic procedures but it would be contentious to argue that mathematical approaches have made an impact or have much to offer in aiding the clinician in his daily round of interviewing patients, arranging for diagnostic tests and deciding upon, commissioning, reviewing and amending treatments.

When we attempt to use mathematics in a medical context, difficulties arise because of the immense variability of biological systems, though within a species the systems function according to the same underlying control criteria but in a rather 'fault tolerant' manner. High precision is not often required for 'normal function' of the body. Hence, in building a tomographic scanner, how do we assess the quality of image obtained? Are improved images valuable and to be aimed at in their own right? Do they ultimately enable more effective treatments to be made? In treatment of a tumour with radiotherapy, how accurately should the treatment volume be defined and how precisely should the treatment plan encompass this volume? In the control of blood sugar concentration in a diabetic, how important is it to maintain target levels? In terms of possible complications of the disease in the longer term, what are the implications of failure to achieve control?

The practice of medicine is a highly individual and experimental science (as individual patients and individual doctors differ so much); subjective valuations of alternative outcomes must be made and thus many questions, such as those above, though highly relevant to clinical medicine, are extraordinarily difficult to answer convincingly. If medicine is to develop and resolve such uncertainties it must come to grips with these essentially quantitative issues.

We now turn to some more general issues concerning the usefulness of quantitative methods. The development of modern science and technology has, on a philosophical level, been characterized by the enrichment and sometimes, though not always to advantage, the replacement of semantic by quantitative reasoning. The language of quantitative reasoning is mathematics. What then are the advantages of quantitative reasoning? Are there problems which are only solvable through the use of mathematics? Is it possible to deal with some problems faster through the use of mathematics? On the negative side, what are the weaknesses of using the mathematical methods?

One of the first points to be made in justification of a more quantitative approach to the present-day practice of medicine is that verbal reasoning alone is not adequate. The history and practice of medicine is rife with wrong conclusions resulting from semantic ambiguities. These can result from using one word to refer to different phenomena, a phenomenon being described by different words and by the inadequacy of semantic language to describe different grades of an occurrence.

Verbal reasoning is limited by the number of items that the mind can cope with simultaneously at one time. It has been suggested that seven items of information represent a 'magical number' beyond which it becomes practically impossible to remember, manipulate and interpret significance. One's attitude to these items of information will usually vary over a range from the dogmatic ('such and such *is* so') through the indeterminate ('such and such may be so') to the completely nescient ('such and such may or may not be so, and we have simply no idea which is the case'). Mathematical formulations help to clarify determinate situations and may also be able to deal with indeterminates, by quantifying the relative plausibilities of the various possible cases and working with probabilities.

Another major justification for the introduction of quantitative reasoning lies in its economy. Rather than having to reason through each event in specific terms, it is possible to apply pre-packaged 'thought modules' or solution algorithms. These algorithms have usually been well worked out and validated and the scientist using such a tool does not have to reinvent the technique each time. By formalizing problems, it often becomes possible to recognize archetypal situations for which solution processes have already been devised. If a clearly wrong conclusion is reached using quantitative reasoning, it is possible to relate it to a source of error in the reasoning process or to assumptions which may have to be challenged. If predicted results deviate from experimental findings it is possible to trace the error or wrong assumption.

One of the most significant features of quantitative reasoning is its ability to allow us to test the completeness of our knowledge. This leads to classical experimental paradigms. By combining a set of known facts using a mathematical procedure, the scientist arrives at a prediction of how a system should behave under given circumstances. He then performs an experiment in which he creates the circumstances and observes the response of the system. Deviations between the predicted and observed results indicate the incompleteness of knowledge. Conversely, however, agreement between prediction and observation does not prove the correctness of the thought or the completeness of the knowledge. It only assures us that, within the range of assumptions and definition of the experiment, no contradiction has been found.

Within a given experimental framework, data measured to reveal features of interest are usually contaminated by 'signal error' or 'noise'. Mathematical techniques make possible the design of special filters which can significantly improve the signal to noise ratio, making use of known features of the true signal such as periodicity. Most diagnostic processes are based on quantifying physical manifestations of biological processes. After a diagnosis has been arrived at, mathematics can assist in devising, designing, describing and optimizing therapeutic interventions. For treatments with low therapeutic indices, such as anticoagulation or radiotherapy, it is crucial to use quantitative techniques in order to reap maximal therapeutic benefit while causing minimal harm.

Most importantly, mathematics allows us to describe, measure and evaluate the effects of diagnostic and therapeutic manoeuvres on the state of health of individuals and groups, that is the field of clinical epidemiology. Health care technology uses the tools of mathematics quite freely in devising diagnostic and therapeutic procedures. However, we can only be confident in assessing their validity if a properly designed trial has been executed. Acquisition of knowledge can be extremely costly. Mathematical reasoning allows us more effectively to bring together and correlate the relevant available information and can enable its efficient and effective use.

We must now equally emphasize the limitations and possible risks inherent in quantitative reasoning or in the application of mathematics in medicine. In today's world we sometimes behave as if conditioned to accept results produced by mathematical reasoning as the truth, and forget the pitfalls. This can give rise to overconfidence in statements derived from mathematical reasoning. Among these are:

(a) Wrong assumptions. The data on which reasoning is based and conclusions drawn are inaccurate or incomplete. The model used to fit the data is not appropriate.

(b) Wrong processing. Simple errors or computational errors have occurred.
(c) Wrong conclusions. The quantitative evidence does not support the conclusions drawn.

A mathematical analysis of clinical decision-making can be both illuminating and helpful to physicians in making better, more informed decisions. However, there are aspects of these decisions for which our mathematical tools are quite inadequate and where human judgement is better able to cope. These are, for example, in the weighing of disparate classes of information, in the recognition of patterns of information and in dealing with essentially human issues.

The art of applied mathematics is to some extent the art of the soluble, and simplification of a mathematical model is often required if the resulting formulation is to be mathematically tractable or capable of solution. A highly precise formulation of a problem is of little value if it cannot be solved either through lack of sufficiently detailed data or because of inherent mathematical complexity.

Before introducing the material contained in the Guidebook, it may be useful to outline in general terms how mathematics becomes involved in attempts to improve our understanding of normal processes and thus, implicitly, of deviations from normality. The investigative process may be described in terms of six idealized steps:

(a) Measurement. A natural variable is observed and transformed onto the set of rational numbers.
(b) Correlation. The measurement of a given variable is usually performed in relationship to one or more other variables and/or controlled conditions.
(c) Idealization. The relationship among the variables is expressed by the simplest plausible mathematical relationship (often a linear one).
(d) Induction. From such apparent relationships one tries to infer a general normative relationship such as the gas laws or the law of gravity in physics.
(e) Prediction/deduction. By combining several inferred results one generates a model that predicts the behaviour of the system studied under given circumstances.
(f) Testing. The model is tested by recreating the circumstances in the system studied and comparing observations with the model predictions. Testing can be done either in a positive sense, where one looks for agreement between the model predictions and the observed system, or in a negative sense, where it is shown that alternative models do not agree with reality.

It would be difficult to fit practical applications of mathematics in medicine and medical research neatly into such an idealized structure. For most people mathematical methods in medicine begin and end with statistical methods, but there are many other analytical techniques which are of well-established and general interest across a range of medical specialities. This volume (Part I) therefore starts from the familiar area of medical statistics and extends from there to discussion of the mainly analytical techniques of signal analysis, compartmental modelling, as applied, for example, to pharmacokinetics, and numerical analysis applied to the modelling of reversible binding of drugs or other endogenous molecular species to protein or other receptor sites. Then we include application of the theory of control mechanisms with the specific clinical examples of the control of drug administration and finally a short presentation of the use of linear graphs in the solution of systems of linear equations, which is particularly useful for sparse systems and is found useful by many non-mathematicians. Interleaved with these chapters on general techniques there are chapters of a more applied kind, which are nonetheless relevant to a number of clinical specialities, on genetics and immunology, analysis of laboratory data and tracer techniques.

Chapter 1 examines basic concepts of medical statistics and, using common medical examples, shows how they are applied in medical investigations. The main relevant formulae are grouped and tabulated.

Chapter 2 examines some of the more advanced techniques of statistics, often essential in practice, again making use of medical examples. It concludes with a discussion of the commonly used computational packages and some discussion of how they should be approached. A very extensive set of references on medical statistics is included at the end of Chapter 2.

Chapter 3 picks up the topic of approaches to the formal analysis of clinical decision-making. This is written primarily for the clinician since it covers the area of his everyday work. The more mathematical issues are introduced and relevant detail pointed to in further general and specific references.

Chapter 4 concerns application of statistical methods in human genetics and introduces the mathematical concepts which are particularly relevant to human immunology and the genetic analysis of disease. The chapter summarizes quantitative methods in this field and gives many worked examples of the techniques in practice.

Chapter 5 considers the mathematical aspects of analysing biological signals. Although some specific examples, notably the electrocardiogram, are considered in detail in the second volume (Part II), this chapter gives an overview of the techniques available, the assumptions made in using them and examples of how these must be tailored to particular applications.

Chapter 6 reviews a mathematical framework relevant to the work of a hospital routine laboratory. A common terminology is defined and particular attention paid to the problems of quality control in laboratory tests.

Chapter 7 discusses mathematical analysis of pharmacokinetics, the absorption, distribution and elimination of pharmacological agents in the body, and the treatment of saturable binding of circulating substances to different classes of ligand molecule. These have relevance to many fields of medicine. Thus, for example, in enzyme kinetics, drug-receptor binding or radioimmunoassay of endogenous hormones, similar mathematical issues arise. The pitfalls of ill-considered applications of textbook methods are highlighted.

Chapter 8 is concerned with the use of tracer techniques in clinical measurement, notably in the area of diagnostic nuclear medicine using injected radioisotopes. This chapter builds on the concepts of compartmental analysis introduced in Chapter 7. It also covers radioactive sample counting and curve processing and gives a variety of worked examples of the techniques from several clinical fields.

Chapter 9 introduces the concepts of control theory which have been exploited in the design of controllers for administration of drugs in a number of clinical specialities such as anaesthesia, intensive care and medical management of diabetes.

Chapter 10 presents an approach to the analysis of systems of linear equations which is based on the technique of linear graphs. This technique has advantages for sparse systems of equations as well as being quite straightforward to understand and apply, and is therefore likely to be of value to medical researchers wanting to develop mathematical models of biological systems.

It is also appropriate in this introduction to discuss the plan of material in the second volume of the Guidebook. There, more emphasis is placed on mathematical models which underlie quantitative understanding in the different fields. The stages in investigation and modelling described above have helped at the most fundamental level towards an understanding of the normal function of body systems. Once 'normal' is understood, causation and course of deviations from normal can be examined quantitatively. On the basis of such knowledge, diagnostic processes may be designed and optimized. However, it is still comparatively rare for these mathematical models, which are mainly deterministic in concept, to find a role in everyday clinical routine, though there is a clearly demonstrable emerging role in medical education where they can be valuable in communicating the essence of how body systems function and are integrated within the body. As discussed above, the general models of control theory, by contrast, are finding a practical role in specific clinical tasks such as the control of nitro-prusside administration to regulate blood pressure in an intensive care unit. The aim of Part II is to take a number of the main clinical areas in which mathematical methods have been widely applied and to show the basis of such application. Inevitably this involves a good deal of discussion of the quantitative frameworks applicable. Although elementary to some, it is our experience that many of the barriers to application of mathematics are at the level of defining a suitable framework of quantification of the systems of interest.

In part II the areas covered include:

Oncology
Diagnostic imaging

Radiology, radiotherapy and radiation protection
Endocrinology and human metabolism
Quantitative aspects of respiration, circulation and kidney function
Clinical management of body fluid volumes and acid–base balance
Anaesthesia
Cardiology
Biomechanical analysis of circulation

With medical research and practice so intertwined and with mathematics playing an increasing role in diagnostic and therapeutic processes, an understanding of mathematical concepts and applications becomes increasingly desirable. Perhaps more effective collaborations between mathematicians, scientists and clinicians holds the main promise for achieving practical benefits from the wide range of mathematical applications in medicine which already exist.

Mathematical Methods in Medicine
Edited by D. Ingram & R. F. Bloch
© 1984 John Wiley & Sons Ltd.

1

Medical Statistics: Basic Concepts and Methods

1.1 INTRODUCTION

In the first two chapters we have aimed to cover most of the commonly used techniques in medical statistics, giving examples of their use and some intuitive explanations of the underlying theory. It is intended that the reader with only a very limited background in statistics will be able to follow most of the material. The more difficult sections have been set in smaller type. References are given, where possible, to available textbooks and to useful medical examples rather than to specialized literature, and these should be consulted together with the *Handbook of Applicable Mathematics* for further details.

In Chapter 1 we introduce the main statistical concepts; several important formulae are collected together in a table at the end of the chapter for easy reference. Chapter 2 introduces more advanced methods such as analysis of variance, multivariate analysis and survival analysis, ending with a discussion of the role of computers. References for the two chapters are grouped together and listed at the end of Chapter 2.

The following rough guide suggests which sections are likely to be most relevant to the various parts of a medical investigation. However, since our overall aim is to enable the reader to gain a 'feel' for medical statistics, the indicated sections are not really intended just to be read in isolation.

Design stage
See Sections 1.1.1, 1.2.6, 1.3.3 and all of Section 1.4.
Analysis
Comparison of two means: Sections 1.3.6, 1.3.7, 1.3.8 and 1.3.11.
Comparison of two proportions: Sections 1.3.10, 1.3.12 and 2.1.7.
More than two means: Sections 2.1.1 and 2.1.3.
More than two proportions: Sections 2.1.7 and 2.1.8.
Adjusting two or more means for bias: Sections 2.1.2, 2.1.3, 2.1.4 and 2.1.6.
Simple correlation and regression: Sections 1.3.13, 1.3.14 and 1.3.15.
Testing a normal distribution: Section 1.2.7.

Computers and calculations in general: Sections 2.4.1, 2.4.2 and 2.4.3.
Interpretation
See particularly Sections 1.3.4, 1.3.15 and 2.4.3.

1.1.1 Variation in biology and medicine

In many of the physical sciences, the variation in measurements is due to fluctuations in the measurement process itself rather than in the value of the quantity being measured. For example, the velocity of light and the gravitational constant are themselves constant and variation in the results is essentially due to experimental error. In biology and medicine we have a different problem: there is real variation in the quantities being measured because the individuals differ in many ways. However accurate the experimental method, the results will vary because of the nature of what is studied, as well as varying due to the experimental method. There is no 'true' single value for the heights of adult males in the United Kingdom. 'Statistics' is a set of methods for describing and quantifying variation and for drawing inferences about variation; as such it has particular relevance to medicine.

For example, suppose we are comparing blood pressure measurements on hypertensive subjects who have been given different treatment drugs. We anticipate different responses to treatment, and we are mainly interested in the deliberately imposed *between-treatment* variation. Unfortunately this will be partly obscured by *inter-subject* variation (variation *between* individual subjects due to differences in age, sex, initial blood pressure before treatment, etc.).

The inter-subject variation is itself difficult to evaluate because of *intra-subject* variation (variation *within* a subject: a given person's blood pressure varies because of changes in his diet, emotional state, etc.). On top of all this will be *measurement error* because of variable laboratory equipment and finally *observer variability* in using the equipment and reading off the measurements.

For a carefully designed study, *statistical analysis* is able to indicate how much of the observed variation is attributable to these different sources, ultimately giving an idea of the real difference between treatments. Any unattributed variation is called *random variation* or random error. Note that the term 'error' in statistics is used to mean essentially 'variation due to causes which have not been explained' and does not necessarily imply that a mistake has been made [see VI, §8.3].

It is particularly important in medical statistics to consider the sources of variation, and we must not mix up inter-subject analysis and intra-subject analysis. For example, if we want to examine the association between blood pressure and dose of hypotensive drug, then we will usually be most interested in the association *within* a particular individual or group ('is treatment good for you?'). Single measurements of the blood pressures and dose levels for several individuals can be totally misleading: people are treated because they are ill, so in the general community higher doses of hypotensive drug may appear to be associated with higher rather than with lower blood pressure. The fallacy is easy to spot in this instance, but may not be so clear elsewhere.

We must try to minimize the effects of sources of variation in which we are not interested by using a carefully *designed* medical investigation: **the statistical aspects of any problem must be considered right from the start.**

1.1.2 The idea of a variable [see II, §§4.1 and 4.2]

A *variable* is some characteristic that differs from subject to subject or from time to time. A variable may be *numerical* (e.g. blood pressure in millimetres of mercury) or not (e.g. primary site of cancer).

Numerical (or *quantitative*) variables may be 'continuous' or 'discrete'. A *continuous* variable is one which can take values anywhere in some continuous range. For example:

(a) Seriousness of burn measured as a percentage of body surface area can take any value from 0 to 100.
(b) Blood pressure in millimetres of mercury or weight in kilograms might take any positive value.
(c) Change in blood pressure after treatment can take any value (positive or negative).

Discrete data usually occur as whole numbers or *integers* (e.g. for expectant mothers, the number of previous pregnancies). In general the possible values for a discrete variable are separate, with intermediate values (such as 2.7 pregnancies) being meaningless.

Non-numeric (or *qualitative*) variables are obtained by classifying data into groups or *categories* (e.g. lung, breast, bowel, other). There may be a natural ordering among the categories: a patient's condition may be assessed as good, fair, poor, serious, critical or dead. We might also have unordered categories (sometimes called *nominal* data) such as blood group (O, A, B, AB) or site of cancer. A particular case is *binary* data where the variable can take one of two values, such as dead/alive, male/female or with/without complications.

The different types of variables are measured on correspondingly different scales. Thus unordered categories constitute a *nominal scale*, binary data a *dichotomy*. If the possible values are ordered then we have an *ordinal scale* (e.g. the patient's condition). An ordinal scale with a well-defined distance between any two possible values is called an *interval scale*. For example, temperature is measured on an interval scale and the statement 'patient A has a temperature 1 Centigrade degree higher than patient B' has a clear meaning whatever patient B's actual temperature. If an interval scale has a true zero, representing 'absence', then it is a *ratio scale*. Thus weight is measured on a ratio scale and someone who weighs 60 kg can be said to be 25 per cent lighter than someone weighing 80 kg.

This is independent of the units of measurement: he would still be 25 per cent lighter if weight were in pounds. By contrast, the zero point for degrees Centigrade is arbitrary (and different from that for degrees Fahrenheit), so temperature as normally used is not measured on a ratio scale.

Our analysis of data depends on the types of variables recorded, although we may legitimately change the type of variable. For example, numerical data may be *grouped* into ordered categories (e.g. age less than 20, 20 to 29, 30 to 39, 40 to 49, 50 +), and we usually analyse categorical data by counting the number of subjects occurring in each category (e.g. the number of cancer patients seen where the primary cancer site is the lung, the breast, the bowel, or some other site) and analysing this count as a discrete numerical variable [see VI, §3.2].

For convenience and simplicity, discrete variables are often analysed as though they were continuous and ordered categories are sometimes analysed as though they were unordered. Note also that in practice 'continuous' data are in effect discrete, since we can only measure to a given accuracy.

Usually each *unit* (i.e. subject, patient or experimental animal) has many variables measured, and it is helpful to distinguish between *response variables* (or *outcomes*) which measure a particular effect (e.g. survival time) and *explanatory variables* (e.g. dose), whose different values may help 'explain' some of the variation in the response variable.

Variables are usually denoted by capital letters (X, Y) and their values by lower-case letters (x, y); if we want to distinguish between individual values we should *index* them $(x_1, x_2$ or, in general, $x_i)$. However, we sometimes bend these rules to make things easier to follow.

1.1.3 Descriptive statistics (1): central tendency or location

'Descriptive statistics' is the art of illustrating the nature of variation and of presenting a summary of that variation in a way that shows the important features of data to the reader. With a set of 100 successive live births in a hospital we would want to be able to summarize the recorded weights at birth rather than list all the weights themselves. An obvious summary is to work out their (arithmetic) *mean*, often simply called their average. This involves adding all the weights together and dividing by 100, the number of observations.

Mathematical shorthand for this equation uses the Greek capital letter for S, sigma, to stand for 'sum all the numbers'. If we use x_i to stand for the weight of the *i*th individual, then the equation for mean weight $(\bar{x})$ is given by

$$\bar{x} = \sum_{i=1}^{100} \frac{x_i}{100},$$

read as 'sum the weights x_i for all values of *i* from 1 to 100 and divide by 100'. In general the mean is given by formula (1.1.1) (see the summary of formulae at the end of this chapter). Sometimes the subscripts and range of summation are dispensed with: $\bar{x} = \sum x/n$ ('sum all the observations and divide by *n*') [see II, §8.1].

To summarize the 100 birth weights we may say that they have a mean of 3,250 grams. On dealing with 100 measurements which do not have any extreme values, the mean will be an adequate summary measure of where the centre is situated. However, if the number of observations is small then a single extreme value (called an *outlier*) can alter the mean dramatically. In such cases it is sensible to put the values into order of increasing size and to take the middle value (or the mean of the two middle values if there is an even number of observations); this middle value is called the *median* and is not affected by outliers [see II, §10.4.2]. This property, known as *robustness*, will be returned to later (Section 1.2.7).

There are many instances in medicine where a median may be much more appropriate than a mean. An important area is where radioactive counting methods are used: extreme values in either direction may occur and using the median is usually better than deciding subjectively which values to ignore. Mean and median are examples of measures of *central tendency* or *location*. Another measure is the *mode*, which is the most frequently occurring value; unfortunately a large number of observations is necessary in order for the mode to be reliable [see II, §10.1.3].

There are other robust measures such as *trimmed means* where equal numbers of the highest and lowest values are ignored and we obtain the mean of the middle values. A similar idea gives *Winsorized means* where the few highest and the few lowest observations are replaced by less extreme values. Some computer packages now produce robust measures of location (e.g. Dixon *et al.*, 1983).

In practice the choice of measure of location is necessarily subjective, and we must be especially careful when deciding whether or not to reject a particular observation as an outlier (e.g. if we are using a trimmed mean). Note, however, that the two extremes of 'no trimming' and 'maximum trimming' give rise to the mean and median respectively, so any trimmed mean is typically just a compromise between the mean and the median.

1.1.4 Descriptive statistics (2): scatter [see II, §§9.1 and 10.4.2]

The summaries of location on their own conceal almost as much as they reveal: they tell us the magnitude of a 'typical' value but give us no idea of the extent of variation in the data. An immediate question is, therefore, 'How close to 3,250 g are the 100 weights?'

The simplest measure of scatter in the data is the *range*, 3,000 g in this case. This is the difference between the largest and the smallest value. The range has the considerable advantages of easy calculation and interpretation, although it is even more informative to quote the minimum and maximum observed values: 'The range is 1,500 to 4,500 g.' However, for the following reasons the range should never be used as the *sole* measure of scatter:

(a) It is *unstable*; minimum and maximum values usually vary enormously between sets of data.

(b) It is *intractable* (awkward to analyse mathematically).

(c) It is *inefficient*, only considering the two most extreme observed values.

(d) It is inappropriate for *comparison* of scatter between different data sets; the more data we have, the more likely we are to see very large or very small values, so the expected value of the range increases with the number of data.

A more efficient measure of scatter will tell us how close most of the values are to 3,250 g; we could, for example, take each value and note how far it is from the mean. Thus 3,000 g is 250 g below the mean and we say that its deviation from the mean (often called a *residual*) is -250 g, while 3,600 has a deviation of 350 g. If we add up all the deviations taking the sign into account we obtain a total of zero. However, if we ignore the signs and divide by 100 we get an average of the absolute deviations from the mean, called the *mean absolute deviation* or *MAD*.

The MAD is given in formula (1.1.2), where the notation is the same as before and the vertical lines mean 'take the absolute value of' [see I, (2.6.5)]. Mathematically this is still not easy to deal with, though some modern techniques using computers do use the MAD.

Another way to get rid of the signs of the residuals is to square them, the average squared residual being called the (sample) *variance*. For technical reasons, mentioned in Section 1.3.5, we usually divide the sum of the squared residuals by $(n-1)$ rather than by n; this makes very little difference unless n is small. The variance is therefore given by formula (1.1.3), which may be rearranged to give formula (1.1.4) (which is sometimes easier to work with).

The variance (like the MAD) has many advantages over the range, being easy to calculate, fairly stable and using information from all the data values [see VI, §§3.1 and 3.3]. Since it also has exactly the same expected value for any sample size n [see VI, §2.3.2] and is much more tractable mathematically, it is generally the best measure of scatter to use in statistical theory.

The *standard deviation* (SD or s.d.), the square root of the variance, has the same units as the original quantity and is therefore more useful than the variance when it comes to presenting results. For example, if the variable concerned is a weight measured in grams, then the mean and s.d. are also in grams, but the variance is in grams squared. An intuitive interpretation of the standard deviation is that roughly two-thirds of the data values lie within one s.d. either side of the mean. Unfortunately this interpretation can be erroneous because the standard deviation is even more sensitive to outliers than is the mean.

We may therefore want a more robust measure of scatter; analogous to the median as a measure of scatter is the *inter-quartile range* (IQR). Here the data values are put in order of magnitude and the value which has 25 per cent of values below it (the *lower quartile*) is noted, as is also the value with 25 per cent of values above it (the *upper quartile*). The interquartile range is the distance between these and includes 50 per cent of all the values.

Measures of scatter are also known as measures of *spread* or *scale*. Of course, sets of data may still be very different even if they have similar location and scatter, so measures of *shape* may be useful. *Skewness* is a measure of asymmetry and *Kurtosis* indicates whether the data are fairly evenly spread or whether the scatter in the data is just due to a few atypical values. Skewness and Kurtosis are given in formulae (1.1.6) and (1.1.7), and are discussed further in Section 1.2.4 [see II, §9.10].

1.2 DISTRIBUTIONS IN THEORY AND PRACTICE

We can use observed values to get an idea of the 'distribution' of a variable (Sections 1.2.1 to 1.2.5). We must consider whether we are justified in doing this (Sections 1.2.6 and 1.2.7) but, if we are, then theoretical ideas such as likelihood (Section 1.2.8) and practical ideas like transformations (Section 1.2.9) may help us.

1.2.1 Distributions, populations and samples

A lot of information can be assimilated and conveyed using purely descriptive statistics (see, for example, Peto, 1979). However, if we want to generalize our findings we need some idea of their reliability, which brings us into the world of probability and statistical distributions.

The *probability* of occurrence of some event (e.g. the death of a patient) may be thought of either as the long-run relative frequency with which the event occurs ('What proportion of patients with this disease have been seen to die as a result of it?') or as a subjective assessment by an informed observer ('What are his chances, Doctor?') [see II, §2.3].

An observed *frequency distribution* is a convenient way of summarizing data, indicating the probability of occurrence of each possible value. For example, Table 1.2.1 gives the number of labelled cells in each of fifty sets of 1,000 cells (eight sets had no labelled cells, thirteen had one, etc.) [see II, §2.2]. If we took another fifty sets of 1,000 cells and so tabulated a second frequency distribution, we would expect this second table to be similar to the first (for example, few of the sets would contain four or more labelled cells) but not identical, because of biological variation.

This expresses the idea that a *sample* of observations (each observation here being 'number of labelled cells per thousand') is taken from an underlying *population* of all possible observations and that the sample is somehow representative of the population [see II, §§3.1 to 3.3]. In other words, the observed frequency distribution is similar to some actual *population distribution* and in particular the observed mean, median, standard deviation, etc., are close to some theoretical values for the mean, median, s.d., etc. The population may be a hypothetical idea, as in our example, or may actually be a physical reality like 'children in the Isle of Wight'.

Table 1.2.1 Distribution of labelled cells.

Number of labelled cells	Frequency
0	8
1	13
2	10
3	7
4	7
5	2
6	2
7	0
8	1
9 or more	0
Total	50

A useful technique is to assume some standard form for the population distribution and then to use the observed sample to specify this assumed distribution exactly. For example, a *Poisson distribution* arises as the count of the number of independent times an unlikely event occurs in a fixed interval [see II, §5.4]. Since labelled cells only appeared occasionally, it might seem reasonable to assume that the variable defined by 'number of labelled cells seen in a sample of 1,000' follows a Poisson distribution.

In general, the *probability distribution* of a variable is a formula or rule giving the probabilities that the variable takes each of its possible values. Probability distributions usually involve symbols called *parameters* which indicate location, scatter or shape; these parameters must be given values before the probabilities can be calculated [see II, §4.3]. For example, to specify a Poisson distribution exactly we need one parameter, the mean (in this context 'mean' stands for 'population mean', or 'expected value'). The observed *sample mean* is 2.24 (the average of eight '0's, thirteen '1's, ten '2's, etc.) so a reasonable guess for the approximate population distribution of labelled cells per thousand is 'Poisson with mean 2.24'.

1.2.2 Discrete distributions, independence [see II, Chapter 5 and §3.5]

The probability distribution of a discrete-valued variable is called a *discrete distribution*; an example is the Poisson distribution (mentioned in Section 1.2.1) which can take the values 0, 1, 2, or any other non-negative integer. If X is a variable distributed as Poisson with mean m, then the probability that $X = n$ (a non-negative integer) is given by

$$P(X = n) = \frac{m^n e^{-m}}{n!},$$

where $e = 2.718$ approximately and $n!$ (*factorial* *n*) means $n \times (n-1) \times (n-2) \times \cdots \times 2 \times 1$ [see II, §5.4]. Thus $4! = 4 \times 3 \times 2 \times 1 = 24$ and factorial zero $(0!)$ is taken to be 1. Hence, for example, if X follows a Poisson distribution with mean 2.24 then the probability that $X = 0$ can be calculated as

$$P(X = 0) = \frac{2.24^0 e^{-2.24}}{0!} = e^{-2.24} = 0.106.$$

Another important discrete distribution arises when we count how often an event occurs in n independent 'trials' where on each occasion the event has probability p of occurring; in this case we have a *binomial distribution* with parameters n and p—sometimes denoted $B(n, p)$ [see II, §5.2.2]. If n is very large and p is small, $B(n, p)$ is practically indistinguishable from the Poisson distribution with mean np.

Binomial distributions and their properties are very useful in practice. For example, if a fair coin is tossed ten times, then the count of the number of heads (i.e. the number of occurrences of the event 'coin showed heads') follows a binomial distribution with $n = 10$ and $p = 0.5$. Similarly, the count of the number of Rh-positives in a sample of 100 people follows a binomial distribution with $n = 100$. The value of p is unknown, but a reasonable guess is the observed proportion, so if we counted 85 Rh-positives we would estimate $p = 0.85$.

The vital (and often forgotten) assumption here is *independence* [see II, §4.4]: two events are independent if the probability that one occurs is unaffected by whether the other occurs or not. Independence is a very nice property because it means we can just multiply probabilities together [see II, §3.5]. For example, if the probability p of an arbitrarily selected person being Rh-positive is 0.85, then the probability of two people independently both being Rh-positive is $(0.85 \times 0.85) = 0.7225$ $(= p^2)$. Similarly, we can work out the probabilities of other combinations: in general the probability that the event occurs exactly r times in n independent trials is

$$P(\text{exactly } r \text{ out of } n) = \frac{n!}{r!(r-r)!} p^r (1-p)^{n-r}.$$

These probabilities are given by using the *binomial theorem* on $[(1-p) + p]^n$ [see I, (3.10.1)]; this is why the binomial distribution is so called.

Suppose, however, that our sample of 100 people includes some from the same family. Then the binomial distribution is inappropriate since the events 'A is Rh-positive' and 'B (a blood relative of A) is Rh-positive' are not independent: the occurrence or non-occurrence of one gives information about the probability of occurrence of the other.

We can similarly define *independent variables* X_1 and X_2 as ones for which the probability of observing any given value of X_2 is unaffected by the observed value of X_1 [see II, §6.6.2]. Almost all statistical analysis is based on the assumption of independent random errors (i.e. the assumption that even if we know the distribution of the random variation, then the actual random error in a particular observation gives us no information about the random error in any other observation). We will return to this assumption in Section 1.3.14.

1.2.3 Distribution of a continuous variable [see II, §10.1]

We can indicate the frequency distribution of *continuous* data by dividing the range into classes and grouping the observed values into these classes (see Section 1.1.2). For example, Table 1.2.2 gives the plasma fibrinogen levels of 209 healthy subjects. If we are to be able to interpret the distribution in terms of probability, the class intervals must be *exhaustive* and *mutually exclusive*: every subject has a fibrinogen level falling in one and only one of the classes. The following points are also important for presentation:

(a) The original readings were taken to the nearest milligram per hundred millilitres, so the grouping limits are also given to this accuracy.
(b) The number of classes shown is usually between 10 and 20 (any fewer than 10 tends to be too coarse a grouping; any more than 20 is difficult for us to assimilate).
(c) The intervals are all of equal width (otherwise to get an idea of the

Table 1.2.2 Distribution of plasma fibrinogen.

Plasma fibrinogen (mg/100 ml)	Number of subjects
< 120	0
120–	2
140–	5
160–	6
180–	21
200–	28
220–	23
240–	36
260–	21
280–	20
300–	27
320–	5
340–	9
360–	4
380–	1
400–	1
420 or more	0
Total	209

distribution we would have to divide the number in each class by its corresponding class interval).

(d) Non-empty open intervals are avoided. Had the last interval been ' ≥ 400' with one fibrinogen level falling in that category, there would have been no information as to whether the value was 414 or (say) 763.

(e) The total number of values is also indicated in the table.

Also note that, for example, the class '120–' contains all readings between 120 and 139. As readings were originally taken to the nearest integer, the true range in this class is from 119.5 to 139.5 with a mid-point of 129.5, **not** 130. This may not be too important for graphical summaries, but is important for calculations.

A glance at the distribution tells us about *location* (if asked to pick a 'typical' value we would guess about 240), *scatter* (most values are between 180 and 320) and *shape* (fairly symmetrical with short *'tails'*: few atypically high or atypically low values). The distribution is made even clearer when the data are drawn up as a *histogram* [see VI, §3.2.2], as shown in Figure 1.2.1.

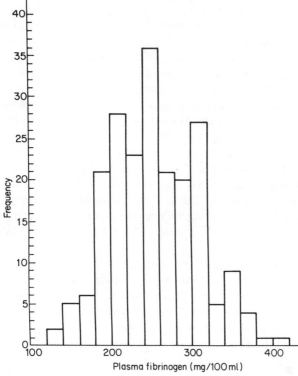

Figure 1.2.1 Histogram of measured fibrinogen levels from Table 1.2.2.

The mean and variance can be estimated from grouped data [see VI, §3.2.2] by assuming that every value falls at the *mid-point* of its class, thus assuming there to be two readings of 129.5, five of 149.5, etc. Therefore we calculate:

$$\sum x = (2 \times 129.5) + (5 \times 149.5) + (6 \times 169.5) + \cdots = 53,005.5,$$

$$\sum x^2 = (2 \times 129.5^2) + (5 \times 149.5^2) + \cdots = 14,048,642,$$

and arrive at approximate values of 253.6 (i.e. 53,005/209) and 54.0 for the mean and standard deviation respectively. These are fairly close to the actual values of 252.5 and 53.8 calculated from the original ungrouped data (not presented here).

1.2.4 The Normal distribution

The most important continuous distribution is the '*Normal*' or '*Gaussian*' distribution [see II, §11.4]. This distribution always has the same symmetrical 'bell' shape, but needs two parameters to specify location and scatter: the *mean* indicates the centre of the distribution and the *standard deviation* gives the scale.

The Normal distribution with mean 0 and standard deviation 1 is called the *standard Normal distribution* [see II, §11.4], and is sometimes denoted $N(0, 1)$. Properties of any Normal distribution can be inferred from the properties of the standard Normal distribution, which are given in tables such as those of Fisher and Yates (1963), Diem and Lentner (1970) or Pearson and Hartley (1970), and also on many electronic calculators. For example, the probability of observing an $N(0, 1)$ value less than 1.96 is approximately 0.975 (i.e. 1.96 is the 97.5 *per cent point* of the standard Normal distribution), so in general the probability of an observation from a Normal distribution being less than 1.96 standard deviations above the mean is also roughly 0.975.

Theoretical analysis involving the Normal distribution is relatively easy to develop and easy to interpret. The *log likelihood* [see VI, §6.2.1] is a useful theoretical measure of how 'likely' is a particular set of observations from a given distribution. For the Normal distribution, the log likelihood is equivalent to a sum of squared deviations, which may be interpreted geometrically as a squared distance. Therefore we can ask, quite literally, 'How far are the observations from what we might expect?'

As well as being convenient, the assumption that a population is Normally distributed can sometimes be justified theoretically. The *central limit theorem* [see II, §11.4.2] can be stated roughly: 'If an observation can be thought of as the sum of a large number of variables, then the distribution of that observation is approximately Normal.' For example, a binomial distribution with n sufficiently large (say greater than both $5/(1 - p)$ and $5/p$) may be approximated by a Normal distribution with mean np and s.d. $\sqrt{np(1 - p)}$.

Suppose we assume that the fibrinogen levels from Section 1.2.2 are Normally distributed. The observed mean and s.d. were 253.6 and 54.0 respectively, so a reasonable guess for the population distribution of fibrinogen level in milligrams per hundred millilitres might be 'Normal with mean 253.6 and standard deviation 54.0'. With this assumption, we can calculate, for example, the probability of observing a fibrinogen level greater than $(253.6 + 1.96 \times 54.0)$ mg/100 ml (roughly 359.5 mg/100 ml) to be $(1 - 0.975) = 0.025$, which agrees well with the observed frequency of 6/209.

The Normal distribution is a convenient standard with which to compare other distributions [see II, §9.10]. It is symmetrical and therefore has skewness zero; by contrast a distribution is *positively skewed* if atypically high values are more likely than atypically low values, or *negatively skewed* if the other way round. Similarly, the Normal distribution has zero kurtosis, but a *'heavy-tailed'* distribution giving rise to more outliers than the Normal has positive kurtosis, and a more compact distribution has negative kurtosis. Unfortunately the measures of skewness and kurtosis given in formulae (1.1.6) and (1.1.7) are very sensitive to outliers and may therefore be inappropriate in the situation where we want to use them. Other ways of comparing distributions are indicated in Section 1.2.7.

Note that the statement 'fibrinogen levels seem to be Normally distributed' describes the shape of the distribution but says nothing about whether or not any particular fibrinogen levels are *medically* normal.

1.2.5 The χ^2, t and F distributions [see VI, §2.5]

As mentioned in Section 1.2.4, it is often convenient to assume that observations are Normally distributed. When we analyse such observations we will obtain variables whose distributions may be derived from the Normal distribution. For example, formula (1.1.4) for the variance of a sample involves $\sum x_i^2$, the sum of the squares of the observations. If the $x_i (i = 1$ to $n)$ arise from independent standard Normal distributions, then the sum $\sum x_i^2$ follows a *chi-squared distribution on n degrees of freedom*, usually written $\chi^2(n)$ or χ_n^2. The idea of degrees of freedom (often abbreviated to *d.f.*) will be discussed later in Section 1.3.5.

The χ_n^2 distribution can be shown to have mean n and variance $2n$, and the range of possible values is zero to infinity. The distribution is also *positively skewed* (see Section 1.2.4). The χ^2 distributions have different shapes for different numbers of degrees of freedom and so cannot be tabulated as exhaustively as the Normal distribution, but most statistical tables give the 90, 95 and 99 per cent points of χ_n^2 for $n \leq 20$. Approximations based on the central limit theorem can be used for large n; details may be found in, for example, Abramowitz and Stegun (1970) or in Diem and Lentner (1970, p. 167).

If Y is a variable with a χ_n^2 distribution it can often be thought of as a 'squared distance'. In this case Y/n is an 'average squared distance' and appears in many statistical formulae. If, for example, X is a variable following a standard Normal distribution independently of Y (i.e. the actual observed value of Y gives no additional information about the likely value of X) then $X/\sqrt{Y/n}$ is an important derived variable, and follows a t *distribution on n degrees of freedom*, often written $t(n)$ or t_n.

The t distributions are symmetrical about zero and bell shaped, but are more spread out than the normal distribution (i.e. they have heavier tails), particularly for a small number of d.f. Consequently, for example, the 97.5 per cent point of the t distribution for any number of d.f. is greater than 1.96 (the 97.5 per cent point of the standard Normal distribution). However, as the number of d.f. increases, the corresponding t distributions come closer to the Normal distribution and the t distribution with infinite degrees of freedom is identical to the standard Normal distribution. Most statistical tables give the 90, 95, 99 per cent, etc., points for various d.f.

A third important distribution arises from the ratio of two sums of squares. If Y_1 follows a $\chi^2_{n_1}$ distribution and Y_2 independently follows a $\chi^2_{n_2}$ distribution, then the ratio $(Y_1/n_1)/(Y_2/n_2)$ follows an F *distribution with n_1 and n_2 degrees of freedom*, often written $F(n_1, n_2)$ or F_{n_1, n_2}. Tables of the F distribution usually present the 90, 95 per cent, etc., points on separate pages, the columns in each table giving n_1 and the rows giving n_2.

1.2.6 Random and non-random samples, randomization

Before diving into formal statistical analysis, we must appreciate that we can *never* be certain that a sample is representative of a population, since individual members of the population are either observed and in the sample or unobserved and therefore nothing is known directly about them.

It is obviously dangerous to draw conclusions about the population if the sample is in some way *biased* (e.g. if we wish to study all people ill with a certain disease, but the sample contains a disproportionate number of males, old people or smokers). We should ensure that such a bias is unlikely and that some correction can be made for any bias that does occur.

The only safe way to find a sample whose characteristics are similar to those of the whole population is by using a *randomization* process whereby a table of random numbers, a computer-generated 'pseudo-random' sequence, or some other chance method is used to decide which individuals appear in the sample. The mechanics of randomization are described in Cox (1958) and Peto et al. (1976) [see II, §§3.3 and 9.3].

One scheme employing randomization is *simple random sampling* in which every possible sample of the required size is equally likely to be chosen. Another possibility is *stratified random sampling*, where the population is divided into categories or *strata* (e.g. males aged under 40, females under 40, males 40 or over, females 40 or over) and we combine random samples from each stratum. See Armitage (1971, Sec. 6.2) for details.

Similarly, suppose we **have** a representative sample and we wish to compare two treatments A and B by assigning a treatment to each individual subject in the sample. Then again we must use randomization to ensure that the only systematic difference between the groups receiving A and B is the actual treatment we give. If we believe (no matter how unjustifiably) one treatment to be better than another then without some *random allocation rule* we may tend to give our preferred treatment to those patients we consider to be in greatest need, thus making it impossible to evaluate the treatments. The importance of randomization is discussed in, for example, Chalmers (1975) and Byar *et al.* (1976).

There are obvious ethical problems in clinical trials with concurrent 'control groups' (Section 1.4.2). However, **if it is ethical to have controls then it is unethical not to randomize**. If for any reason a particular subject is ineligible for any of the studied treatments, then he is by definition not a control and should not appear in the study unless we use special (and perhaps dubious) methods of statistical analysis. Conversely, if randomization is not used, the results may be largely due to unrepresentative sampling or unfair allocation of treatment: the work is worthless and in the long run more patients will suffer.

1.2.7 Robustness and 'Normality'

We saw in Sections 1.1.3 and 1.1.4 above that a mean and standard deviation can be heavily affected by outliers, whereas the median and inter-quartile range are not affected. This property of robustness is very important in dealing with medical data: we frequently have small sample sizes and very asymmetric or other non-Normal distributions, so we should use measures which are not adversely affected in such situations. This is known as robustness of *validity*. The median is a valid measure of location in a variety of different circumstances; it is valid for a Normal distribution and also for very asymmetric distributions.

Three different situations are shown in Figure 1.2.2 and the mean and median are shown on them, together with the standard deviation (s.d.) and inter-quartile range (IQR). The data are from a series of birth weights. In (a) the mean and s.d. are perfectly adequate. In (b) the mean is shifted to the right by 15 per cent while the standard deviation is increased by 340 per cent (because of a data error). In (c) the mean and median are closer but the standard deviation is increased by 385 per cent due to outliers on both sides of the mean.

A convenient pictorial summary showing the median, IQR and range of a set of data is the '*box and whisker*' plot; see, for example, Wade and Wingate (1980). Full details are in Tukey (1977) and McGill, Tukey and Larsen (1978).

Robust methods give reliable answers under a wide variety of conditions, and many of these techniques have been developed recently; they have become more practical with the ease of access to computers. These methods often involve *ranking* (sorting the data into ascending order, giving rank 1 to the smallest observation, rank 2 to the next smallest, etc.) [see VI, §14.4.2].

Many distributions encountered in practice have a roughly Gaussian shape in

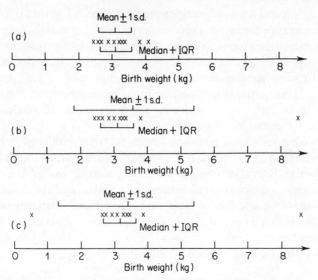

Figure 1.2.2 Diagram of birth weights showing effect of outlier
values.

the middle, but have heavier tails than the Normal distribution itself. This
provides the underlying justification for using trimmed or Winsorized means
(Section 1.1.3) and for the related '*M-estimates*' described in Huber (1981) and
produced by some computer programs.

It can be difficult to check whether data follow a roughly Gaussian
distribution. Examining a histogram of the data is not sufficiently precise and a
better approach is to plot a *cumulative frequency distribution* of the number of
observed values less than each possible value [see II, §4.3.2]. Thus for the plasma
fibrinogen levels in Table 1.2.2, none fall below 120 mg/100 ml, 2 are below
140 mg/100 ml, $(2 + 5) = 7$ are below 160 mg/100 ml, etc. Then a fitted Normal
distribution can be computed using the sample mean and standard deviation and
its cumulative distribution also plotted. A judgement by eye of the goodness of fit
may be sufficient but a formal statistical test is possible using the one-sample
Kolmogorov–Smirnov statistic [see VI, §14.2] to see if the difference in
cumulative frequency is greater than that expected by chance; details of how to
do this are in Siegel (1956, pp. 47–52) or Conover (1980, pp. 344–356). Conover
gives two other tests for Normality due to Lilliefors and to Shapiro and Wilk. The
UNIVARIATE procedure in the SAS computer package (see Chapter 2,
Section 2.4.2) provides the Kolmogorov–Smirnov test for Normality as an
option.

For a Normal distribution, 50 per cent of values should lie on either side of the
mean. A test of whether the number of values below the mean is different from the
number of values above provides a simple test for symmetry, and if the

distribution is not symmetric then it is certainly not Gaussian. Details of how to use the binomial distribution to carry out this test are given on page 161 of the *Documenta Geigy Tables* (Diem and Lentner, 1970). The same reference gives details on page 164 of the chi-square test for non-Normality [see VI, Chapter 7], though it should be noted that a Kolmogorov–Smirnov test will be more sensitive. The description of fitting a Normal curve which is given there is relevant to both these tests.

1.2.8 Likelihood and sufficiency

As mentioned in Section 1.2.1, the probability distribution of a variable tells us the probability of the different possible data values. As we try different parameter values we get different distributions, and for each of these distributions we can calculate the *likelihood*: the overall probability of the data we actually observed [see VI, §6.2.1]. In general, the lower the likelihood for a parameter value, the smaller is the probability of getting our observed data, so the less plausible is that value for the parameter.

Any mathematical formula evaluated from the data (e.g. the sample mean) is called a *statistic*, and often the likelihood only depends on the data via certain summary statistics. For example, when sampling from a Normal distribution, we only need know the sample mean and variance in order to reconstruct the likelihood function. In this case the mean and variance (or equivalently the mean and s.d.) are called *sufficient statistics* since **if our assumption of an underlying Normal distribution is valid**, they give us all the information from the sample about the population [see VI, §3.4].

Therefore for analysis or description of Normally distributed data we can 'forget' the original data and just keep a record of the sample mean and standard deviation. Other distributions have other sufficient statistics: for a 'nearly' Normal distribution, the mean and s.d. are 'nearly sufficient'. Unfortunately, as pointed out in Section 1.2.7, for a far from Normal distribution the mean and s.d. are far from sufficient!

Likelihood is also a very important concept when calculating *conditional probabilities* (probabilities of occurrence of events given the occurrence or non-occurrence of other events [see II, §3.9]), as in the following simple example.

Suppose a patient is known to have one of three diseases (indexed by parameter $d = 1, 2$ or 3) and a test is carried out giving three possible responses, A, B and C. Suppose also that the *prior* probabilities (i.e. before the test) of diseases 1, 2 and 3 were 0.2, 0.1 and 0.7 respectively, that the probabilities of each response given the disease are known from previous experience to be as shown in Table 1.2.3 and that the observed response was C.

The events 'patient has disease d' and 'test result is C' clearly are not independent, so we should update the probabilities of the given diseases to incorporate our knowledge of the test result. *Bayes' theorem* [see II, §16.4, and VI,

Table 1.2.3 Probabilities of different responses.

	Response			
	A	B	C	Total
Disease 1	0.82	0.15	0.03	1
Disease 2	0.07	0.09	0.84	1
Disease 3	0.21	0.56	0.23	1

§15.2] says that the *posterior* probabilities (i.e. after the test) of diseases 1, 2 and 3 are calculated by multiplying together the prior probability and the likelihood, and are therefore in the ratio

$$0.2 \times 0.03 : 0.1 \times 0.84 : 0.7 \times 0.23,$$

i.e.

$$0.006 : 0.084 : 0.161.$$

So, after dividing by $(0.006 + 0.084 + 0.161)$ to make the probabilities sum to one, the posterior probabilities of diseases 1, 2 and 3 are 0.024, 0.335 and 0.641 respectively. This idea can be developed to give a 'Bayesian' approach to medical diagnosis (see Chapter 3 in this Guidebook and, for example, Leaper *et al.*, 1972).

1.2.9 Transformations

All statistical analysis is based on certain assumptions, so it is logical to transform the data to make the assumptions more nearly valid. Interpretation is easier if the transformation is physically meaningful (e.g. the square root of the area of a lesion represents its 'diameter', the reciprocal of the R–R interval is the heart rate), but this is not always possible.

Note that only transformations *monotone* in the appropriate range (i.e. preserving the order of the values, or exactly reversing them, but not mixing them up [see IV, §2.7]) are likely to be useful or sensible. Examples of monotone transformations are [see IV, §2.11, and I, §§3.2 and 3.3]:

$$\log(x), \sqrt{x} \quad \text{for} \quad x > 0,$$

$1/(x + c)$ for some constant c and for all $x > -c$.

Usually the feature of most interest in a population is the magnitude of a 'typical' value. For a symmetric distribution (such as the Normal) the obvious value to take is the point of symmetry, but for an asymmetric distribution there is seldom such an obvious choice. Therefore any transformation which makes the data more symmetrically distributed often makes analysis, interpretation and presentation easier. If the transformed values are Normally distributed, so much the better (Sections 1.2.4 and 1.2.8). A transformation that produces a Normal distribution is called a *Normalizing* transformation [see II, §2.7.3].

For example, many medical measurements such as hormone levels are always greater than zero and their distributions are positively skewed; atypically high values can occur. A log transformation (which effectively converts multiplication into addition) may help cure this since values of 1, 10, 100 and 1,000 become equally spaced on a log scale. Usually for theoretical work we use logs to base e (*natural logs*, sometimes written $\log_e$ or ln), but in practice it is easier to use logs to base 10 (*common logs*, $\log_{10}$). Natural logs are just common logs multiplied by $\log_e(10)$, 2.303 [see I, §3.6]. If the distribution of values after a log transformation is exactly Normal, then the original untransformed data are said to have a *lognormal* distribution [see II, §11.5].

However, note that 'robust' statistical techniques are less affected by transformations; in particular, the *ranks* are by definition unaltered by a monotone transformation. The median of a set of data is therefore essentially the same as the median after the most 'meaningful' transformation possible.

Often a more serious problem than non-Normality is the fact that different groups of values have different degrees of scatter, making comparison of their locations difficult if not meaningless. The solution is to use a *variance stabilizing* transformation. For example, if the variable X follows a Poisson distribution with mean m, then X has the theoretical standard deviation $\sqrt{m}$ [see II, §5.4]. However, the transformed variable $Y = \sqrt{X}$ has approximate s.d. 1/2, no matter what the value of m. Therefore the square root transformation is variance-stabilizing for the Poisson distribution (the transformation $Y = \sqrt{X} + \sqrt{X+1}$ is in fact even better).

Tukey (1977) gives many guidelines for choosing appropriate transformations (or, as he calls them, reexpressions). A particular transformation may be chosen for many reasons (see, for example, Box and Cox, 1964), but the important criterion is that it gives good results in practice.

1.3 INTRODUCTION TO STATISTICAL INFERENCE

Statistical inference is the process of drawing conclusions about a population based on the results from a sample. Inference is traditionally considered under the headings estimation (Section 1.3.1) and testing (Section 1.3.2).

Test results must be interpreted carefully (Sections 1.3.3 and 1.3.4), but we can easily devise 't-tests' for well-behaved numerical data (Sections 1.3.5, 1.3.6 and 1.3.7), 'robust' tests for any numerical data (Section 1.3.8) and 'χ^2 tests' for qualitative data (Sections 1.3.9 and 1.3.10). We can also estimate the likely range of values of a parameter or a variable (Section 1.3.11). Qualitative data can often be analysed in terms of proportions (Section 1.3.12). Finally, we can investigate the association between two numeric variables (Sections 1.3.13, 1.3.14 and 1.3.15).

These are the basic techniques used in statistical analysis and examples are given in many standard books such as Armitage (1971), Colton (1974) and Hill (1977). It is advisable to check with a capable statistician what techniques are appropriate for a given problem and whether more sophisticated methods such as those in Chapter 2 are necessary. However, it is usually possible to go a long way with relatively simple analysis after careful consideration of the relevant sources of variation, as in many of the examples given by Cox and Snell (1981).

There are many approaches to any statistical problem (Section 1.3.16); we should always consider whether our chosen approach is reasonable. If two methods give completely different answers then (at least) one of them is based on wrong assumptions (see, for example, Prentice and Marek, 1979). Colquhoun (1971) is a good book for reminding us of the assumptions that are all too often made uncritically in statistical analysis.

1.3.1 Estimation (point estimation)

We often want to examine some characteristic quantity in a population (e.g. the mean fibrinogen level). An *estimator* is just a statistic that should give a value 'near to' the quantity we want [see VI, §3.1]. The estimator itself has a frequency distribution since repeated sampling will give repeatedly different values of the estimator—different *estimates* of the population quantity [see VI, §2.2].

The standard deviation of this distribution is called the *standard error* (s.e.) of the estimator [see VI, §4.1.2]; it is in the same units as the estimator and gives an idea of precision. The standard error could be estimated by observing the distribution of the estimator in repeated sampling. However, the standard error can usually be estimated from just one sample, using whatever assumptions we have made about the parent population.

For example, in estimating the mean of a population, the natural estimator is the mean of the sample. The frequency distribution of this estimator—the *sampling distribution of the mean*—has the following properties [see VI, §§2.2 and 2.3.1]:

(a) The *expected value* (i.e. the theoretical mean value) of the sample mean is the population mean. Such an estimator is called *unbiased*.
(b) The standard error of the mean $= \sigma/\sqrt{n}$ where σ is the population standard deviation; thus the standard error decreases as n increases (more observations mean higher precision). The standard error of the mean can therefore be estimated by formula (1.3.1).
(c) The shape of the distribution is approximately Normal, whatever the shape of the distribution of the parent population. This is a consequence of the *central limit theorem*, and the distribution tends closer to Normality as the sample size increases [see II, §2.5.3(*b*)].
(d) If the parent population is Normally distributed, then the distribution of the sample mean is also Normal. Similarly, if some transformation of the original values (e.g. logarithm of weight) is found to make the observed frequency distribution more nearly Gaussian, then the distribution of the mean of these transformed values will also be closer to Normality and so statistical methods

based on the properties of a Normal distribution are likely to be more accurate.

Estimates are very useful for conveying information as succinctly as possible. For example, Table 1.3.1 gives data on the heights and weights of seventy-seven male medical students: a few individual measurements are given (the students appearing in no particular order), followed by summary totals.

If we are interested in the weights (y) of male medical students and are prepared to assume that the underlying distribution is Normal, then we can completely summarize the observed frequency distribution by quoting the *sufficient statistics* (Section 1.2.8) for the Normal distribution:

$$\text{Mean} = \frac{\sum y}{n} = 68.2\,\text{kg},$$

$$\text{Variance} = \frac{\sum y^2 - (\sum y)^2/n}{n-1} = 97.9\ \text{kg}^2.$$

The standard deviation is therefore $\sqrt{97.9} = 9.9$ kg and the standard error of the mean is estimated by $(9.9/\sqrt{77}) = 1.1$ kg (see property b above).

As a rough rule for presenting results, give the standard error to two significant figures (i.e. 1.1 kg rather than 1.13 kg) and give the mean to the same precision as

Table 1.3.1 Summary of data on male medical students.

Height, cm (x)	Weight, kg (y)
161	61.5
177	69.0
173	58.5
177	62.5
196	90.0
...	...
...	...
174	58.5

Totals	
n	$= 77$
$\sum x$	$= 13{,}575$
$\sum y$	$= 5{,}248$
$\sum xx$	$= 2{,}397{,}520$
$\sum xy$	$= 365{,}124$
$\sum yy$	$= 929{,}126$

its standard error (here 0.1 kg). The mean and its standard error, particularly for the distribution of a response variable, are often presented together by saying that the mean is '68.2 $\pm$ 1.1 kg'. Unfortunately, standard deviations and confidence limits (Section 1.3.11) are also sometimes presented in this way, so it must be made clear whether '1.1 kg' is the standard deviation, the standard error of the mean or something else entirely.

Even if the distribution of weights is not Gaussian (and in practice no distributions are exactly so), we know from the sampling distribution of the mean (property c) that '68.2 $\pm$ 1.1 kg' should still be a good estimate of the mean and s.e. The main problem is not 'have we a good estimate of the mean?' but 'is it worth estimating the mean anyway?'. It may be more informative to estimate the *median* of the population, the natural estimator being the median of the sample (which is actually 66 kg, the thirty-ninth weight 'from the bottom').

Many problems can be reduced to estimating the mean of a distribution, but the sampling distribution of other statistics (e.g. the sample median or the sample variance) can also be determined and used in statistical inference [see VI, § 3.1]. A useful formula to remember when analysing sampling distributions in general is given in formula (1.3.2).

1.3.2 Hypothesis testing [see VI, Chapter 5]

We often want to answer questions like 'Is treatment A better than treatment B?'. We can carry out a hypothesis test (or *significance test*) by making some simplifying assumption, called the *null hypothesis*, about the parent population. For example, the null hypothesis could be 'treatment A is no better than treatment B'. The general method of testing is to form a statistic whose distribution is known if the null hypothesis is true, and we can use the sample to see whether this assumption seems reasonable or not.

In general the *null distribution* of a test statistic looks like Figure 1.3.1 (though in many instances it is symmetric). The null distribution is the distribution implied by the null hypothesis. The likeliest values are in the middle of this null distribution; conversely, the further the test statistic is in the tails, the less likely is the observed result. Extreme values of the test statistic are therefore evidence against the null hypothesis, and this idea is made mathematically exact by the concept of *significance*. For example, a *significance level* $P = 0.04$ means 'if the null hypothesis is valid, the probability of obtaining such a result or one even more extreme is 0.04' [see VI, §5.2.1(f)].

If the null hypothesis is of the form 'treatment A is no better than treatment B', then the test statistic will be some measure of how good A is compared to B, and only high positive values of the test statistic provide evidence against the null hypothesis (large negative values indicating that A is worse than B). Such a situation is called a *one-tailed test* [see VI, §5.2.3] since we are only interested in one tail of the distribution of the test statistic.

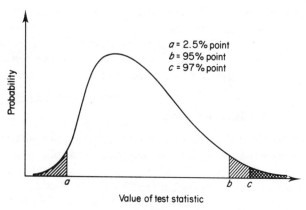

a = 2.5% point
b = 95% point
c = 97% point

Probability

Value of test statistic

Figure 1.3.1 Null distribution of a test statistic.

As a simple example, suppose we are looking for evidence that a person's blood alcohol level is over 80 mg/100 ml, and our measuring technique is known to have errors that are Normally distributed with mean 0 and standard deviation 5 mg/100 ml. The null hypothesis is that 'the person's alcohol level is no greater than 80 mg/100 ml' so if we observe a value of 90 mg/100 ml, this is two standard deviations above 80 mg/100 ml (the closest value consistent with the null hypothesis) and has an associated one-tailed probability $P = 0.023$ (from tables of the standard Normal distribution).

If the null hypothesis is of the form 'treatment A and treatment B are equally effective' then we have a *two-tailed test* [see VI, §5.2.1] since both very high and very low values of the test statistic are evidence against the null hypothesis. In practice we usually adopt two-tailed tests in case we obtain an extreme value of the test statistic in the 'wrong' direction, when interpretation would be difficult for a one-tailed test.

Traditionally, $P < 0.05$ (*the 5 per cent significance level*) is regarded as 'significant', $P \geq 0.05$ as 'not significant' or 'NS'. Thus in a one-tailed test, the null hypothesis would be *rejected* (i.e. tentatively regarded as implausible) for any value of the test statistic greater than b in Figure 1.3.1, since in only 5 per cent of tests of a valid null hypothesis would we obtain such an unlikely result. Otherwise the null hypothesis is *accepted* (i.e. tentatively regarded as being consistent with the data). This approach means that we are prepared to accept a chance of 1 in 20 of incorrectly rejecting a true null hypothesis; see Section 1.3.4 for further comments.

Similarly, in a two-tailed (or *two-sided*) test, the null hypothesis would be rejected 'at the 5 per cent level' or '$P < 0.05$' for any value of the test statistic less than a or greater than c (see Figure 1.3.1). Many test statistics have distributions that are *symmetric about zero*: $a = -c$.

Whether or not a given null hypothesis is rejected, it is important to report how large a difference was actually observed and how large a difference seems plausible given the data (see Freiman *et al.*, 1978). Note that testing implicitly involves estimation: to test whether something is significantly different from its presumed value we must first estimate its actual value. McPherson *et al.* (1978) is an example of medical data communicated in terms of estimates.

1.3.3 Type I and type II errors, power

Section 1.3.2 introduced significance tests and illustrated the *null distribution* of a test statistic. Now we must look at what happens if the null hypothesis does not hold.

A *type I error* occurs if we reject something that is actually correct [see VI, §5.12.2]. The probability of committing a type I error is often denoted by α. If we base our decisions on whether or not a significance level is less than 5 per cent (in other words, accept a null hypothesis if $P \geq 0.05$, reject if $P < 0.05$), then α, the probability of a type I error, is by definition 0.05.

A *type II error* occurs if we erroneously accept something false. The probability of committing a type II error is often written as β, and the *power* of a test $(1 - \beta)$ is the probability of avoiding a type II error [see VI, §5.3.1]. The more powerful a test, the less likely we are to commit a type II error and the more likely we are to reject a false null hypothesis.

These two types of error are illustrated in Figure 1.3.2.

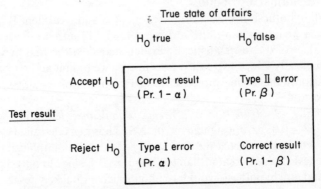

Figure 1.3.2 Types of error in test of a null hypothesis H_0.
Pr. denotes probability.

In the artificial example from Section 1.3.3 (testing whether a person's blood alcohol level is over 80 mg/100 ml), suppose we fix $\alpha = 0.01$ (ensuring that anyone with a level less than 80 mg/100 ml has no more than a 1 in 100 chance of being judged over the limit of 80 mg/100 ml). What is the power of the test to detect someone whose blood alcohol level is actually 95 mg/100 ml?

The observed level in milligrams per hundred millilitres is Normally distributed with standard deviation 5, and the 99 per cent point for the standard Normal distribution is roughly 2.33. Consequently, we would reject the null hypothesis (denoted H_0) of 'not over 80 mg/100 ml' if we observed any level greater than the *critical value* $(80 + 5 \times 2.33) = 91.6$.

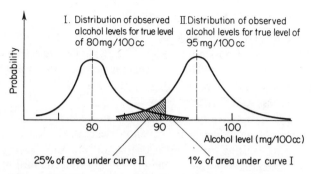

Figure 1.3.3 Hypothetical distribution of blood alcohol concentration assuming means of 80 mg/100 cc (H_0) and 95 mg/100 cc (H_A) and standard deviation of 5 mg/100 cc in both cases to illustrate the concept of power of a test.

The probability of observing a value greater than this from a Normal distribution with mean 95 and s.d. 5 is found by considering

$$z = \frac{91.6 - 95}{5} = -0.68,$$

which corresponds to the 25 per cent point of the standard Normal distribution. Therefore $\beta = 0.25$ for the particular *alternative hypothesis* (H_A) that the actual alcohol level is 95 mg/100 ml (see Figure 1.3.3), and the power of the test is $(1 - \beta) = 0.75$.

Similarly, β can be calculated under other alternative hypothesis and the power can be plotted as a function of the actual alcohol level. Plotting *power curves* using $(1 - \beta)$ or *operating characteristic curves* using β in this way can help us to decide which of several plausible statistical tests we should use [see VI, §5.3.1]. Unfortunately this is complicated in practice because we never know the exact form of random errors (what is their standard deviation and are we justified in assuming a Normal distribution?), but we can compare possible tests on large samples by considering their efficiencies (the relative sample sizes for the tests to have equal power).

Note that in the above example if we want to increase the power of the test and reduce β, then we must lower the critical level from 91.6. But then more people with blood alcohol levels below 80 mg/100 ml will erroneously appear to be over the critical level, and α is increased. This trade-off between the risks of committing type I and type II errors is unavoidable. The only way to reduce both risks simultaneously is by decreasing the standard error of the test statistic, either by making more precise measurements or by increasing the sample size.

Using a legal analogy, H_0 is that the accused is truly innocent, H_A is that the accused is truly guilty. The jury can acquit or convict. When an innocent man is convicted there is a type I error and when a guilty man is set free there is a type II error. Decreasing the probability of a type I error by, for example, requiring unanimous verdicts to convict will automatically increase the probability of a type II error. Decreasing the probability of a type II error by, for example, allowing confessions to be obtained without a lawyer present will increase the probability of a type I error. The only way to reduce both is to have further relevant evidence available.

1.3.4 Interpretation of statistical significance

There is nothing special about the 5 per cent significance level, so the actual *P-value* should be quoted if possible [see VI, §5.2.1(f)]. Two test results, $P = 0.04$ and $P = 0.06$ both correctly indicate that there is reasonable but not convincing evidence against the null hypothesis; $P < 0.05$ and NS give the misleading impression of success and failure.

Straightforward acceptance or rejection may, however, be useful if we decide the significance level **beforehand** (as in sequential designs, Section 1.4.5). This idea can be extended to *decision theory* (Section 1.3.16) [see VI, Chapter 19].

Note that $P = 0.03$ does **not** mean 'the probability that the null hypothesis is true is 0.03', since any specific null hypothesis is almost certainly false (e.g. there is bound to be some difference between the effectiveness of two treatments, but it may be so small as to be unnoticeable in practice). For similar reasons, if we say we 'accept' the null hypothesis, we implicitly add 'for convenience, for the moment, since as yet there is insufficient evidence against it'. Schwartz, Flamant and Lellouch (1980) provide an important discussion of the meaning and relevance of type I and type II errors in practice.

Bear in mind that 'statistically significant' may not mean 'medically important', 'useful' or even 'surprising'. The peak response to a placebo will be higher than the baseline, since peaks are by definition higher than baselines. The average age of second generation sufferers from a disease will be less than that of first generation sufferers, since sons and daughters are younger than parents. Equally, because the sample sizes are too small, a medically important result may not be 'statistically significant' (see Section 1.3.3).

A 'significant result' might also be due to sources of variation we have not considered. Suppose that the null hypothesis, 'there is no difference between the effects of treatment A and treatment B', is rejected. This just tells us that the observed difference between A and B is unlikely to be due to **chance**. It is up to us to ensure that our result was unlikely to be caused by inherent differences between the group given treatment A and the group given treatment B, or to differences in the way the groups were handled (see Section 1.4.2). Problems with interpretation are amply illustrated in Burch (1978) and the ensuing discussion.

In particular, remember that statistical significance does not necessarily imply a causal relationship [see VI, §5.2.1(g),(h)]. However, if we are satisfied that all sources of variation other than those under study have been accounted for, we may regard 'significance' as evidence of some association between different treatments and different results.

1.3.5 One-sample *t* test, degrees of freedom [see VI, §5.8.2]

A *t test* is designed for data measured on an interval or ratio scale, and is based on a statistic of the form

$$t = X/\text{s.e.}(X),$$

where

X = something whose expected value is zero when the null hypothesis is valid,

s.e.(X) = the estimated standard error of X.

The idea is to get a test statistic with a distribution close to the standard Normal distribution (with mean 0 and s.d. 1). Unfortunately there is variability in both X and s.e.(X), so the distribution of t is rather more complicated and involves the idea of *degrees of freedom* (often abbreviated to d.f.), which is the number of independent values used to estimate a population quantity such as the standard error of X.

In general, to estimate a standard error we must estimate the variance of some population by using the sample variance. But the population variance represents scatter about the *unknown* population mean μ, so we first have to estimate μ by the sample mean, $\bar{x}$.

In the simplest case ($n = 1$), where the sample contains only one observation x, we estimate $\mu = \bar{x} = x$ and there is no information about scatter. In other words, the act of calculating the mean from the data leaves no independent values to form the variance, and the number of degrees of freedom is 0.

For $n = 2$ and two observations x_1, x_2, the formula for the mean $\bar{x}$ ensures that one observation is as far below $\bar{x}$ as the other is above $\bar{x}$. The only quantity we can use to calculate the variance is this one value (the difference between the mean and one of the observations), and hence there is one degree of freedom.

In general, the number of degrees of freedom is given by

d.f. = total number of independent observations
      − number of other population quantities estimated.

For the variance of n observations, we have estimated one other parameter (the mean), so the number of degrees of freedom is $n - 1$.

In fact, the distribution of the sample variance of n observations from a normally distributed population with unknown mean can be shown to be proportional to a variable with a χ^2_{n-1} distribution, and (if the null hypothesis is valid) the t statistic $X/\text{s.e.}(X)$ has a t distribution on $n - 1$ degrees of freedom (the χ^2 and t distributions were introduced in Section 1.2.5).

The simplest example of a t test is the *one-sample t test*.

The following numbers are the serum cholesterol levels in milligrams per hundred millilitres for fifteen males aged between 20 and 29. Is it reasonable to assume a population mean of 200 mg/100 ml?

159, 133, 223, 218, 291, 226, 240, 174, 165, 180, 223, 137, 175, 121, 183

The null hypothesis states that 'the population mean cholesterol level for males in this age group is 200 mg/100 ml'. If the null hypothesis is valid, and if we are prepared to assume that the cholesterol levels are Normally distributed, then the formula.

$$t = \frac{\text{observed mean} - \text{hypothesized mean}}{\text{standard error of the mean}}$$

will have a t distribution on $(n-1) = 14$ degrees of freedom (see formula 1.3.3). For our cholesterol values the mean and standard deviation are 189.9 mg/100 ml and 46.3 mg/100 ml respectively, so

$$t = \frac{189.9 - 200.0}{46.3/\sqrt{14}} = -\frac{10.1}{12.0} = -0.82.$$

From tables, the 90 per cent point of the t_{14} distribution is 1.345, so the probability that t is outside the range $(-1.345$ to $1.345)$ is 0.2, and $t = -0.82$ therefore corresponds to a two-tailed significance level $P > 0.2$. Note that the sign of t is irrelevant in a two-tailed test.

These values are therefore reasonably consistent with a population mean cholesterol level of 200 mg/100 ml and the null hypothesis is accepted (with all the qualifications mentioned in Section 1.3.4).

Remember that a t test makes the implicit assumption that the numerator is Normally distributed. This is often a reasonable approximation because of the central limit theorem, but can be unduly optimistic for a small number of degrees of freedom. We can check whether a sample distribution is close to a Gaussian distribution by using, for example, the Kolmogorov–Smirnov test (Section 1.2.7) and if the assumption of 'Normality' seems inadequate then we can try transforming the data (Section 1.2.9) or using more robust methods such as the non-parametric tests in Section 1.3.8.

1.3.6 Two-sample t test [see VI, §5.8.4]

Often we want to compare the means of two separate populations (e.g. to test whether there is a difference on average between the effects of two treatments, A and B). Our null hypothesis is that the population means are equal, and the test statistic is therefore based on the difference between the sample means, which has the expected value zero if the null hypothesis is valid.

To derive a t test, we need to divide by the standard error of the difference between two means. Unfortunately, the distribution of the resulting statistic is complicated unless we make the additional assumption that the variances of the two populations are equal, as in the following example.

Anorexics are randomly assigned to one of two treatments. The gains in weight measured in kilograms after 3 months (written for convenience in order of magnitude) are:

Drug A -1.9, -0.7, 0.4, 1.4, 1.8, 2.2, 3.7, 5.0
              (number $n_A = 8$, mean $\bar{x}_A = 1.49$, s.d. $s_A = 2.25$),

Drug B   0.7, 2.5, 3.9, 4.5, 4.9, 5.2, 5.6, 6.3
              (number $n_B = 8$, mean $\bar{x}_B = 4.20$, s.d. $s_B = 1.82$).

If the variation in results is the same under each treatment (which seems reasonable since the standard deviations are similar) the best estimate s of the common population standard deviation σ is the *pooled* sample s.d., obtained from a weighted mean of the two variances (formula 1.3.4). For our example we obtain:

$$s = \sqrt{\frac{7 \times 2.25^2 + 7 \times 1.82^2}{14}} = 2.05.$$

The standard error of the observed difference $(\bar{x}_A - \bar{x}_B)$ can be found by using formula (1.3.2), and the t statistic is then calculated from formula (1.3.5) to be

$$t = \frac{-2.71}{1.02} = -2.65 \qquad \text{on 14 d.f.}$$

which has an associated two-tailed significance level of $P < 0.02$.

If we believe that the two treatment groups were initially similar and were representative of anorexics in general, that the only difference between the ways the two groups were treated was in the drug given and that weight gain is an appropriate measure of treatment value, then we can interpret this result as meaning that the drugs are not equally effective and (by looking at the sign of the difference $\bar{x}_A - \bar{x}_B$) that in fact drug B is more effective than drug A.

If the variances σ_A^2 and σ_B^2 are markedly **unequal** then we can estimate the standard error of $\bar{x}_A - \bar{x}_B$ by formula (1.3.6) (which again is a special case of formula 1.3.2). The main problem now is to decide how many d.f. to use for a t test. If $\sigma_A^2 = \sigma_B^2$, we know that the number of d.f. is $(n_A + n_B - 2)$, as above. However, if $\sigma_A = 0$, then $\bar{x}_A$ is a constant and we effectively have a one-sample t test on $(n_B - 1)$ d.f.; similarly, if $\sigma_B = 0$ but σ_A is non-zero then we have a t test on $(n_A - 1)$ d.f.

There are many ways of coping with unequal variances; one technique is to note that if Y is a variable following a χ_n^2 distribution, then kY (k some constant) has mean kn and variance $2k^2n$ (using formula 1.3.2 and remembering that Y has mean n and variance $2n$). But s_A^2 can be written in the form kY, where $k = \sigma_A^2/(n_A - 1)$ and Y follows a χ_{n-1}^2 distribution; s_B^2 can be written in a similar fashion. A little algebra then shows that we can estimate the sampling variance of $V = (s_A^2/n_A + s_B^2/n_B)$ as

$$\frac{2s_A^4}{n_A^2(n_A - 1)} + \frac{2s_B^4}{n_B^2(n_B - 1)}.$$

We can now approximate $V = \text{Var}(\bar{x}_A - \bar{x}_B)$ itself by a variable of the form kY, choosing k and n (the number of degrees of freedom of Y) so that kY has the same mean and variance as V, finally giving formula (1.3.7) for $\hat{n}$. This is known as *Satterthwaite's approximation* and gives a useful general method of approximating the distribution of a non-negative variable which has a known (or well-estimated) mean and variance. Note that n will probably not be an integer, but we can look up the nearest integral d.f. t distribution in statistical tables.

Using formula (1.3.7) and (1.3.8) on our example,

$$t = 2.65 \qquad \text{on 13.4 d.f.}$$

which is close to the result assuming equal variances, not surprisingly since here the sample standard deviations were similar.

We can actually test for equality of two observed variances (assuming both samples are Normally distributed) by comparing their ratio with the F distribution (Section 1.2.5). If the larger variance is v_1 with sample size n_1 and the smaller is v_2 with sample size n_2, then v_1/v_2 is clearly at least one and can be compared with the tabulated 95, 99 per cent, etc., points of the $F(n_1 - 1, n_2 - 1)$ distribution [see VI, §5.8.6].

1.3.7 Paired t test [see VI, §5.8.2]

Another particularly useful form of t test occurs when every observation in one sample has a corresponding observation in the other sample so that the two values in each such pair will tend to be both high or both low.

Sometimes each subject 'acts as his own control' (each patient is tried on both of two treatments to compare his responses). This idea is further elaborated in Section 1.4.4 on *crossover trials*. Alternatively, pairs of subjects may be *matched* in some way (Section 1.4.2), and one of each pair is given treatment A, the other being given treatment B (the particular treatment allocation within a pair being decided randomly).

A source of variation in which we are not interested and which can be removed is that *between pairs*. We just need to perform a one-sample t test on the differences within each pair to see if the mean difference can be assumed to be zero.

For example, suppose we want to see whether there is evidence that drug A in the previous section is of any value in treating anorexics. The original data (weights before and after treatment) are given in Table 1.3.2, and weights of a given patient should obviously be paired together. The mean (1.49) and standard deviation (2.25) of the differences within each pair were given in Section 1.3.6.

The paired t statistic (formula 1.3.9) is given by

$$t = \frac{\text{mean difference (weight after} - \text{weight before)}}{\text{standard error of mean difference}},$$

$$= \frac{1.49}{2.25/\sqrt{8}} = 1.87 \quad \text{on 7 d.f.}$$

which corresponds roughly to a two-tailed significance level of $P = 0.1$, suggesting that drug A may be of some value, but not consistently enough to be demonstrated on only eight patients.

1.3.8 Simple non-parametric methods [see VI, Chapter 14]

The statistical methods used so far have made assumptions about the underlying distributions (e.g. 'Normality') and have then estimated the parameters of these distributions. *Non-parametric* or *distribution-free* methods make fewer distributional assumptions. Thus the t tests typically compare observations x_A and x_B

Table 1.3.2 Weights of anorexic subjects using
drug A.

Initial weight, kg	Final weight, kg	Increase, kg
36.1	37.5	1.4
40.3	42.1	1.8
35.2	40.2	5.0
38.6	36.7	− 1.9
36.6	38.6	2.2
39.0	39.4	0.4
35.5	34.8	− 0.7
29.7	33.4	3.7

from populations A and B by looking at the distribution of $(x_A - x_B)$ and seeing whether the mean of this distribution is significantly different from zero. Non-parametric equivalents do the same for the *median* of this distribution; in other words, they ask whether $(x_A - x_B)$ is equally likely to be positive or negative.

For two independent samples the *Mann–Whitney U test* (which is exactly equivalent in logic and result to the *Wilcoxon rank sum test* but differs in the arithmetical calculations) is based on ranking the two samples jointly and obtaining the sum of ranks for each sample separately [see VI, §14.6.2]. For small sample sizes there exist tables of critical values of the test statistic U for P values of 0.1, 0.05, 0.01, 0.001 in many textbooks, and for larger samples the distribution of U may be approximated by a Gaussian distribution. However, the answers obtained in almost all realistic large samples (say $n > 50$ in each sample) will be the same as those from t tests.

For two paired samples we obtain a single sample of differences (with sign) between the members of each pair. The *Wilcoxon matched pairs signed ranks test* [see VI, §14.4.2] then tests whether these differences are symmetric about zero by ranking the *absolute values* of the differences from low to high. The sum of the positive ranks and the sum of the negative ranks are compared; the critical values for small samples sizes are again available in tables with approximations for large samples.

A simpler but generally less sensitive test for paired samples just counts the number of positive and negative differences to see whether these numbers are roughly equal. This is known as the *sign test* [see VI, §14.4.1] and we can work out significance levels from the binomial distribution with $p = 0.5$.

The t tests and their non-parametric equivalents examine the locations of two distributions and test if they are the same. However, the *Kolmogorov–Smirnov test* [see VI, §§14.2.1 and 14.2.2] mentioned in Section 1.2.7 is a non-parametric test which is sensitive to differences in location and/or scatter and/or shape. Its interpretation is not always easy unless, as in its use in that section to test for Normality, the particular difference can be identified. It can be unsatisfactory simply to say that there is a difference, but not to be able to specify the nature of the difference.

Many elementary statistics books give the formulae and tables for these non-parametric tests (see, for example, Siegel, 1956, and Phillips, 1978). Colquhoun (1971) emphasizes the importance of non-parametric methods in biology and gives many examples, while Randles and Wolfe (1979) give a lot of the underlying theory and illustrate how we can devise our own non-parametric tests (particularly '*U tests*') and estimators.

Distribution-free methods are often used for hypothesis-testing, but can be inconvenient for estimation or simple data description. For example, the overall mean and standard deviation of two samples can be calculated directly from the individual means and standard deviations, but this is impossible for the median and inter-quartile range.

1.3.9 The chi-squared test on observed counts [see VI, Chapter 7]

The chi-squared (χ^2) test provides a method of analysing the numbers of subjects falling into given categories to see if the observed frequencies are in line with the theoretical proportions.

First we make a null hypothesis about the expected probabilities of a single observation falling into each of the several categories or *cells* (e.g. the probability of a fair die landing on each of its faces is 1/6). From these expected probabilities we calculate the expected numbers of observations in each category (e.g. in sixty throws of a fair die the expected numbers of ones, twos, etc., are each ten). Note that the expected numbers, being hypothesized mean values, need not in general be integers.

The deviation in each category is then the difference between the observed number and the expected number of observations falling in that category. These deviations are scaled to have approximately the same variance, and the sum of squared scaled deviations gives the X^2 *statistic* (formula 1.3.10).

If the null hypothesis is valid and the deviations are purely due to random variation, the X^2 statistic will roughly follow a χ^2 distribution (Section 1.2.5), with the number of degrees of freedom being the number of categories minus the number of restrictions implicit in the null hypothesis. The larger the value of X^2, the worse is the fit and the more evidence there is against the null hypothesis. Significance levels arising from this χ^2 *test* are only approximate, but are accurate enough provided the expected numbers are sufficiently large (say, provided that nearly all the expected frequencies are over 5 and none less than 2 [see VI, §7.3]). For example, in Section 1.2.1 we suggested that the data in Table 1.2.1 might follow a Poisson distribution with mean 2.24, and Section 1.2.2 showed that there is a probability of 0.106 of a count of zero arising from a Poisson distribution with mean 2.24. Therefore the expected number of zeros in a sample of fifty is (50 × 0.106), i.e. 5.3.

Table 1.3.3 Data from Table 1.2.1 retabulated for a χ^2 test.

Number of labelled cells	Observed frequency	Expected frequency	$\dfrac{(O - E)^2}{E}$
0	8	5.3	1.38
1	13	11.9	0.10
2	10	13.4	0.86
3	7	10.0	0.90
4	7	5.6	0.35
5 or more	5	3.8	0.38

The expected number of ones, twos, etc., can similarly be calculated and are given in Table 1.3.3. Note that the categories '5', '6', '7', '8' and '9 or more' have been combined so that all the expected values are reasonably large. The value of the X^2 statistic is therefore

$$X^2 = \sum \frac{(O - E)^2}{E} = 1.38 + 0.10 + \cdots + 0.38 = 3.97.$$

The number of degrees of freedom can be guessed from the minimum number of categories necessary to perform the test. Here if there were only two categories ('0 labelled cells' and '1 or more'), we could always fit a Poisson distribution to make the expected frequencies equal to the observed frequencies, which would force the X^2 statistic to be zero. This suggests that the number of degrees of freedom is $(n - 2) = 4$. More formally, we can say that there are two restrictions implicit in the null hypothesis:

(a) The sum of the expected frequencies must equal 50, the total number of observed counts. This restriction always holds for a χ^2 test.
(b) The theoretical mean of the assumed Poisson distribution was calculated from the data.

Only high values of X^2 represent evidence against the null hypothesis, so the significance level is calculated from the upper tail of the χ^2 distribution. An X^2 of 3.97 on 4 degrees of freedom corresponds to a significance level of $P > 0.2$, so the observed frequencies are fairly consistent with a Poisson distribution.

It is common practice to talk of the χ^2 test statistic and X^2 statistic synonymously, and this approach will be taken from hereon.

1.3.10 Chi-squared on 'contigency tables' [see VI, §7.5]

The χ^2 test is particularly useful when the categories are different possible combinations of qualitative variables. In the following example, two treatments are used against an illness that is often rapidly fatal.

Out of 45 patients on treatment A, 34 survive.
Out of 70 patients on treatment B, 64 survive.

We want to know whether treatments A and B can be assumed to be equally effective in terms of keeping the patient alive over the critical period. The null hypothesis is 'the proportion surviving one year after treatment A is the same as that surviving after treatment B', i.e. that the two *attributes*, 'treatment used' and 'success rate', are independent.

The data can conveniently be represented in a table with two rows and two columns: a 2 × 2 *contingency table* (also known as a *fourfold table* since there are four categories altogether). Each of our 115 patients appears in one of the four possible categories:

	Survived	Died	
Treatment A	34	11	Observed frequencies
Treatment B	64	6	

If the success rate is equal for both treatments, the estimate of this common rate is given by the observed overall success rate:

$$\text{Probability of survival} = \frac{\text{total surviving}}{\text{total treated}} = \frac{98}{115} = 0.852$$

So the expected number surviving after treatment A is $(0.852 \times 45) = 38.3$. The other expected frequencies are calculated similarly to give the following table:

	Survived	Died	
Treatment A	38.3	6.7	Expected frequencies
Treatment B	59.7	10.3	

giving a value $X^2 = \sum \frac{(O-E)^2}{E} = 5.48$.

Here there are three independent constraints:

(a) The total of the expected counts = sum of observed counts = 115;
(b) Total number under treatment A must be the same (45) in each table (consequently the total number under treatment B must be the same);
(c) The total number of survivors must be the same (101) in each table (consequently the total number of deaths must be equal).

Therefore the number of degrees of freedom is $(4 - 3) = 1$.

A χ^2 value of 5.48 on 1 d.f. corresponds to a significance level $P = 0.02$, indicating that the observed differences in survival rates are unlikely to have arisen purely by chance. Looking at the differences $(O - E)$ in each category (or, better still, the *scaled deviations* $(O - E)\sqrt{E})$ suggests that, other things being equal, treatment A is less effective than treatment B. Note that although we are only considering the upper tail of the χ^2 distribution we are in effect performing a two-sided test, since the null hypothesis is 'no difference'.

The null hypothesis of this χ^2 test assumes that the relative probabilities of falling in each cell are the same for every individual in the population. This is unlikely to be true and we may be able to exploit other information: as a start we should analyse males and females separately. Similarly, we must modify the analysis if the data are paired in some way (see Section 1.3.12).

The fact that the number of d.f. is 1 has an important consequence: once one of the expected frequencies under **any** null hypothesis has been calculated, the others can be written down almost directly. For example, having calculated that the expected number of survivors under treatment A is 38.3, we know that the expected number of survivors under treatment B must be 59.7, since we have observed 98 survivors altogether.

For a general contingency table with r rows and c columns, the number of d.f. is $(r - 1)(c - 1)$ [see VI, §7.5.2]. For example, if we want to test whether proportions of blood groups (O, A, B and AB) are the same in each of three cities, we might draw up a table with four rows and three columns counting the number of people of each blood group in samples from each city. The number of degrees of freedom in the corresponding χ^2 test is $(4 - 1)(3 - 1) = 6$.

The χ^2 test is the simplest way to compare proportions; further details may be found in Section 1.3.12 and Chapter 2. Remember that the O and E in the formula represent **counts**, not percentages, means or anything else.

1.3.11 Confidence limits (interval estimation) [see VI, §4.2]

Confidence limits (CLs) give a range (the *confidence interval*) which is likely to include the actual value of some unknown quantity. Thus 95 *per cent confidence limits* are formulae giving two values in such a way that we can say 'if our underlying assumptions (Normality or whatever) are correct, then in the long run as we calculate confidence limits from different samples, the quantity will lie between these two limits for 95 per cent of the samples'.

Confidence limits are usually obtained simply by manipulating the formulae for estimators and their standard errors. This is the same principle as significance tests, and in fact 95 per cent confidence limits give precisely the parameter values that would be 'accepted, $P \geq 0.05$' if specified as a null hypothesis. For example, in Section 1.3.5 when we tested the observed mean cholesterol level against a hypothesized value we used a t test on 14 degrees of freedom. Therefore to obtain *confidence limits for the mean* we again use the t distribution on 14 d.f., and the confidence limits are the minimum and maximum values that are not significantly different ($P \geq 0.05$) from the observed mean cholesterol level.

The tabulated value for t_{14} corresponding to a two-tailed significance level

$P = 0.05$ is $t = 2.145$, and the cholesterol levels had a mean of 189.9 mg/100 ml. Therefore the upper confidence limit, U, is obtained from

$$\frac{U - 189.9}{12.0} = 2.145,$$

since any value less than U corresponds to $t < 2.145$ and any value greater than U corresponds to $t > 2.145$. This gives

$$U = 189.9 + 2.145 \times 12.0 = 215.6 \text{ mg/100 ml.}$$

The lower limit is similarly given by $(189.9 - 2.145 \times 12.0) = 164.2$ mg/100 ml. Formula (1.3.11) gives the general method of calculating confidence limits for the mean. In our example, the 95 per cent confidence interval for the mean cholesterol level is (164.2 to 215.6) mg/100 ml, corresponding to $\alpha = 0.05$ in formula (1.3.11).

Similarly, using the observed standard deviation 46.3 mg/100 ml, we could estimate that 95 per cent of cholesterol levels of men aged between 20 and 29 lie between $(189.9 - 2.145 \times 46.3) = 90.6$ mg/100 ml and $(189.9 + 2.145 \times 46.3) = 289.2$ mg/100 ml. However, we can get more accurate 95 *per cent limits for a single observation* if we notice that the distribution of cholesterol levels is positively skewed, but that taking logarithms appears to give a more nearly Normal distribution.

Taking logs to base 10 [see I, §3.6] gives values with a mean of 2.266 and standard deviation 0.106, which correspond to 95 per cent confidence limits for a single observation of (2.039 to 2.493). We can then take antilogs of these values, since if 2.5 per cent of log cholesterol levels lie below 2.039 then 2.5 per cent of unlogged levels lie below antilog (2.039). This gives 95 per cent confidence limits for a single observed cholesterol level of (109.3 to 311.2) mg/100 ml.

We could similarly use the mean and s.e. of the mean of log cholesterol values to get confidence limits for mean log cholesterol, which translates back to confidence limits for the *geometric mean* [see IV, §21.2.4] of the original data. This is not so important statistically because the distribution of the mean unlogged values is nearly symmetrical anyway (Section 1.3.1).

Confidence limits can be used for other distributions: suppose we want 99 per cent limits for the variance V of cholesterol levels. If we assume that $V = kY$ where k is some constant and Y has a χ^2_{n-1} distribution (this is approximately so if the original data are roughly Normally distributed), then we can ask 'what is the largest variance U which, if specified in a null hypothesis for a two-tailed test, would correspond to $P \geq 0.005$?'.

If U is the hypothesized variance then k (defined in the previous paragraph) $= U/(n-1) = U/14$ (using properties of χ^2_{n-1} as in Section 1.3.6). U corresponds to $P = 0.005$ if the observed value of V (i.e. 2,142) corresponds to Y having an observed value of 4.07, the 0.5 per cent point of the χ^2_{14} distribution. Hence $4.07 \times U/14 = 2,142$, or

$$U = \frac{2142 \times 14}{4.07} = 7,368.$$

Similarly the lower limit is calculated using the 99.5 per cent point of the χ^2_{14} distribution (31.32) and is found to be $(2142 \times 14/31.32) = 957$.

We would take the square root of these limits to get 99 per cent confidence limits for the s.d. of cholesterol means. The general equations for the *confidence limits of a variance* are given in formula (1.3.12).

Note that to calculate the **upper** confidence limit we used the **lower** tail of the χ^2 distribution, and vice versa. If the null distribution is symmetrical and does not change shape for the different null hypotheses (as we assumed when finding confidence limits for the mean cholesterol level) then we do not need to worry about this rather convoluted logic, which is theoretically necessary because confidence limits rely on what **might** have happened under different null hypotheses.

Methods giving distribution-free confidence intervals are described in textbooks such as Hollander and Wolfe (1973) and Conover (1980), and computer programs make the calculations easier.

Although confidence limits are a rather artificial answer to the straightforward question 'what is the likely range of values?', they are particularly useful when, as for cholesterol levels, some transformation on the data is advisable. Thus plotting the 68 per cent confidence limits for a parameter is equivalent to plotting 'mean ± standard error' for symmetrical distributions, and is informative even for skewed distributions.

1.3.12 Analysis of proportions

Many medical measurements can be summarized as binary data: dead/alive, hypertensive/normotensive, etc. Binary data are often conveniently coded 1 or 0, and for simplicity the two possible values are often referred to as positive and negative responses.

The simplest case arises when all members of the population have the same probability p of a positive response. The observed number of responses in a sample of size n has a binomial distribution (Section 1.2.2) with parameters n and p, sometimes written $B(n, p)$ [see II, §5.2.2]. The binomial distribution can be thought of as the sum of n observations, each being 1 (with probability p) or 0 (with probability $q = 1 - p$). Simple probability theory shows that each observation has mean p and variance pq [see II, §5.2.1]; the sum of n such observations has mean np and variance npq [see II, Example 8.1.2]. Therefore the observed **proportion** of positive responses has mean p and variance pq/n.

The central limit theorem (Section 1.2.4) tells us that, for large n, the binomial distribution is similar to a Normal distribution [see II, §11.4.7]. This means, for example, that if $n = 45$ and $p = 0.852$, then the probability of observing a value between, say, 33.5 and 34.5 is nearly the same for a binomial distribution with parameters n and p as for a Normal distribution with mean $np(= 38.34)$ and s.d. $\sqrt{npq}(= 2.38)$. Therefore the probability of observing the value 34 from $B(45, 0.852)$ is roughly the same as the probability of observing a value from the standard Normal distribution $N(0, 1)$ between $(38.34 - 34.5)/2.38 = 1.61$ and $(38.34 - 33.5)/2.38 = 2.03$. From statistical tables [see II, §11.4.6] this probability is $(0.979 - 0.946) = 0.033$; the actual probability calculated from the binomial distribution is 0.03268. This approximation is good provided that neither np nor $n(1 - p)$ is too small (say neither is smaller than 5).

Similarly we can estimate the probability of observing a value 34 or more from $B(45, 0.852)$ by adding the probabilities of observations being between 33.5 and 34.5, between 34.5 and 35.5, etc. Therefore (as above) this probability is roughly the same as the probability of observing a value higher than 1.61 from $N(0, 1)$.

Note that $1.61 = (|np - 34| - 0.5)/\sqrt{npq}$, where the vertical lines about $np - 34$ as usual mean 'the absolute value of', i.e. neglect the sign of $np - 34$. The 0.5 in the formula is a *continuity correction* [see II, §11.4.1], used because we are approximating a discrete distribution which can only take integer values (the binomial) by a continuous distribution (the Normal). Now that tables of the binomial distribution are readily accessible (both in book form and making use of functions available on calculators and computers), the importance of approximations of this kind is diminishing.

Continuity corrections are also useful when **comparing** proportions. The underlying mathematics involved in the χ^2 test in Section 1.3.10 (from which the above figures were taken) is in fact identical to that involved in comparing the two proportions by using the Normal approximation to the binomial, but without any continuity corrections. Subtracting 0.5 from the absolute deviation in each cell of a 2×2 table as a correction for continuity is called *Yates' correction* [see VI, §7.5.1], which is discussed further in Section 2.1.7 of Chapter 2. Yates' correction is recommended for hypothesis-testing, and using the example from Section 1.3.10 gives a value of

$$X^2 = \sum \frac{(|O - E| - 0.5)^2}{E} = 4.29 \qquad (P = 0.04).$$

We can also use *Fisher's exact test* (see, for example, Siegel, 1956), on 2×2 tables [see VI, §5.4.2]. This test sums the exact probabilities which are only approximated by the χ^2 test, giving a *one-sided* test (e.g. 'does treatment B result in significantly fewer deaths than treatment A?'). For our example Fisher's exact test gives $P = 0.020$; note that this is half the P-value for the *two-sided* corrected χ^2 test given above. Fisher's test is generally recommended when any of the expected cell frequencies is below 5.

A disadvantage of the χ^2 test is that it gives no direct estimate of the size or nature of the differences between proportions (though this is more important for tables larger than 2×2). Another approach uses the Normal approximation to the binomial directly, estimating the standard error of the observed proportion p by $\sqrt{pq/n}$. In our example the overall success rate out of 115 was 0.852, so the s.e. of this proportion is $\sqrt{0.852 \times (1 - 0.852)/115} = 0.033$. Similarly, under the null hypothesis of 'no difference between treatments' the s.e. of the differences between the observed success rates $p_A(34/45)$ and $p_B(64/70)$ is

$$\text{s.e.} (p_A - p_B) = \sqrt{0.852(1 - 0.852)\left(\frac{1}{45} + \frac{1}{70}\right)} = 0.068.$$

We can now use standard methods (Sections 1.3.5, 1.3.6 and 1.3.11) to derive confidence limits and t tests for proportions; slight difficulties arise because of continuity corrections and the fact that different proportions have different standard errors (see, for example, Colton, 1974, Chapter 5). The *arcsine* (or *angular*) transformation [see VI, §2.7.2(c)] can be useful here since it stabilizes variances (see, for example, Armitage, 1971).

A very common mistake is to analyse paired binary data as though they were unpaired. The paired t test (Section 1.3.6) looked at differences **within** pairs; we must use a similar method for binary data. The usual approach is to say that pairs in which each member has the same response give us no information about differences within pairs; therefore we just look at pairs in which the members showed different responses (*discordant pairs*). There are two sorts of discordant pair (say AB or BA); we can test whether these are equally likely by referring the number of discordant pairs of type AB(n_{AB}) to the binomial distribution with $p = 0.5$ and $n =$ (total number of discordant pairs, $n_{AB} + n_{BA}$).

An equivalent approach is to draw up a 2×2 table containing just the discordant pairs: this is known as *McNemar's test* and is illustrated in Siegel (1956). Further discussion may be found in, for example, Pike and Morrow (1970) and Miller (1980).

1.3.13 Simple linear regression

Usually several variables of interest are measured on each subject and we will want to know how these variables are interrelated—perhaps to predict one particular variable (e.g. 'ideal weight') given others (sex, age, height, etc.). The technique of seeing how one numerical variable depends on others is called *regression*.

The simplest case is where we have two variables, X (e.g. height) and Y (e.g. weight), and we want to know 'what happens to Y as X varies'. As a first step it is always useful to plot the data in a *scatter diagram* to see what sort of relationship, if any, might be present. Figure 1.3.4 is a plot of the data from Table 1.3.1. It often seems adequate to assume that the relationship follows a straight line, $Y = a + bX$ (+ random variation), and the usual way to fit this *linear model* is by *least squares*, which means minimizing the sum of squared deviations, $\sum$ (observed y − fitted y)^2 [see VI, §§3.5.2 and 8.1].

Always bear in mind the following points:

(a) The relationship between X and Y is assumed to be *linear*. However, even if this is known to be untrue, it may be a very good approximation for X in the range under investigation. This should, however, be checked by visual inspection of the scatter diagram. For example, if we are interested in the relationship between height and weight, we might expect weight to increase more rapidly with height for taller people (since weight is likely to be more closely related to volume than to height). However, if we are looking at adults

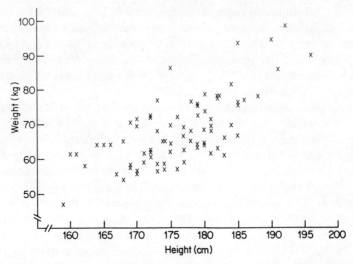

Figure 1.3.4 Scatter diagram of heights and weights of male medical
students.

then we are most interested in heights from 1.5 to 2 metres, over which
comparatively small range approximate linearity seems plausible. **This
emphasizes that the fitted line is only appropriate for values of x in the range
covered by the sample.**

(b) If we intend to predict the value of Y corresponding to a given value of X, the
random variation is assumed to be contained in the Y variable. Y is then
called the *dependent* or *response* variable and X the *independent*, *explanatory*
or *predictor* variable. It often happens that one of the variables selects itself as
the X variable. For example, it is natural to think of weight (Y) depending on
height (X) or height (Y) depending on age (X), rather than age depending on
height or height on weight. If both variables are subject to random variation
then some more sophisticated analysis is generally necessary (e.g. Riggs,
Guarnieri and Addelman, 1978).

(c) Pairs of observations (x, y) should be independent [see II, §6.6.2]. If we are
looking at height/weight relationships on a number of children over
successive years we can expect interrelationships between the observations
on a given child. Such interdependence between pairs of values means that
simple linear regression analysis is inadequate: multivariate methods
(Section 2.2 of Chapter 2) may be appropriate instead.

(d) The data should be *homoscedastic*, which means that the standard deviation
of observed y for given x should be the same for any x within the sample range
[see VI, §6.5.1].

To check the above assumptions, plots of residuals (see Section 1.3.14) are very helpful. If the assumptions are not satisfied then we can try transformations or use the more sophisticated regression methods in Chapter 2.

Note that standard errors for the *regression coefficients* a and b can be calculated by repeatedly using formula (1.3.2), and we can use t tests to test, for example, whether $b = 0$ (i.e. to see if there is no linear dependence of y on x) or whether the slopes b_1 and b_2 of two regression lines can be assumed to be *parallel* ($b_1 - b_2 = 0$). Examples of such tests may be found in, for example, Armitage (1971).

Similarly, we can obtain confidence limits for a and b or for predicted y values [see VI, Example 4.5.5]. The confidence limits for y get wider apart as x moves away from its observed mean (so as might be expected we are less sure of the probable y values at the extremes of the x range). This again indicates the danger in attempting to use the regression line to predict y for a value of x outside the sample range.

A summary of linear regression is given in formulae (1.3.13) to (1.3.17). Regression analysis on the data in Table 1.3.1 to investigate how weight (Y) varies with height (X) gives the following results:

$$\text{Slope } b = \frac{\sum (x - \bar{x})(y - \bar{y})}{\sum (x - \bar{x})^2} = 0.917 \qquad \text{(standard error 0.110)};$$

$$\text{Intercept } a = \bar{Y} - b\bar{X} = -93.5. \qquad \text{(standard error 19.4)}.$$

Hence for every centimetre difference in height between two male medical students, we would expect a difference in weight of 0.9 kg (the taller student weighing more, since b is positive).

Often the relationship between two variables is clearly non-linear but can be straightened by a *transformation to linearity*. Simplifying the structure of a relationship is the single most important function of transformations in statistics. For example, suppose the pairs (x, y) lie close to a smooth curve through the origin (such a curve might in fact hold for heights and weights over a wide range of values since a height of zero is obviously associated with zero weight). Then we might do better to use Y/X as the response, or alternatively to use $\log(Y)$ as the response and $\log(X)$ as the explanatory variable. Note, however, that transforming the response variable will change the nature of the random variation and we may need *weighted regression* as discussed in Section 2.1.5 of Chapter 2. If the data can not be transformed to give a reasonable straight line then it is possible to use *non-linear regression*, as used, for example, by Draper and Smith (1981, Chapter 10) [see VI, §8.2.5].

Various techniques for robust and distribution-free regression are also available; these are able to deal with ordinal data (Section 1.1.2) or other cases where not all the assumptions for standard linear regression hold. A useful and simple example is to take all possible pairs of points and obtain a slope and intercept for each pair. The median of all the slopes may be used as the slope of the

line and the median of the intercepts as the intercept. Approximate standard
errors may be obtained for these and we can derive significance tests and
confidence intervals (see, for example, Conover, 1980).

These and other more sophisticated techniques, as in Huber (1981) or Maritz
(1981), will probably be used more when they become widely available on
computers.

1.3.14 Residuals [see VI, §8.2.4]

In regression a *residual* is defined as the vertical distance of a measured point from
the line of best fit to all the data. Thus the residuals $(y_{obs} - y_{fit})$ are defined in terms
of the observed (y_{obs}) and the predicted (y_{fit}) values of the dependent variable Y.
The predicted value y_{fit} of the dependent variable is in general obtained from
whatever *model* we fit to the data: in simple regression our model is the equation
$y = a + bx$. Similarly, when we do a simple independent sample t test we implicitly
assume the model $y = x_i (i = 1, 2)$ where x_1 is the mean for group 1 and x_2 is the
mean for group 2; x_1 is thus the 'predicted' value for group 1 and residuals may be
seen as the deviations from the appropriate group mean.

In more complex situations we may have more complex models for the data
but we can still define residuals as 'observed − fitted'. The assumption in most
parametric statistical tests is often stated as 'the data have a Gaussian
distribution', whereas it is really the *random variation* that is taken to be Normally
distributed. We should therefore investigate this assumption by looking at
residuals rather than at the original data; two particularly useful techniques are
Normal plots and *residual plots* [see VI, § 10.3].

Normal plots and variants of them can be used to check the distribution of the
data (see, for example, Healy, 1968). We obtain a cumulative frequency
distribution of the data or residuals and plot this on *Normal probability graph
paper* [see VI, §3.5.1]; the resulting plot should be a straight line if the
underlying distribution is Gaussian. Figure 1.3.5 shows the Normal plot of the
data from Table 1.2.2, formed by noting the number (R) of subjects with levels less
than 120, less than 140, etc., denoting the total number of subjects (209) by N and
plotting $y = (3 \times R - 1)/(3 \times N + 1)$ on Normal probability graph paper against
the corresponding fibrinogen level. This y is a slight modification of the observed
cumulative proportion (R/N) to treat both tails symmetrically and to avoid
proportions 0 or 1.

Alternatively, the cumulative percentages may be converted to *Normal scores*
by finding the corresponding percentage points of the standard Normal
distribution (e.g. a cumulative percentage of 2.5 per cent has a Normal score of
− 1.96) and we can plot the observed Normal scores against their corresponding
theoretical values (see, for example, Pearson and Hartley, 1970). Many computer
programs use this technique.

A variant of the normal plot is the *half-Normal plot*, where we assume the

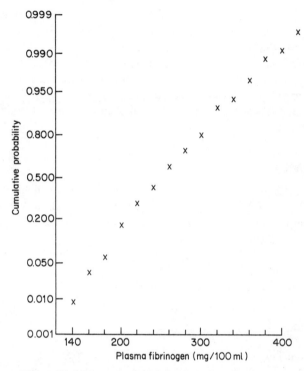

Figure 1.3.5 Normal plot of the data from Table 1.2.2.

distribution is symmetric and therefore take the absolute values of the residuals to see if the distribution is non-Gaussian. Many examples of Normal and half-Normal plots are given in Daniel and Wood (1980).

Residual plots are useful for checking independence (Section 1.2.2) and other assumptions such as equal variances. For example, after having chosen a model to fit the data we can plot the residuals against the predicted values (y_{fit}) of the dependent variable. This plot will indicate whether the equation is a good fit over the whole range of the data or whether a more complex form of equation might be necessary.

Another useful check is to plot the residuals against the explanatory variables in the model (e.g. to check linearity) or against variables which are not in the model, to see whether there is any possibility of a relationship with them. Many examples are given in Draper and Smith (1981). In practice all these plots are very useful to check for errors in the data. There are other more subtle methods (such as *Cook's distance* and plots due to Andrews and Pregibon) which can be used to detect outlying values of importance in a regression equation (see, for example, Draper and Smith, 1981, Sec. 3.12).

Graphical techniques are well illustrated in Healy (1968). A particularly useful way to check for trends in residuals is the CUSUM plot; this is used (with varying degrees of enthusiasm!) in Mitchell, Collins and Morley (1980) and Rosa, Fryd and Kjellstrand (1980).

The general importance of residuals is illustrated in Anscombe (1961), Anscombe and Tukey (1963) and Draper and Smith (1981). Residuals can equally well be defined as distances from the median (or indeed any fitted value) rather than from the mean (see Tukey, 1977). As Tukey himself says: 'Forget the fit, just look at the residuals!'.

1.3.15 Correlation

The *correlation coefficient r* (formula 1.3.18) is a measure of the degree of linear relationship between X and Y [see VI, §§2.1.2(d) and 16.2.5]. A typical scatter diagram is elliptical in shape and the thinner the ellipse for a given slope, the higher is the correlation.

If there is no linear relationship between X and Y, then $r = 0$ (X and Y are *uncorrelated*).

If there is an *exact* linear relationship, then

$r = 1$ if X and Y increase together,

$r = -1$ if Y increases as X decreases.

For the student height and weight data used in Section 1.3.13,

$$r = \frac{\sum (x - \bar{x})(y - \bar{y})}{\sqrt{\sum (x - \bar{x})^2 \sum (y - \bar{y})^2}} = 0.694.$$

Some manipulation of the formula for r suggests a t test, given in formula (1.3.19), to test the null hypothesis of no linear interrelationship between X and Y (i.e. $r = 0$). The number of degrees of freedom is $(n - 2)$ where n is the number of pairs (x, y). Note that if there are only two pairs, then the correlation is forced to be either $+1$, -1 or undefined.

For the student data,

$$t = 0.694 \sqrt{\frac{77 - 2}{1 - 0.694^2}} = 8.35 \qquad \text{on 75 d.f. } (P < 0.00001).$$

Thus the rather artificial null hypothesis of no correlation between height and weight of the medical students is extremely unlikely to be true. It should be noted that this test for zero correlation is exactly the same t test as that for testing whether the regression slope is zero (Section 1.3.13).

This t test is invalid and the correlation coefficient is inappropriate if the random variation in the data does not follow a Normal distribution (in particular, if there are a few outliers). We can, however, use robust measures of correlation: *Spearman's rho* is simply the correlation between the ranks of x and y [see VI, §14.9.1], *Kendall's tau* looks at pairs (x_i, y_i) and asks 'if x_i is bigger than x_j, is y_i bigger than y_j?' [see VI, §14.9.2]. Formulae and examples are given in, for example, Siegel (1956) and Hollander and Wolfe (1973).

Correlation can be helpful in purely observational studies, but is usually meaningless if we can somehow choose X or Y values. Correlation coefficients have often been used inappropriately (for discussions see, for example, Westgard and Hunt, 1973, and Gore and Altman, 1982). The interpretation of a genuine correlation depends on intuition and previous experience; it may be that X influences Y or that Y influences X, or perhaps something else influences both X and Y and there is no direct causal link between them (see Section 1.3.4).

It should be emphasized that the height and weight data are for illustration only: we know that height and weight are related, so there is little value in testing their correlation other than as an exercise. A few P-values do not make a paper automatically respectable, and reporting the results of pointless statistical tests is liable just to blind the reader with bad science.

1.3.16 Different approaches to statistical inference

(a) The classical approach [see VI, §3.1]

This is the most widely used philosophical approach to statistics and was largely developed by E. S. Pearson and R. A. Fisher. It is based on the *frequentist* interpretation of probability (i.e. as a long-run relative frequency) and uses criteria based on sampling distributions to quantify the relative merits of different estimators and of different significance tests.

There are still many plausible criteria for good estimation of a parameter. For example, *unbiasedness* says 'don't consistently over- or under-estimate the parameter' [see VI, §3.3.2]; *maximum likelihood* says 'estimate the parameter by its most likely value' [see VI, §6.2]. Often these ideas clash (e.g. the maximum likelihood estimator of the variance is biased) and often we ignore them (the usual estimator of standard deviation is neither unbiased nor maximum likelihood). The maximum likelihood approach is particularly useful for the more complicated statistical methods introduced in Chapter 2, since it is relatively easy to compare the likelihoods under different sets of assumptions (hence deriving *likelihood ratio* tests [see VI, §5.5]). It is also easy to program a computer to find the maximum of a likelihood function.

If we have two *consistent* estimators (i.e. we can estimate the parameter to any required accuracy by taking a large enough sample [see VI, §3.3.1]) and wonder which to use, one possible criterion is the *asymptotic relative efficiency* (ARE). For example, both the sample mean and the sample median are consistent estimators of the centre of a Normal distribution, but, if we use the median to estimate the centre of a large sample, its s.e. is as large as that of the mean of only 64 per cent as many observations. Therefore for a Normal distribution the median is only '64 per cent as efficient' as the mean. For some other symmetric distributions the median is more efficient than the mean—for most distributions they are estimating different things anyway. The ARE is discussed in, for example, Randles and Wolfe (1979, Chap. 5).

Classical statistical methods emphasize the concepts of efficiency, often assuming 'Normality' by invoking the central limit theorem. However, the Gaussian distribution may be a poor approximation, particularly in small samples of real medical data (note that 'asymptotic' means roughly 'something that is never reached'!). Consequently, we want measures and statistics which do not lose much efficiency when the Gaussian assumption holds, but which are still efficient for other distributions. For a fuller discussion of the issues involved see Mosteller and Tukey (1977).

Note, by the way, that some distributions (e.g. the t distribution on 1 d.f., sometimes called the 'Cauchy' [see II, §11.7]) do not even **have** a mean: the sample mean will not converge no matter how large a sample we take. This is not just a theoretical point: we sometimes want to estimate where two nearly parallel lines intersect, e.g. when analysing enzyme kinetic data using the 'direct linear plot' of Cornish-Bowden and Eisenthal (1974). The distribution of the observed point of intersection may be even more 'badly behaved' than the Cauchy; in such circumstances medians may be reasonable, but means are nonsensical.

(b) Decision theory [see VI, Chapter 19]

The second main approach to statistics is *decision theory*, which reduces the emphasis on estimating parameters or carrying out significance tests, and instead examines the practical implications of making decisions. This approach was begun by Wald (1950). In the modern formulation of decision theory, we set out formally the possible outcomes and their relative advantages (or *utilities*), how we might try to get the outcome we want (the *decision space*) and how likely we feel the different possible outcomes to be (the *prior probabilities*). The prior probabilities and utilities can be combined to give the *risks* associated with each possible decision.

An obvious medical application of decision theory is in deciding what treatment to give to a particular individual, (see, for example, Pauker and Kassirer, 1980, and Chapter 3 in this Guidebook). Possible methods of assessing utilities are reviewed in Spiegelhalter and Smith (1981); unfortunately the utilities may appear very different to the patient, to the patient's relatives and to the clinician (not to mention the Government). However, it is at least instructive to find the optimal decision under different utilities and prior probabilities; even if decision theory is not in practice the best approach to a specific medical problem, it may be the best way of investigating our approach.

(c) *Bayesian inference* [see VI, Chapter 15]

In *Bayesian* inference our ideas about parameter values are modelled by *subjective probabilities* (Section 1.2.1), so in effect the parameters themselves have probability distributions. This is a different philosophical basis from the classical or frequentist approach, in which parameters are supposed to have 'true' (but usually unknown) values. Subjective probability distributions can be updated after observing data by using Bayes' theorem, which was introduced in a rather more traditional context in Section 1.2.8.

Bayesian methods have the advantage of automatically including our previous knowledge about a problem and the disadvantage of automatically including our prejudices (see, for example, Leaper *et al.* (1972)). If we have no information (*prior ignorance*) then we usually get similar results to those given by the 'classical' methods illustrated here. Box and Tiao (1973) give a detailed survey of Bayesian methods, an example of Bayesian analysis in medicine being given by Darby and Fearn (1979). Bayesian methods make use of likelihood and can be easily and naturally extended to a decision theoretic approach.

(d) *Other approaches*

Another method of some appeal is to emphasize likelihood itself as the only valid measure of the support for different hypotheses. This has been formalized by defining *support* as the natural logarithm of the likelihood ratio, notably by Edwards (1972). Likelihood inference involves the relative heights of ordinates of distributions rather than their tail areas, and it does not allow probability statements to be attached to hypotheses, only allowing a comparison of hypotheses.

A very clear discussion of alternative methods of inference and of their practical differences is given by Barnett (1982), and Box (1980) stresses the importance of combining ideas from these different statistical ideologies. The methods tend to give similar answers in most circumstances; as Lindley (1965, p. xii) says: 'Intuition has saved the statistician from error.'

Some other approaches such as 'cross-validation' in Stone (1974), 'bootstrapping' in Efron (1979), non-parametric methods (Section 1.3.8) and the books on data analysis by Tukey (1977) and Mosteller and Tukey (1977) make fewer assumptions about distributions. Efron (1981) compares several different distribution-free approaches to estimating standard errors.

1.4 DESIGN OF MEDICAL INVESTIGATIONS

Sections 1.1 to 1.3 introduced the main statistical techniques and have put us in a better position to design medical experiments, surveys and trials. In order to consider what we want to know (Section 1.4.1) we usually need some baseline for comparisons (Section 1.4.2). We must also consider how large a trial is needed to have a reasonable chance of getting results (Section 1.4.3). *Crossover designs* (Section 1.4.4) and *sequential designs* (Section 1.4.5) are used in medicine and require special statistical techniques.

The design of clinical trials is a major topic in its own right and is discussed in, for example, Byar *et al.* (1976), Peto *et al.* (1976), Friedman, Furberg and DeMets (1981), Gore and Altman (1982) and Pocock (1983), while Peterson and Fisher (1980) give a list of useful references. Many examples of clinical trials are given in Hill (1962), and Gilbert *et al.* (1975) is a good example of how difficult it can be to run and analyse a trial in practice.

Cox (1958) covers planning and conduct of experiments in general and Abramson (1979) considers the particular problems encountered in medical studies. Anderson *et al.* (1980) give many examples of the statistics we might use.

1.4.1 Asking the right questions

Clinical trials and other medical studies have the ultimate aim of 'making or keeping people healthier'. We need to know what is meant by 'healthier' and to what group of people the results may be applicable.

For example, suppose we aim to reduce the prevalence of hypertension. First we need clear unambiguous definitions of hypertension and how we are to determine its presence. We must be clear whether our *study population* (the collection of people who might appear in our study) is representative of the population in which we are interested; this may not be true even if we try to look at the whole population, as in Cox *et al.* (1977). Note also that 'diagnosed as having the disease' is not the same as 'having the disease' and that patients in a centre with research facilities may not be representative of patients in general (see, for example, Ellenberg and Nelson, 1980).

A particular study is designed to answer questions, so if the results are to be *reliable* and *reproducible* these questions must be clearly stated. Abramson (1979) discusses the aims of medical investigations and the importance of clear definitions throughout, while Feinstein (1977a) discusses the difficulties.

For example, if we decide that our aim is specifically to reduce diastolic blood pressure to under 100 mm Hg and we want to know how best to do this, then we should think about the proportion of treated patients with diastolic BP under 100 mm Hg, not about the mean blood pressure of all patients receiving that treatment. If we simply perform a *t* test on treatment means, then we are answering an interesting question, but not the one we have asked.

Note also that in the real world we can always discontinue an ineffective treatment, so by 'comparison of treatments' we implicitly mean comparison of **decisions**: 'which treatment should we try **first**?'. Consequently, if we put a patient on treatment A but because he shows little improvement we switch him to treatment B, he should appear in the 'treatment A' group in any statistical analysis. Similarly, if some patients (group G_1) are automatically given the standard treatment but others (G_2) are given a **choice** of treatments, as in the design proposed by Zelen (1979), then we must not combine the subjects in G_1 with those from G_2 who opt for the standard treatment.

This approach is known as 'analysis by decision to treat' and is one of the facets of what is known as the *pragmatic* approach to clinical trials. By contrast, the *explanatory* approach emphasizes the physiological basis for comparison and aims to achieve ideal conditions. A full exposition is given in Schwartz, Flamant and Lellouch (1980) translated by Healy.

1.4.2 The use of controls

In medical research we are usually mainly interested in *comparison*. It is less important to know the chance of recovery using a new treatment or the risk of leukaemia in a certain occupation than it is to know whether the chances are improved (and, if so, to what extent?) or the risk is higher than normal (and, if so, by how much?). A *control group* represents the standard with which to compare the treatments or characteristics being studied.

Many investigations are designed to look for a relationship between a response and some other variable (such as 'treatment'). The most direct method is a *controlled comparative trial* where we allocate treatments to subjects in a suitably random manner (see Section 1.2.6). If we are investigating a new treatment then the control group may be given an existing recommended treatment, a placebo or no treatment at all depending on what comparisons we wish to make.

However, for ethical reasons or because of lack of resources, we may have to use some other method, e.g. if the response variable is 'subject develops leukaemia' and the other variable is 'number of years working with radiation'. *Observational* studies (looking for cause–effect relationships without being able to control the cause) may be classified according to the sampling mechanism by which individuals are included in the study.

A *cross-sectional* study takes a sample from the susceptible population and looks for an association between the hypothesized cause (or *risk factor*) and the effect (or *outcome*). However, in our example it would obviously be very wasteful to investigate random sample of people to find those few who have leukaemia and/or have worked with radiation.

A *cohort* study compares the outcomes of individuals with different degrees of risk. Thus we could collect suitable numbers of subjects with different degrees of exposure to radiation (such as groups of people in different occupations) and compare the outcomes (whether or not they develop leukaemia).

A *case-control* study compares the degrees of risk of individuals who have different outcomes. We could compare the history of radiation exposure of a group of leukaemia patients with that of a suitable group of subjects without leukaemia. Such studies are particularly useful in studying rare diseases but always need careful interpretation; a classic paper is Mantel and Haenszel (1959). A useful recent survey is given by Horwitz (1979) and a comprehensive discussion of appropriate statistical methods is given by Breslow and Day (1980). Hayden, Kramer and Horwitz (1982) review the problems of interpretation, with many examples and references.

Details of cross-sectional, cohort and case-control investigations may be found in, for example, Anderson *et al.* (1980). Cohort studies are often called *prospective* and case-control studies *retrospective*, but these terms have been used ambiguously and are misleading since cohort studies can easily be based on past records; similarly data can be collected and stored for a future case-control study. For further discussion of the use of controls and the different aspects of prospective and retrospective research see Feinstein (1977b, Chaps 13 and 14). Abramson (1979) also gives further details of different types of medical investigation.

Controlled trials, cohort studies and case-control studies all require us to assemble different groups of subjects; these groups should be as similar as possible apart from the features in which we are interested (e.g. the particular treatment given). Comparing a new treatment solely with past results (*historical controls*) is inadvisable since standards of medical care will be different, diagnostic criteria may be different and we may be looking at a different strain of disease anyway. Similarly, it can be misleading to compare one treatment in one hospital with another treatment in a second hospital (see, for example, Fleiss, 1981, Chap. 11, and Byar *et al.*, 1976).

Sometimes there is a natural choice of control group: e.g. if more than one treatment can be tried on each subject then each subject can act as his own control, as in a *crossover trial* (Section 1.4.4).

Alternatively, we can assemble a control group by *individual matching* (every member of the treated group being similar in what the investigator decides are 'all important respects' to a corresponding member of the control group) or *group matching* in which the distributions of these 'important respects' (or *controlled variables*) are similar for each group. Naturally these controlled variables (age, sex, severity of illness, etc.) should always be recorded for every subject so we can check the adequacy of the matching and try to correct for any bias that does occur (see, for example, Rubin, 1979, and Section 2.1.6 in Chapter 2). Different ways of matching are described in Anderson *et al.* (1980), together with hazards such as 'over-matching'.

It may not be easy to get comparable groups in a study; see Sackett (1979) for a detailed discussion of different types of bias. For example, suppose we are investigating the aetiology of disease A in hospital patients and decide to use as controls patients from the same hospital with an unrelated disease B. If the admission rates for diseases A and B are different then spurious differences may appear between the two groups of patients. In particular, we will see associations with a third disease C that may also require hospitalization, even if there is no such association in the general population (a person with disease A being as likely as one with B to have disease C as well). This is known as *Berkson's bias* after Berkson (1946), and the problem arises because some patients entering hospital with disease C are found to have A or B as well, thus inflating the 'A and C' or 'B and C' groups, but inflating them to a different extent because of the different admission rates.

The effect of Berkson's bias on some genuine medical data is shown in Roberts *et al.* (1978). Similar difficulties can appear whenever the groups under investigation are not representative samples of the population in which we are interested.

Randomization (Section 1.2.4) must be used whenever applicable (e.g. to decide which of a matched pair of subjects should be assigned to which treatment). Randomization is generally more important than matching for assembling comparable groups (see Peto *et al.*, 1976). Ideas like *double blindness* (neither the subject nor the investigator knowing the allocated treatment until all measurements have been made) are important during the course of the investigation.

Results from a particular study should always be compared with previous findings. For example, an apparent improvement of treatment might be partly explained if the control group happens by chance to have fared worse than would be expected (see Peto *et al.*, 1977, Example I).

The *ethics* of using controls in a clinical trial are discussed in, for example, Hill (1963) and Meier (1975). A major ethical problem arises because what is good for the community is not necessarily good for the individual; the same difficulty arises with vaccination. For a controversial view of this problem see Burkhardt and Kienle (1978) and the ensuing correspondence. However, the medical profession has just three options when a new treatment appears: to ignore it completely, to use it exclusively or to use it on some subjects and not on others. The first option means that we will never know whether the treatment is effective, the second means that a large number of people are automatically put at risk, the third means that we have a clinical trial with a control group. Any help that statistical theory can give in bringing about the greatest good of the greatest number as quickly as possible should not be ignored.

If a seemingly effective new treatment suddenly appears where there was none before it would be unethical to have a control group and we may have to use historical controls as in Gehan and Freireich (1974). However, there will always be suspicions that something other than the new treatment is responsible for any observed improvement.

1.4.3 Deciding sample size for *t* tests and other tests

We can use the formulae for *t* statistics to get a rough idea of how large a sample is needed. For example, suppose we want to compare a new treatment A for anorexia with a standard (control) treatment B. We might assume that the weight increases in kilograms over a certain time will follow a Normal distribution with different means μ_A and μ_B for treatments A and B respectively, but with standard deviation 2 in each case. This seems reasonable from the example in Section 1.3.6. If we are only interested in showing that A is better than B, we may decide to carry out a one-tailed two-sample t test with n anorexics in each of the two treatment groups.

We may decide that we want an estimate of n which, with α set at 0.05, will give us a power $(1 - \beta)$ of 0.9 for $(\mu_A - \mu_B) = 1$. In other words, we decide to accept the null hypothesis 'treatment A is no better than treatment B' if we find a one-tailed $P > 0.05$, but we want to have a 90 per cent chance of picking up a true treatment improvement of 1 kg.

For the moment, let us approximate the test statistic

$$t = \frac{\bar{x}_A - \bar{x}_B}{s\sqrt{1/n + 1/n}} = \frac{\bar{x}_A - \bar{x}_B}{s\sqrt{2/n}},$$

by a Normal distribution (since n is as yet unknown, we must make some such assumption). The 95 per cent point of the $N(0, 1)$ distribution is 1.645, so we will reject the null hypothesis if $t > 1.645$.

Therefore for $(\mu_A - \mu_B) = 1$ we want a 90 per cent chance that we will observe $t > 1.645$. The numerator $(\bar{x}_A - \bar{x}_B)$ of t has mean 1 and the 10 per cent point for the $N(0, 1)$ distribution is -1.282, so our requirement (giving s its assumed value of 2) is that

$$\frac{1}{2\sqrt{2/n}} - 1.282 > 1.645,$$

i.e.

$$\frac{n}{8} > (1.282 + 1.645)^2 \qquad \text{or} \qquad n > 69 \text{ approximately.}$$

This calculated value of n is quite large, giving some justification for our approximating a t distribution by the standard Normal distribution.

In general, if we propose a *two-sample one-tailed t test* on two samples of equal size n, each with assumed standard deviation σ, and we specify a type I error of α and, for mean treatment difference $d = |\mu_A - \mu_B|$, a type II error β, then the above method will estimate the required number in each sample as

$$n > 2\left[\frac{(z_\alpha + z_\beta)\sigma}{d}\right]^2,$$

where z_α is the 100α per cent point of the standard Normal distribution. Note that by symmetry $z_\alpha = -z_{1-\alpha}$.

Similarly, if we propose a *two-tailed t test* (and assume that a genuine treatment improvement will never appear as a statistically significant deterioration, or vice versa!) we end up with the estimated sample size given by formula (1.4.1).

In the above example with $\sigma = 2$ and $d = 1$, $\alpha = 0.05$ and $\beta = 0.2$, we obtain

$$Z_{\alpha/2} = -1.96, \quad Z_\beta = -1.282,$$

and therefore $n > 85$. This estimated sample size gives only a very rough guideline since it is based on estimating $\sigma = 2$ and it also uses essentially arbitrary values for β and for the treatment difference (1 kg) that we would regard as medically important.

We can similarly estimate the sample sizes required for other statistical tests by manipulating the formulae for the test statistics; it is often good enough to say that standard errors go down roughly in proportion to the square root of the number of observations (Section 1.3.1). Fleiss (1981) gives examples of recommended sample sizes for analysis of proportions based on χ^2 with Yates' correction. However, this procedure may well overestimate the required sample size, and a simpler estimate without the continuity correction is given in formula (1.4.2) (see Pocock, 1982). Again this estimated sample size is only a very rough guide, so discussion over the use of the continuity correction is not particularly important.

Although the actual values of α and β are up to the investigator, it is useful to find the size of trial required for some conventional choice like $\alpha = 0.05$ and $\beta = 0.2$ for whatever treatment difference is felt to be **medically important**. The advisable sample sizes are often depressingly large, emphasizing the value of cooperation between different research centres, although multicentre trials have their own problems (see, for example, Wermuth and Cochran, 1979, and the Cancer Research Campaign Working Party Report, 1980). Conversely, if a difference is reported as 'not significant' it may just mean that the study was too small (see Section 1.3.4 and, for example, Freiman *et al.*, 1978).

Large trials are particularly necessary when rare events are under consideration. For example, in following up patients who have survived a myocardial infarction the proportion who subsequently die within one year is small, so large numbers are necessary to compare the death rates in two or more treatment groups.

Note also that if a clinical trial which did not reach significance on 10,000 patients had instead been split up into 100 trials each on 100 patients, we would expect about 5 to be reported as reaching significance 'with $P < 0.05$', and probably more than 5 if the underlying assumptions (Normal distributions, equal variances, similar handling of different treatment groups, etc.) are invalid. The larger the sample size, the more reliable is the reported significance level (see Peto *et al.*, 1976).

1.4.4 Crossover trials

In a *crossover trial* each subject receives all the treatments under test. Given two treatments A and B and two treatment periods, half the subjects receive A then B and the others receive B then A. The general argument in favour of crossover trials is that patients differ greatly in their responses to treatment between themselves but that responses for a given patient are consistent from treatment to treatment.

As a specific example, let us consider two treatments for hypertension. The variation of a single individual's blood pressure from one occasion to another is very much less than the variation between different individuals. Thus a trial which uses blood pressure itself as the response variable is likely to gain considerably if it uses a crossover design. In other words, the strong correlation between measurements on two occasions makes the crossover design worth while, (see, for example, Cox, 1958, Chap. 13, and John and Quenouille, 1977, Chap. 11).

However, most trials of hypotensive drugs do not use blood pressure itself but rather **change in blood pressure** as the outcome variable. Because a change is used, the crossover design loses its attraction for two major reasons:

(a) The correlation between changes in blood pressure from one occasion to another is substantially reduced, and may be close to zero (or even negative), making the design almost worthless by comparison with independent samples.

(b) There is a major problem in deciding which change to use for the second time period. For the first time period the change is clearly the difference between the baseline (pre-treatment) value and the last value for that treatment. For the second time period the last value from the first time period is the only logical value to use as a baseline, but this has clear disadvantages. A 'washout' period between the two treatments has considerable gains, both for minimizing pharmacological interaction between the two treatments and also for allowing a new baseline value to be obtained.

Unfortunately, the results (the difference between A and B) from the second time period may be different from those of the first time period. This discrepancy might, for example, be due to pharmacological interaction or to 'carryover' effects from one or more previous treatments. This is described in statistical terms as an *interaction* [see VI, §9.8.1], whatever its cause; see Section 2.1.3 in Chapter 2 for more details. If such a time period difference is found, then the interpretation of the trial becomes rather difficult: interpretation depends more on the medical than on the statistical pre-suppositions. As a technical point, the statistical test to tell whether the results differ in the two time periods is not very powerful, so that merely deciding the difference between results is 'not statistically significant' may be misleading.

As a further problem, withdrawals and missing data cause considerable problems in the analysis and reduce what effectiveness the design had at the beginning. A full discussion of the two-period crossover trial may be found in Hills and Armitage (1979), Armitage and Hills (1982) and in Barker *et al.* (1982).

If the outcome variable is a binary response (treatment success or failure) which only occurs once at most, then interpretation is difficult when the outcome (e.g. death) occurs at the very beginning of the second time period. Again, a long 'washout' period may be the only answer but there will be problems if the outcome event occurs in that period!

Finally, all these problems can be made much worse when testing three or more treatments. However, it may be possible to use more treatment periods than there are treatments (although this has rarely been done in clinical trials). As an example, with four treatment periods and a multiple of four patients to test two drugs A and B, the sequences ABAB, ABBA, BABA and BAAB may be used. See Kershner and Federer (1981) for a discussion of many possible designs for two-treatment crossover studies. Cox (1958) discusses *Latin squares* [see V, §9.5] and some other designs for several treatments.

1.4.5 Sequential methods

For ethical and/or economic reasons it may be important to assess the results obtained at various times during the course of an investigation (this may of course be impossible if the response to treatment only become apparent after some years). For example, in comparing two treatments we may have overestimated the variability of response to a particular treatment or we may have underestimated the actual difference between mean treatment response. In either case we will have overestimated the required sample size. Alternatively, we may find that the observed difference in response to the treatments is so small that to gain any reliable information our estimated sample size must be increased to a prohibitive extent.

A *sequential* study is one in which the sample size depends on the results obtained up to a given time [see VI, Chapter 13]. For example, we may define a *stopping rule* which after each observation gives one of three options:

(a) Stop sampling and reject the null hypothesis.
(b) Stop sampling and accept the null hypothesis.
(c) Continue sampling since the results so far are insufficient but promising.

To illustrate that special methods are necessary for *sequential hypothesis testing*, suppose we have a series of subjects, each of whom receives two treatments A and B in a suitably randomized and balanced order. We might disregard patients for whom there is no observable difference and perform a *sequential sign test*, pausing after every subject to see if the proportion of the times that A appears better is significantly different (at the 5 per cent level) from a half.

After six subjects we would reject the null hypothesis of 'no treatment difference' if we had seen either A better each time (denoted AAAAAA) or B better each time (BBBBBB), since the probability of either of these occurring under the null hypothesis is 2/64 or 0.03125. After nine subjects we would regard as significant any sequence with 0, 1, 8 or 9 A's (a combined probability of 20/512 or 0.03906). However, using our sequential test we would also have rejected a sequence like AAAAAABBB without actually observing the seventh, eighth or ninth subjects. The total number of sequences that would cause rejection of the null hypothesis is in fact 28 out of 512, with a probability of 0.0547, and if we were to sample up to 100 subjects we would have a probability of 0.227 of rejecting equally effective treatments as being different 'at the 5 per cent level ($P < 0.05$)', whereas by definition the probability should be at most 0.05.

Consequently, for a given *overall* significance level (α error) we need much higher significance levels (lower α errors) for the **individual** tests at different times in the study. Calculations similar to those above can be used to derive sequential tests with specified overall α errors.

The sequential nature of the study is irrelevant in a *Bayesian* analysis (Section 1.3.16), which depends on the likelihood function and is unaffected by the stopping rule or the order in which the observations occurred. However, even in a Bayesian analysis, if none of the postulated models appear adequate then interpretation may be influenced by the sequential nature and by considerations like randomization (see Box, 1980).

Other aspects of the study, such as the relative sizes of the treatment groups, may also be decided sequentially (see, for example, Simon, 1977, and Efron, 1980a). Armitage (1975) is a standard work which provides sequential plans specially for use in medicine; other developments are in, for example, Pocock (1978). Sequential trials have very seldom been used in practice, but a discussion of the many problems may be found in George (1980).

SUMMARY OF FORMULAE

Mean $\bar{x}$ of $x_1, x_2, \ldots, x_n$ (Section 1.1.3)

$$\bar{x} = \sum_{i=1}^{n} x_i/n = \sum x/n, \text{ for short.} \tag{1.1.1}$$

Mean absolute deviation (Section 1.1.4)

$$\text{MAD}(x) = \frac{\sum |x - \bar{x}|}{n}. \tag{1.1.2}$$

Variance (Section 1.1.4)

$$\text{Var}(x) = \frac{1}{n-1} \sum (x - \bar{x})^2, \tag{1.1.3}$$

$$= \frac{\sum x^2 - n\bar{x}^2}{n - 1}. \tag{1.1.4}$$

Standard deviation (Section 1.1.4)

$$\text{s.d.}(x) = \sqrt{\text{Var}(x)}. \tag{1.1.5}$$

Skewness (Section 1.1.4)

$$\text{Skew}(x) = \frac{\sum(x - \bar{x})^3}{[\text{s.d.}(x)]^3}. \tag{1.1.6}$$

Kurtosis (Section 1.1.4)

$$\text{Kurtosis}(x) = \frac{\sum(x - \bar{x})^4}{[\text{s.d.}(x)]^4}. \tag{1.1.7}$$

Standard error of the mean of n observations (Section 1.3.1)

$$\text{SEM} = \frac{s}{\sqrt{n}}, \tag{1.3.1}$$

where s is the sample standard deviation, $\sqrt{\sum(x - \bar{x})^2/(n - 1)}$.

Combination of variances (Section 1.3.1)

$$\text{Var}(k_1 X_1 + k_2 X_2) = k_1^2 \text{Var}(X_1) + k_2^2 \text{Var}(X_2), \tag{1.3.2}$$

where k_1 and k_2 are constants (positive or negative) and X_1 and X_2 are independent (or, more generally, uncorrelated; see Section 1.3.13).

One-sample t test of the hypothesis 'mean = μ' (Section 1.3.5)

$$t = \frac{\bar{x} - \mu}{s/\sqrt{n}} \qquad \text{on } n - 1 \text{ degrees of freedom,} \tag{1.3.3}$$

where $n =$ the size of the sample,
$\bar{x} =$ the sample mean,
$s =$ the sample standard deviation.

Pooled standard deviation from two samples, A and B (Section 1.3.6)

$$s = \sqrt{\frac{(n_A - 1)s_A^2 + (n_B - 1)s_B^2}{n_A + n_B - 2}}. \tag{1.3.4}$$

Two-sample t test of the hypothesis '$\mu_A = \mu_B$', assuming $\sigma_A^2 = \sigma_B^2$ (Section 1.3.6)

$$t = \frac{\bar{x}_A - \bar{x}_B}{s\sqrt{1/n_A + 1/n_B}} \qquad \text{on } n_A + n_B - 2 \text{ d.f.,} \qquad (1.3.5)$$

where s is defined by formula (1.3.4).

Standard error of $\bar{x}_A - \bar{x}_B$, assuming $\sigma_A^2 \neq \sigma_B^2$ (Section 1.3.6)

$$\text{s.e.}(\bar{x}_A - \bar{x}_B) = \sqrt{s_A^2/n_A + s_B^2/n_B}. \qquad (1.3.6)$$

Approximate number of degrees of freedom for t in formula (1.3.6) (Section 1.3.6)

$$n = \frac{(s_A^2/n_A + s_B^2/n_B)^2}{s_A^4/[n_A^2(n_A - 1)] + s_B^4/[n_B^2(n_B - 1)]} \qquad \text{approx.} \qquad (1.3.7)$$

Two-sample t test, assuming $\sigma_A^2 \neq \sigma_B^2$ (Section 1.3.6)

$$t = \frac{\bar{x}_A - \bar{x}_B}{\sqrt{s_A^2/n_A + s_B^2/n_B}}. \qquad (1.3.8)$$

Paired t test (Section 1.3.7)

$$t = \frac{\bar{d}}{s/\sqrt{n}} \qquad \text{on } (n - 1) \text{ d.f.,} \qquad (1.3.9)$$

where n = number of pairs,

$\bar{d}$ = mean difference,

s = s.d. of the n differences.

χ^2 test (Section 1.3.9)

$$X^2 = \sum \frac{(O - E)^2}{E}, \qquad (1.3.10)$$

where O = observed count,

E = expected count,

and the sum is taken over *all* categories. The sum X^2 is commonly denoted by χ^2 (see text).

Confidence limits of $100(1 - \alpha)$ per cent for the mean of a Normal distribution (Section 1.3.11)

$$\bar{x} = \pm t_{n-1, 1-\alpha/2} s/\sqrt{n}, \qquad (1.3.11)$$

where $\qquad n =$ the size of the sample,

$s =$ the sample standard deviation,

and $\qquad t_{n-1,1-\alpha/2}$ is the $100(1-\alpha/2)$ per cent point of the t_{n-1} distribution.

Confidence limits of $100(1-\alpha)$ per cent for the variance of a Normal distribution (Section 1.3.11)

$$\text{Lower:} \frac{n-1}{\chi^2_{n-1,1-\alpha/2}} s^2,$$

$$\text{Upper:} \frac{n-1}{\chi^2_{n-1,\alpha/2}} s^2,$$

(1.3.12)

where $\qquad n =$ the size of the sample,

$s^2 =$ the sample variance,

and, for example, $\chi^2_{9,0.975}$ is the 97.5 per cent point of the χ^2_9 distribution.

Residual sum of squares (RSS) from the 'least squares' regression line $Y = a + bX$ (Section 1.3.13)

$$\begin{aligned} \text{RSS} &= \sum (y - a - bx)^2 \\ &= \sum (y - \bar{y})^2 - \frac{[\sum (x - \bar{x})(y - \bar{y})]^2}{\sum (x - \bar{x})^2}. \end{aligned}$$

(1.3.13)

Slope b of least squares regression line $Y = a + bX$ (Section 1.3.13)

$$b = \frac{\sum (x - \bar{x})(y - \bar{y})}{\sum (x - \bar{x})^2},$$

(1.3.14)

$$\text{s.e.}(b) = \frac{s}{\sqrt{(x - \bar{x})^2}},$$

(1.3.15)

where $s = \text{RSS}/(n-2)$ is the *residual mean squared error*.

Intercept a of least squares regression line $Y = a + bX$ (Section 1.3.13)

$$a = \bar{y} - b\bar{x},$$

(1.3.16)

$$\text{s.e.}(a) = s\left[\frac{1}{n} + \frac{\bar{x}^2}{\sum (x - \bar{x})^2} \right],$$

(1.3.17)

where $s = \text{RSS}/(n-2)$.

Correlation coefficient (Section 1.3.15)

$$r = \frac{\sum (x - \bar{x})(y - \bar{y})}{\sqrt{\sum (x - \bar{x})^2 \sum (y - \bar{y})^2}};$$ (1.3.18)

The t test of hypothesis $r = 0$, *i.e. 'no correlation' (Section* 1.3.15)

$$t = r \sqrt{\frac{n - 2}{1 - r^2}} \qquad \text{on } n - 2 \text{ d.f.}$$ (1.3.19)

Estimated sample size required for a two-sample t test (Section 1.4.3)

$$n = 2 \left[\frac{(z_{\alpha/2} + z_\beta)\sigma}{d} \right]^2,$$ (1.4.1)

where n is the number required in each sample,
            d is the difference in means that is thought clinically important,
            α is the significance level to be used (e.g. 0.05),
            $1 - \beta$ is the required power to detect a difference of size d,
            $z_{\alpha/2}$ is the $100\alpha/2$ per cent point of the standard Normal
            distribution (e.g. $z_{\alpha/2} = -1.96$ for $\alpha = 0.05$),
            z_β is the 100β per cent point (e.g. $z_\beta = 0$ for $\beta = 0.5$).

Estimated sample size required for a χ^2 test (Section 1.4.3)

$$n = \frac{P_A(100 - P_A) + P_B(100 - P_B)}{(P_A - P_B)^2}(z_{\alpha/2} + z_\beta)^2,$$ (1.4.2)

where P_A, P_B are the estimated percentage success rates on treatments A and B
respectively, and n, $z_{\alpha/2}$ and z_β are as defined in formula (1.4.1). Neither P_A nor P_B
should be close to 0 per cent or to 100 per cent for this formula to give sensible
answers (10 to 90 per cent is reasonable).

J. E. H. S.
S. J. W. E.

Mathematical Methods in Medicine
Edited by D. Ingram & R. F. Bloch
© 1984 John Wiley & Sons Ltd.

2

Medical Statistics:
Advanced Techniques and Computation

2.1 BUILDING STATISTICAL MODELS IN MORE COMPLEX SITUATIONS

Statistical methods for more complicated situations than those in Chapter 1 are usually based on *model building*: taking account of as many sources of variation as seems reasonable. Often we can use analysis of variance, or *ANOVA* (Sections 2.1.1 to 2.1.4), particularly for a carefully designed study. Multiple regression (Section 2.1.5) is necessary if we have several numerical explanatory variables. Analysis of covariance, or *ANCOVA* (Section 2.1.6), combines ANOVA with multiple regression in an attempt to reduce bias and improve precision. Special techniques are necessary for a qualitative response variable (Sections 2.1.7 and 2.1.8).

A simple example of a model was provided by linear regression in Chapter 1. All the comments and caveats found there and throughout Chapter 1 about the importance of robustness, transformations, checking assumptions, careful consideration of sources of variation and careful interpretation of statistical significance should be borne in mind when building models.

Examples of most of the methods in Section 2.1 may be found in books such as Snedecor and Cochran (1980) and Armitage (1971). Two particularly useful books with examples of several statistical techniques applied to real data are Miller *et al.* (1980) and Cox and Snell (1981).

2.1.1 Analysis of variance (ANOVA) [see VI, Chapter 8]

The analysis of variance is a general formal method of comparing different models for a set of data. For example, Section 1.3.6 of Chapter 1 presented data on weight gains for two treatment groups, each containing eight anorexics. Suppose we assume that there is no underlying difference between groups A and B, so that only random variation causes the observed mean weights to differ from a single common value, which we can estimate to be the observed overall mean (2.845). We can give as a measure of lack of fit the *total sum of squares* about the mean:

$$\text{TSS} = (-1.9 - 2.845)^2 + (-0.7 - 2.845)^2 + \cdots + (6.3 - 2.845)^2$$
$$= 87.90.$$

The number of degrees of freedom associated with this sum of squares is $(16 - 1) = 15$, since we have fitted one parameter by assuming that the population mean equals the sample mean. Therefore the average lack of fit per observation is estimated to be $(87.9/15) = 5.86$, the *mean square*. For this simplest model the mean square is actually the variance of all sixteen observations.

We may now consider the alternative model that the group means are different. We estimate the group means by their observed values, 1.49 and 4.20, so the lack of fit is now given by the *residual sum of squares*:

$$\text{RSS} = (-1.9 - 1.49)^2 + (-0.7 - 1.49)^2 + \cdots + (5.0 - 1.49)^2$$
$$+ (0.7 - 4.20)^2 + (2.5 - 4.20)^2 + \cdots + (6.3 - 4.20)^2$$
$$= 58.47.$$

The number of degrees of freedom for the residual sum of squares is 14, since we have fitted two population parameters (the group means). The *residual mean square* is now $(58.47/14) = 4.18$.

Therefore, by fitting different means to groups A and B we have reduced the residual sum of squares by $(87.90–58.47) = 29.43$. The number of degrees of freedom has been reduced by 1, so this 1 d.f. is linked with the difference between treatments, and the *mean square for treatments* is $(29.43/1) = 29.43$.

To test whether there is a significant difference between the mean responses to the different treatments we see whether this reduction in lack of fit is larger than is reasonable by chance. If the *full model* of the unequal group means is no better than the *reduced model* of a single overall mean, then the mean square for treatments (29.43) and the residual mean square under the full model (4.18) should be independent estimates of the same quantity (the *residual variance*), and their ratio should be close to 1. High values of this *variance ratio* suggest that the fit with different treatment means is better than that with a single overall mean.

If the random errors in the observations are Normally distributed when there is no underlying difference between mean treatment responses, then this variance ratio should in fact come from the F distribution on 1 and 14 d.f. (written here as $F(1, 14)$) [see VI, §2.5.6]. Tables of the F distribution are usually presented with columns representing the d.f. of the numerator and rows the d.f. of the denominator (see Section 1.2.5 in Chapter 1). For example, the table of 95 per cent points for various F distributions shows the 95 per cent point of $F(1, 14)$ to be 4.6.

Large F values are evidence against equality of group means, so we perform a one-tailed test. Our observed variance ratio is $(29.43/4.18) = 7.05$ which corresponds to the 98 per cent point of the $F(1,14)$ distribution, and the null hypothesis of equal treatment means is rejected $(P = 0.02)$.

The results of dividing the total sum of squares into components correspond-

Table 2.1.1 Analysis of variance table for anorexic groups A and B.

Source of variation	Degrees of freedom (d.f.)	Sum of squares (s.s.)	Mean square (m.s.)	F
Treatment	1	29.43	29.43	$7.05 (P < 0.02)$
Residual	14	58.47	4.18	
Total	15	87.90		

ing to different sources can be presented formally in the *analysis of variance* (*ANOVA*) *table*, shown in Table 2.1.1.

In practice we calculate the entries in the ANOVA table from the *fitted sums of squares* rather than from the residual sums of squares:

Total SS (uncorrected for mean)

$$= (-1.9)^2 + (-0.7)^2 + \cdots + (6.3)^2 \qquad = 217.3; \qquad (2.1.1)$$

SS fitting different group means

$$= (1.49)^2 + (1.49)^2 + \cdots + (4.20)^2$$
$$= 8 \times (1.49)^2 + 8 \times (4.20)^2 \qquad = 158.9; \qquad (2.1.2)$$

SS fitting a common mean

$$= (2.84)^2 + (2.84)^2 + \cdots + (2.84)^2$$
$$= 16 \times (2.84)^2 \qquad = 129.0; \qquad (2.1.3)$$

and, apart from rounding errors, the RSS is given by $(2.1.1) - (2.1.2)$ and the treatment SS by $(2.1.2) - (2.1.3)$. We can use such shortcuts in the arithmetic for all *orthogonal* designs (see Section 2.1.4) and the calculations are made still easier by using formulae like:

$$(\text{Number in group}) \times (\text{group mean})^2 = \frac{(\text{sum of values in group})^2}{\text{number in group}}.$$

The above analysis is equivalent to the two-sample t test given in Section 1.3.6 of Chapter 1, apart from rounding errors in the arithmetic. For example:

$$\text{Residual mean square} = 4.18 = (2.04)^2 = (\text{pooled s.d.})^2$$
$$\text{and } F = 7.05 = (2.66)^2 = t^2$$

However, unlike the t test, this *one-way analysis of variance* [see VI, Example 8.2.6] (so called because our data were classified in just one way, according to the treatment given) can easily be generalized to more than two groups. Suppose another five anorexics had been given treatment C and we observed weight increases of 1.3, 1.8, 3.8, 5.6 and 6.5 kg, then the mean for group C

Table 2.1.2 Analysis of variance table for groups A, B and C.

Source	d.f.	s.s.	m.s.	F
Treatment	2	32.92	16.46	3.74 ($P < 0.05$)
Residual	18	79.25	4.40	
Total	20	112.16		

is 3.80 kg and the mean for all twenty-one observations is 3.07 kg. Therefore the sums of squares are:

$$TSS = (-1.9 - 3.07)^2 + (-0.7 - 3.07)^2 + \cdots + (6.5 - 3.07)^2$$
$$= 112.16,$$

$$RSS = 58.47 + (1.3 - 3.8)^2 + \cdots + (6.5 - 3.8)^2$$
$$= 79.25,$$

and we can draw up the ANOVA table in Table 2.1.2. We can then reject the null hypothesis 'all three treatments produce the same mean weight increase' with $P = 0.05$ because the 95 per cent of the $F(2, 18)$ distribution is 3.55, compared with our observed ratio 3.74.

We can examine the residuals $(-1.9 - 1.49)$, $(-0.7 - 1.49)$, etc., and if our assumptions of Normally distributed random errors and of equal variances within each group seem unreasonable then we can transform the original data and try another one-way ANOVA on the transformed values. Here the assumptions seem sensible, so we can continue analysing the data by looking at the treatment means and their standard errors (calculated from the *pooled within group s.d.* $= \sqrt{4.40} = 2.10$):

Treatment	Mean	s.e. (mean)
A	1.49	$2.1/\sqrt{8} = 0.74$
B	4.20	$2.1/\sqrt{8} = 0.74$
C	3.80	$2.1/\sqrt{5} = 0.94$

A *linear contrast* is any linear combination of the group means which would take the value zero if all means were equal. For example, if A is the control treatment and B and C are different brands of a new drug, we may want to see whether the average weight gain from B or C is higher than the average weight gain from A. We can form the contrast

$$L = 0.5 \times (4.20 + 3.80) - 1.49 = 2.51,$$

with standard error

$$s.e.(L) = \sqrt{(0.5)^2 \times (0.74^2 + 0.94^2) + 0.74^2} = 0.95,$$

and look at the statistic $t = (2.51/0.95) = 2.64$ on 18 d.f. (18 degrees of freedom since that is the number of d.f. for the pooled standard deviation). Similarly, we can form confidence limits for the value of L.

A more revealing formula for the standard error of L involves the pooled s.d., the numbers in each group and the coefficients defining L:

$$\text{s.e.}(L) = 2.1 \times \sqrt{\frac{(0.5)^2}{8} + \frac{(0.5)^2}{5} + \frac{(-1)^2}{8}} = 0.95.$$

If we examine several contrasts (e.g. the mean differences between A and B, between A and C and between B and C) then we are making *multiple comparisons* [see VI, §10.2]. Each individual test is valid by itself, but because we are carrying out several t tests simultaneously, the probability of finding at least one $P < 0.05$ by chance is greater than 0.05, and considerably so for more than three groups.

There are many conservative techniques (due to Newman, Duncan, Scheffé and others) to avoid inflated significance levels; formal methods of carrying out multiple comparisons are reviewed in, for example, Winer (1971, Secs 3.8 to 3.10) and in Wallenstein, Zucker and Fleiss (1980). These methods may still give misleading conclusions, so the simplest reasonable way to present results is probably to quote the group means and standard errors along with any important contrasts, allowing the reader to interpret the nominal significance levels for himself.

2.1.2 Two-way ANOVA and other options [see VI, §§10.1 and 11.3]

The data in Table 2.1.3 show the changes in heart rate for five rabbits each given four experimental treatment drugs. Again we can use ANOVA to compare possible models for the data. We would expect each of the twenty responses to depend partly on the treatment applied (e.g. treatment 1 seems to produce the largest decrease in heart rate) and partly on which rabbit we are using (e.g. rabbit 5 shows larger decreases than rabbit 2). We therefore have two *factors* (qualitative

Table 2.1.3 Change in heart rate (beats per minute) after treatment.

| | | \multicolumn{4}{c}{Treatment number} | |
		1	2	3	4	Row total
Rabbit	1	−41	11	−18	−2	−50
	2	−14	17	1	−5	−1
	3	−17	−1	−10	9	−19
	4	−28	11	20	−7	−4
	5	−18	−22	−1	−23	−64
Column total		−118	16	−8	−28	−138
Mean		−23.6	3.2	−1.6	−5.6	−6.9

variables whose values, or *levels*, are used to classify the data): factor 1 (treatment) has four levels and factor 2 (rabbits) has five. The factors are *crossed* [see VI, §10.1.5], which means that the first value in each treatment group corresponds to the same rabbit (by contrast, the treatment groups in Section 2.1.1 contain different individuals, and we say that anorexics are *nested* within treatments). We can use a *two-way analysis of variance* to compare possible models.

The overall mean response is (− 138/20) = − 6.9 and the mean for treatment 1 is (− 118/5) = − 23.6; therefore we estimate the *effect of treatment* 1 to be [− 23.6 −(− 6.9)] = − 16.7. Similarly, the other treatment effects are 10.1, 5.3 and 1.3; note that the four treatment effects sum to zero.

In the same way, since the mean response of rabbit 1 is (− 50/4) = − 12.5, we estimate the rabbit 1 effect to be [− 12.5 − (− 6.9)] = − 5.6. Again we can calculate residual sums of squares for different models. We consider the *full model* (a) and various *submodels* (b, c and d):

(a) The **full model**. An observed value depends on the row and column in which it occurs; these effects are *additive*. Therefore, for example, the fitted value for row 1, column 1 (rabbit 1 under treatment 1) is (− 6.9 − 16.7 − 5.6) = − 29.2, and the residual is [− 41 − (− 29.2)] = − 11.8.

(b) If there were no differences between treatment effects then the fitted value for row 1, column 1 would be (− 6.9 − 5.6) = − 12.5 with residual − 28.5.

(c) If treatments differed but there were no consistent variation between rabbits then the fitted value would be (− 6.9 − 16.7) = − 23.6 with residual − 17.4.

(d) Finally, if there were no differences between rabbits or between treatments, we would fit each value by the overall mean − 6.9, so the residual for row 1, column 1 would be − 34.1.

The sums of squares are calculated most easily by considering the fitted sums of squares, as in Section 2.1.1. For example, after fitting the mean (model 4 above) we have the fitted sum of squares $20 \times (− 6.9)^2$, or, equivalently,

$$\frac{(− 138)^2}{20} = 952.2.$$

Similarly, the fitted sum of squares for model 3 is:

$$\frac{(− 118)^2}{5} + \frac{(16)^2}{5} + \frac{(− 8)^2}{5} + \frac{(− 28)^2}{5} = 3,005.6.$$

Therefore the sum of squares for treatments is:

$$(3005.6 − 952.2) = 2053.4.$$

The full analysis of variance table is shown in Table 2.1.4 and suggests that there are significant differences between treatments $(F(3,12) = (684.5/167.3) = 4.09, \ P < 0.05)$ but not between rabbits $(F(4,12) = (197.8/167.3) = 1.18,$

Table 2.1.4 ANOVA table for rabbit heart rate data.

Source	d.f.	s.s.	m.s.	F	
Treatments	3	2,053.4	684.5	4.09	$(P < 0.05)$
Rabbits	4	791.3	197.8	1.18	$(P > 0.2)$
Residual	12	2,007.1	167.3		
Total	19	4,851.8			

$P > 0.1$). In other words, the variation within a given rabbit is large enough to hide any genuine consistent differences between rabbits, but not large enough to mask the differences between treatments. The standard error for each treatment effect is $\sqrt{167.3/5} = 6.47$, and as in Section 2.1.1 we can form contrasts to investigate the ways in which treatments differ.

An experiment in which we try to improve precision by classifying subjects into groups, or *blocks*, of similar units and comparing treatment responses within each block is sometimes called a *randomized block design* [see VI, §§9.4 and 9.5] and generalizes the paired *t* test in the same way as one-way ANOVA generalizes the two-sample *t* test. In these terms, each rabbit is a block! We will return to the interpretation of such experiments in Section 2.1.3.

Treatments should be allocated randomly within a block, which here means that the order in which treatments are given should be random. We might also try to balance out the order of treatments; e.g. with five treatments on five rabbits we could use a *Latin square* design [see VI, §9.11.1] with columns representing the order of treatment and rabbits being randomly assigned to different rows. Examples may be found in books such as Cochran and Cox (1957).

Unfortunately, for various reasons the treatments here were given in the same order for each rabbit. This means that our estimates of the treatment effects are probably *biased*: external conditions such as room temperature will be different and any apparent differences between treatments may just be due to these other factors. In other words, the treatment effect is *confounded* with the order effect (this is in addition to the problems with possible after-effects, mentioned in Section 1.4.4). Although we can never be sure that we are taking account of all important external factors, we can try to reduce this bias, correcting for external factors by an *analysis of covariance* (Section 2.1.6).

We might also carry out a *non-parametric ANOVA* to test for differences between treatments. We can rank the observed responses for each rabbit and look at the sum of ranks for each treatment; thus the sum of ranks for treatment 1 is $(1 + 1 + 1 + 1 + 3) = 7$, whereas the expected value if all ranks are equally likely is $(5 \times 2.5) = 12.5$. This generalization of the sign test is called the *Friedman two-way ANOVA* and examples are given in Siegel (1956) and Colquhoun (1971), which also cover other non-parametric techniques such as *Kruskal–Wallis one-way*

ANOVA, a generalization of the Mann–Whitney–Wilcoxon test mentioned in Section 1.3.8 of Chapter 1.

Hollander and Wolfe (1973) give further practical examples of non-parametric methods. Such methods are robust provided that with small treatment groups we use the *exact* distributions of the test statistics; however, they can be difficult to extend to more complicated problems like those in Sections 2.1.3, 2.1.4 and 2.1.6.

Tukey (1977) shows how to estimate the various effects by medians rather than by means (*median polishing*). This descriptive approach is useful as an automatic first step in the analysis; we can then look at the residuals and decide whether an analysis based on means, Normal distributions, etc., is justifiable (possibly after transforming the response) or whether we should just report the median effects without attempting to build a probabilistic model. Maritz (1981) indicates some methods of building more sophisticated models in a distribution-free way.

2.1.3 Interpretation of ANOVA for more complicated designs

ANOVA tables are usually produced using standard computer programs (see Section 2.4.2), so we have not placed much emphasis on the calculations. Many standard textbooks such as Cochran and Cox (1957) give formulae and several numerical examples for sums of squares in various experimental designs.

We still need to know how to interpret ANOVA tables. Table 2.1.5 shows a computer-produced ANOVA for an experiment in which two drugs were compared, each at three concentrations, for their ability to reduce allergic reactions. Two observations were made on each of ten patients for all six (drug, concentration) combinations, the whole experiment being carefully designed ('double-blindness' and randomization). We have a *many-way classification* with a total of $(2 \times 3 \times 10 \times 2) = 120$ observations.

Experiments like this with all factors crossed (i.e. observations made for all

Table 2.1.5 Example of many-way ANOVA.

Source	d.f.	s.s.	m.s.
Drug	1	33.8	33.77
Concentration	2	162.7	81.37
Patient	9	79.0	8.78
D × C	2	1.8	0.92
D × P	9	42.2	4.69
C × P	18	94.1	5.23
D × C × P	18	52.9	2.94
Residual	60	128.5	2.14
Total	119	595.0	

possible factor combinations) are called *factorial experiments* and here we have two *replicates per cell* (two observations for each factor combination) [see VI, §§9.8 and 11.3.6].

As well as looking for *main effects* (differences between drugs, between concentrations and between patients) we can examine the *interactions*. For example, if the difference between drug effects varies from patient to patient then we have a *drug × patient interaction* (D × P), and we can test whether this *two-way* (or *first-order*) interaction is larger than would be expected by chance.

Similarly, the *three-way* (or *second-order*) interaction drug × concentration × patient (D × C × P) indicates whether the D × P interaction is similar for all three drug concentrations. Interactions are illustrated geometrically in Winer (1971, Sec. 5.11).

The best way to interpret the ANOVA table is to begin with the highest order interaction. Here the interaction D × C × P is tested by $F(18,60) = (2.94/2.14) = 1.38$. This value is easily accounted for by chance ($P = 0.2$), so we can simplify the table and our interpretation of the results by including the three-way interaction in the residual error variation; we calculate:

$$\text{Residual mean square} = \frac{128.5 + 52.9}{60 + 18} = 2.33 \text{ with 78 d.f.}$$

which may be a more accurate estimate of the residual variance (it certainly has more degrees of freedom).

To test the drug × patient interaction D × P, we compare the ratio $(4.69/2.33) = 2.01$ with the F distribution on $(9, 78)$ d.f. Most tables give the 98 per cent points for $F(9, 60)$ and $F(9, 120)$, which are 2.04 and 1.96 respectively. The 95 per cent point for $F(9, 78)$ will therefore be about 2, and the significance of the D × P interaction is $P = 0.05$. Similarly, the significance of C × P is $P = 0.02$ and that of D × C is $P > 0.5$.

When we look at the main effects (or in general any effects other than the highest order interaction in the model) we must be careful. We are interested in comparing the drugs and the different drug concentrations, and have fixed the drug and concentration for any given observation. They are factors with *fixed effects* and if we repeated the whole experiment we would use the same drugs at the same concentrations. However, we could use a different set of patients. We are not interested in the patient effects as such since the patients are a sample from a population: 'patient number' is a factor with *random effects* and represents a source of variation that we would like to remove.

When we test the drug effects we want to know if the mean drug effects differ **in the population** from which our ten patients are a sample. If there is no such difference we would expect the observed difference between drug means to be due to the random variation in the relative responses for individual patients, which is measured by the *D × P interaction*. Therefore the variance ratio for testing the main drug effect is:

$$F(1,9) = \frac{33.77}{4.69} = 7.20 \qquad (P = 0.025).$$

Similarly, the variance ratio for testing concentrations is:

$$F(2,18) = \frac{81.37}{5.23} = 15.56 \qquad (P < 0.001).$$

If we wanted to test for differences between mean patient responses we could calculate $F(9,78) = (8.78/2.33) = 3.77$ $(P < 0.001)$. The denominator here is the ordinary residual mean square since each patient has observations taken at combinations of fixed effect factors only (D × C), and there is no additional random error in estimating each patient mean.

Experiments like this where several treatments are applied to each experimental subject, 'experimental subject' being a random effect, are sometimes called experiments with *repeated measures*. They occur frequently in medical research and several examples are given in Winer (1971). Note that the 'randomized block' experiment on rabbit heart rates in Section 2.1.2 involved 'rabbit' as a random effect, but because only one observation was made for each (rabbit, treatment) combination we could not estimate the rabbit × treatment interaction. The ANOVA is the same as for two fixed effects, but the interpretation (differences between rabbits indicating the variability of response in the rabbit population, and differences between treatments being referred to the rabbit population rather than to the five particular experimental rabbits) is different.

We could continue the analysis of the drugs and concentrations in many ways. For example, simple ANOVA is only valid with *unordered* qualitative explanatory variables (factors). Here the drug concentrations are ordered (low < medium < high) and we should take account of this by examining the contrasts on drug concentrations:

$$-1 \times \text{(low level)} + 0 \times \text{(medium)} + 1 \times \text{(high)}$$

and

$$-1 \times \text{(low)} + 2 \times \text{(medium)} + -1 \times \text{(high)}$$

and thus dividing up the sums of squares for drug concentration to represent *linear* and *quadratic* effects. This would be meaningful on a log scale since the high concentration is in fact ten times the medium and a hundred times the low concentration.

A general method to investigate *equality of variance* involves taking logs of estimated variances. If s^2 is a variance estimate with $(n-1)$ d.f. then $\log(s^2)$ to base e has the approximate variance $2/(n-1)$. Unfortunately, such an analysis is very sensitive to non-Normality in the original data and is unreliable unless the d.f. for all the s^2 are fairly large. However, we could, for example, calculate the variances of the residuals for each (drug, level) combination and analyse the logarithms of these six variances in a two-way ANOVA. Since the residual sum of squares has 78 d.f. we can assume that each variance v has $(78/6) = 13$ d.f. and we would expect each $\log_e(v)$ to have variance $2/13 = 0.154$ (and therefore standard error $\sqrt{0.154} = 0.392$). More robust methods of testing for equal variances are available and are produced by some computer programs.

The F tests are fairly robust to unequal variances, at least for equal numbers in each group (see Box, 1954). If, however, we found very widely differing variances (say by a factor of 3), then we could use weighted regression analysis with dummy variables (see Section 2.1.5). Draper and Smith (1981, Chap. 9) illustrate regression applied to ANOVA.

If the distribution of the *residuals* appears non-Normal or if patterns in the residuals suggest that the terms in the model are not additive then we could try transforming the data. A transformation to a more appropriate scale of measurement may also remove some interactions; e.g. if the drug with the higher mean response also showed more difference between concentrations, then there would be a drug × concentration interaction which might be removed by a log or square root transformation. A useful check for such an interaction is given by *Tukey's test for non-additivity* (see, for example, Winer, 1971, Sect. 5.20). Tukey's test can be used to suggest a suitable power transformation of the response variable; related procedures may be found in Box and Cox (1964) and in Tukey (1977, Sect. 10F).

Interactions always make interpretation more complicated (see, for example, the sex × treatment interaction in an investigation described by the Canadian Cooperative Study Group, 1978). If there is an interaction between fixed effects, then the corresponding main effects are usually meaningless, so the means and standard errors should be reported for **each** factor combination. If there were a D × C interaction in our example then we ought to report the mean response for all six (drug, concentration) combinations. Note that a crossover trial is a factorial experiment with time as a factor, and time × treatment interactions are almost inevitable.

If we are prepared to lose information about some of the interactions (i.e. if we think their effect is small or irrelevant) then we could use a more sophisticated design such as a Latin square. Designs like this which aim to use as few experimental units as possible are fully discussed in Cox (1958).

2.1.4 Dangers of non-orthogonal ANOVA, missing values

Suppose that in the rabbit heart rate example (Section 2.1.2) we had two readings of change in heart rate for rabbit 1 with treatment 1, but only one reading for the other combinations. We would then have a more precise estimate of the effect of treatment 1 on rabbit 1, so random errors in the rabbit 1 readings would have less effect on our estimates of the mean response under treatment 1 than on the other treatment means. Therefore the errors in our estimates of treatment differences would be correlated with the errors in our estimates of factors other than treatment. Such an experiment is said to have a *non-orthogonal* design [see VI, § §8.2, 12.1.5 and 12.2.5].

Orthogonal means 'at right angles' and for an orthogonal design we can divide sums of squares directly into components corresponding to different factors in the same way as Pythagoras' theorem splits a squared distance into two right-angled components. All our ANOVA examples so far have had orthogonal designs, and other well-balanced designs such as those based on Latin squares are also orthogonal.

Non-orthogonal designs have many disadvantages compared with orthogonal designs: they are more sensitive to non-Normality and other invalidity in the assumptions, and interpretation of results is more difficult, particularly with random effects. Standard ANOVA is invalid since the mean squares are not independent and 'sums of squares' may even be negative. The correct analysis is complicated and some computer programs may produce misleading results without warning.

Even if all our assumptions are justified, an orthogonal design is more *efficient* than a non-orthogonal design (the standard errors of estimates from the orthogonal design are typically smaller than those from a non-orthogonal design with the same number of observations); important treatment differences may be missed because of a poor experimental design.

Non-orthogonality is often caused by *missing values*. If the reason for a value being missing is related to its size (e.g. if a value is too small to register or if we suspect that a particular person would show a dangerous response to the highest drug level so we miss out the highest level on this subject) then it is difficult to interpret the remaining *uncensored* data. Section 2.3 illustrates ways of tackling censored data of certain kinds, but ideally we want to avoid such difficulties by using sensitive measuring equipment, reasonable drug levels, etc.

However, if data are missing from a designed experiment for reasons unrelated to their actual values then we can simplify the analysis by calculating fitted *dummy* values for the missing data in such a way that the residuals corresponding to these fitted values after the analysis are all zero. Since the residuals of these dummy values are automatically zero, the estimated treatment effects depend **only** on the observed data, and the total number of d.f. is the number of genuinely observed values. We can build up an ANOVA table by fitting dummy values separately for every model (note that if the residuals under the full model are zero, the residuals under any sub-model are typically non-zero). We may need to *iterate* (repeat the analysis using better and better fitted values until the residuals disappear). Usually, of course, all this is done for us by a computer program (Section 2.4.2).

This technique is just a simple but correct general method of analysing 'nearly orthogonal' designs using standard ANOVA (therefore assuming in particular that the explanatory variables are unordered categories). Cochran and Cox (1957) give many examples of formulae to fit such values to missing data. Similar techniques are useful elsewhere; e.g. Dawid and Skene (1979) combine clinicians' assessments by assuming that the 'true' case history is missing.

Another problem is that of outliers; if we decide that some of our data are too extreme to be included in the analysis then we might use methods akin to trimming or Winsorization (Section 1.1.3) (see Huber, 1981). Unfortunately any approach to handling possible outliers will be open to some criticism.

2.1.5 Multiple linear regression [see VI, §8.2]

In multiple regression we investigate how the expected value of one variable (Y) depends on the values of a set of other quantitative variables (X_1, X_2, etc.). We will want to know which of the X_i are important and how important they are. Perhaps we actually want to *predict* the value of the response variable Y as, for example, in Armitage and Gehan (1974), or perhaps we hope to identify risk factors as in Pocock *et al.* (1980).

The assumptions and methods are similar to those for simple linear regression: we assume that all the random variation occurs in Y, that the relationship between Y and each X_i is linear and that the errors in Y are independent and have constant variance throughout the whole range of the values of the X_i.

The coefficients in this *linear model* are again fitted by least squares to see whether each individual coefficient is significantly different from zero (in other words, to see which of the X_i are important in the model) and to estimate these coefficients. See Section 2.4.1 for warnings on numerical accuracy.

The data in Table 2.1.6 show the maximum breathing rates of twenty subjects (data from several sources). We might expect this rate (MBC) to be related to build and health, which in turn are related to sex, age, height and weight. Experience with similar data suggests taking logs of weight and MBC, and we can then investigate the data by multiple regression with the model:

$$Y = b_0 + b_1 X_1 + b_2 X_2 + b_3 X_3 + b_4 X_4 + \text{error},$$

where Y is log (base 10) of MBC,

            b_0 is some constant,

            X_1 is 0 for males, 1 for females,

            X_2 is age in years,
            X_3 is height in centimetres,

            X_4 is log (base 10) of weight,

and b_1, b_2, b_3 and b_4 are the *regression coefficients*.

Note that X_1 is a *dummy variable* coding two categories. To code a qualitative

Table 2.1.6 Maximum breathing capacity (MBC) of twenty seated subjects.

Sex	Age, year	Height, cm	Weight, kg	MBC, litre/min
M	23	173	64	191
M	25	180	71	138
M	26	168	63	130
M	31	175	78	177
M	34	182	75	107
M	35	179	66	125
M	37	171	69	93
M	42	170	67	112
M	48	164	54	79
M	48	175	83	113
F	21	152	44	104
F	24	153	45	90
F	24	170	69	136
F	28	167	54	99
F	28	175	64	137
F	30	171	49	135
F	35	178	78	152
F	38	156	60	110
F	39	156	55	95
F	44	160	48	71

variable that takes n values we need $(n - 1)$ dummy variables and can code the n values as $(0, 0, \ldots, 0)$, $(1, 0, \ldots, 0)$, $(0, 1, \ldots, 0)$, $\ldots$, $(0, 0, \ldots, 1)$.

The mathematical solution to a multiple regression problem is best understood in terms of *matrix algebra* [see I, Chapter 6]; in practice we feed the data into a computer and obtain fitted values and standard errors for $b_0, \ldots, b_4$:

$$b_0 = 0.66 \pm 0.45, \qquad t = 1.46 (= 0.66/0.45);$$
$$b_1 = 0.011 \pm 0.040, \qquad t = 0.27;$$
$$b_2 = -0.0078 \pm 0.0021, \quad t = 3.78;$$
$$b_3 = 0.0021 \pm 0.0031, \qquad t = 0.67;$$
$$b_4 = 0.73 \pm 0.35, \qquad t = 2.10.$$

The t statistics suggest whether the coefficients are significantly different from zero, and hence indicate whether we can simplify the model by neglecting, for example, the differences in subjects' heights. The overall lack of fit is shown by the residual sum of squares, 0.0736 (on 15 d.f. since we have fitted five parameters to the model for the twenty responses y_i).

After trying a few other models, the simplest adequate model neglects X_1 and

X_3 and fits:

$b_0 = 0.751 \pm 0.336,$

$b_2 = -0.00826 \pm 0.00188,$

$b_4 = 0.886 \pm 0.191,$

with the residual sum of squares 0.0761 on 17 d.f.

The s.d. of the y_i about their fitted values is estimated by $\sqrt{0.0761/17} = 0.067$. A difference of 0.067 on the $\log_{10}$ scale may be interpreted as corresponding to a percentage error in the original data of roughly

$$[\text{antilog}(0.067) - \text{antilog}(0)] \times 100\% = 17\%.$$

We can use an F test on the residual sums of squares to see whether the model with five parameters is better than the model with three (here of course we are assuming Normally distributed random errors):

$$F = \frac{(0.0761 - 0.0736)/2}{0.0736/15} = 0.25 \qquad \text{on } (2, 15)\text{d.f.},$$

which being less than one is certainly not significant. This indicates, for example, that although the original data suggest a high correlation between height and MBC, the relationship almost disappears when we allow for the fact that height, age and weight are interrelated. Such apparent relationships often disappear when we look at the joint effect of several variables (see, for example, Hulley *et al.*, 1980).

Figure 2.1.1 attempts to show graphically the relationships between MBC, weight and age. Note in particular the increase in MBC with weight and the fact that, for people of a given weight, the older ones appear to have lower MBCs. Some different methods of plotting more than two variables simultaneously are illustrated in Barnett (1981, Pt. III).

Partial correlation [see II, §13.4.6(iii)] can be used to express the linear relationship between two variables, allowing for the fact that both may be related to other variables. Another concept is *multiple correlation* [see II, §13.6], which is the square of the correlation between the observed y and the best corresponding fitted values. Multiple correlation expresses roughly how much one variable is related to a set of other variables, but remember that all relationships are assumed to be linear.

With only twenty subjects (and with no information on, for example, smoking history) we should not read too much into the data, but we might consider including extra terms in the model. For example, the interaction $X_1 X_4$ could be included to investigate whether the linear dependence of log(MBC) on log(weight) is the same for both sexes. Similarly, we might include X_2^2 to investigate non-linear dependence of log(MBC) on age.

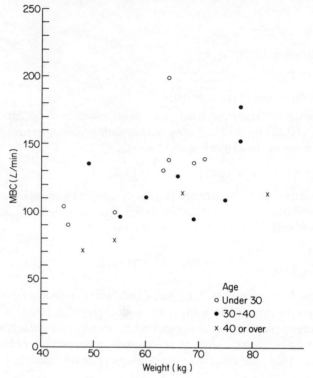

Figure 2.1.1 Relationship between MBC, weight and age in
Table 2.1.6.

As usual we should analyse the residuals; e.g. Figure 2.1.2 shows a Normal plot of the residuals from fitting log(weight) and age to log(MBC). Draper and Smith (1981) give many examples of residual analysis and of regression in general.

Several computer packages include programs for multiple regression, often with options like *stepwise regression* [see VI, §12.3.5] to choose a model automatically. Automatic methods should be handled carefully; an adequate model with a natural biological interpretation is more useful than a slightly better fitting but meaningless model. Another possible option is *ridge regression* which aims for stable estimation, typically finding fewer non-zero regression coefficients b_i on the basis that simpler models are usually more reliable for prediction. Hocking (1976) and Draper and Smith (1981) give examples of these different approaches.

A special case of multiple regression is *polynomial regression* [see VI, §8.2.5], in which we try to fit the response variable by a polynomial in an explanatory variable (X) by setting $X_1 = X$, $X_2 = X^2$, etc., as, for example, in Joossens and Brems-Heyns (1975) [see III, §6.1.3]. Polynomial regression is useful to check

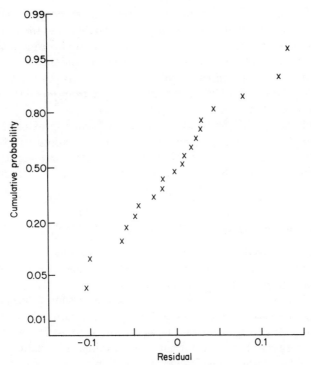

Figure 2.1.2 Normal plot of residuals from fitting log (MBC).

whether simple linear regression is adequate, but is often difficult to interpret and we would usually do better to transform the variables or to divide up the range of the explanatory variable. For example, if a response increases with drug dose concentration up to a certain dose and then drops, we are probably looking at one drug effect for low concentrations and another effect at high concentrations; describing such a response by a quadratic is misleading. If our aim is to fit a smooth curve through the points without postulating a theoretical model, then *splines* are usually more reliable than polynomials [see III, §6.5]. See also Wold (1974) for a useful introduction to splines and Largo *et al.* (1978) for a medical example.

Weighted regression [see III, §6.1.7, and VI, §6.5.2] can be used when the variances are not constant. If we assume that the error in y_i has standard deviation s_i, then we can analyse the data by transforming to $z_i = y_i/s_i$ (equalizing the variances) and using straightforward least squares to fit the model:

$$\frac{y_i}{s_i} = b_0 \frac{1}{s_i} + b_1 \frac{x_{1i}}{s_i} + \cdots + \text{error}.$$

For example, logarithms of MBC were used partly because the standard deviation of MBC was thought to be roughly proportional to the value of MBC. However, by assuming an additive model for log(MBC) we are implicitly fitting a *multiplicative* model to MBC. If we decided this was invalid then we could analyse the original data by weighted least squares with $s_i = (MBC)_i$ and thus develop a linear additive model for MBC. We might then try to improve the weights by setting $s_i = (fitted \ MBC)_i$ and repeating the analysis.

Weighted least squares can be used in this way as an approximate method of fitting *general linear models* in which the random variation may be far from Normally distributed and a crude sum of squares may be inappropriate as a measure of lack of fit (see Nelder and Wedderburn, 1972). A particular case is *logistic regression* (see Section 2.1.7).

2.1.6 Analysis of covariance (ANCOVA) [see VI, §10.1.7]

ANCOVA can be used when some explanatory variables are qualitative and classify the response variable but others (called *covariates*) are quantitative. For example, consider the rabbit data tabulated in Section 2.1.2. The change in heart rate (Y) will depend partly on the initial rate (X), and we should allow for this fact in the analysis of treatment effects. Table 2.1.7 gives the initial heart rates for each y. The simplest way to adjust for initial heart rate is to assume a similar linear relationship between Y and X for all rabbits under all treatments. We can investigate this assumption by fitting the same form of model to the covariate values x as we have done to the responses y; thus if we use the full model from Section 2.1.2 (response = overall mean + rabbit effect + drug effect) then we fit the x values also by a full model. We can then plot the y residuals (observed response − fitted response) against the corresponding x residuals (observed

Table 2.1.7 Initial heart rates (beats per minute) corresponding
to Table 2.1.3.

		Treatment number			
		1	2	3	4
Rabbit	1	281	251	253	253
	2	258	273	236	247
	3	258	238	233	234
	4	232	228	196	200
	5	283	304	276	268
Total		1,312	1,294	1,194	1,202
Treatment mean − overall mean		12.3	8.7	− 11.3	− 9.7

initial value − fitted initial value) and look for a trend. Linear regression in fact indicates that as x increases by 1, the y residual (y − fitted y) decreases by 0.483.

It is now possible to estimate what the responses y would have been had they all been measured with the same initial heart rate, which we may as well take to be the overall mean, $\bar{x}$:

Adjusted response = observed response − slope $(x - \bar{x})$.

Thus the adjusted treatment means are given by

Treatment	Old mean	−	correction	=	adjusted mean
1	− 23.6	−	(−.483 × 12.3)	=	− 17.7
2	3.2	−	(−.483 × 8.7)	=	7.4
3	− 1.6	−	(−.483 × − 11.3)	=	− 7.1
4	− 5.6	−	(−.483 × − 9.7)	=	− 10.3

and we can see that, for example, the apparently large difference between treatments 1 and 3 may have been partly due to the differences in initial heart rates. Similarly, the estimated difference between treatments 2 and 3 has changed from 4.8 to 14.5.

In general if the mean of a covariate differs between different groups, and the covariate is correlated with the response variable, then the unadjusted mean response will be biased. Analysis of covariance is then vital to the correct interpretation of the data.

Note that in this example we would expect an automatic correlation between response and covariate, since here the covariate (initial rate) is used in calculating the response (rate after treatment − initial rate) and any random errors in the covariate also appear in the response. This means that the regression estimate (− 0.483) is itself biased (see, for example, Cox and Snell, 1981, Example E) so it would be misleading to give any physiological interpretation to the regression estimate.

We can form an *ANCOVA table* for y in which each sum of squares is adjusted for the covariate by regression of the y residuals under the particular model on the x residuals under the corresponding model. The calculations involve forming ANOVA tables to split up the sums of squares and *cross-products*:

RSS for x $= \sum (x \text{ residual})^2$

RSS for y $= \sum (y \text{ residual})^2$

Residual sum of cross-products $= \sum (x \text{ residual}) \, (y \text{ residual})$

The ANCOVA table for change in rabbit heart rate is shown in Table 2.1.8. Adjusting for the initial rate has probably reduced bias in the estimates of

Table 2.1.8 ANCOVA for rabbit heart rates.

Source	d.f.	s.s.	m.s.	F
Treatments	3	1,653.9	551.3	3.56
Rabbits	4	380.0	95.0	0.61
Covariate	1	301.0	301.0	1.94
Residuals	11	1,706.1	155.1	
Total	19	4,041.0		

treatment effects but in this case has not caused a significant reduction in the sum of squares ($F(1,11) = 1.94$). For other sets of data we find that ANCOVA leaves estimated treatment effects unaltered (e.g. if we have used matched controls there should be very little bias) but reduces the standard errors of the estimated effects and so improves precision.

Details of the calculations may be found in, for example, Cochran and Cox (1957), but such analysis will normally be done by a computer, particularly if we want to adjust for several covariates simultaneously (by multiple regression of the *y* residuals). ANCOVA is simply a way to combine ANOVA and regression; further examples are in, for example, Anderson *et al.* (1980) and Snedecor and Cochran (1980, Chap. 18).

As mentioned above, when the covariate is some sort of baseline we may have problems of analysis and interpretation similar to those encountered with crossover designs (see Section 1.4.4 in Chapter 1). Often it is not very clear what variables we should use as the response and as the covariate(s) in such circumstances (see Anderson *et al.* 1980, Chap. 12, for a discussion).

2.1.7 Further Analysis of Proportions and Rates

Simple analysis of binary data was introduced in Section 1.3.12 of Chapter 1, but we need to develop more sophisticated statistical techniques to estimate the probability *p* of a positive response in complicated situations. The methods may be less convenient than the analogous ones for quantitative data but they are just as important.

For example, we may want to see how the proportion of women developing breast cancer varies with smoking and drinking alcohol. However, the probability of developing cancer obviously varies with age, and the age distributions of various smoking/drinking groups may be very different. We must therefore estimate what the proportions would be if each group had the same standard distribution. This technique of *standardization* is analogous to analysis of covariance and is discussed in, for example, Anderson *et al.* (1980, Chap. 7) and Fleiss (1981, Chap. 14). Standardization is probably best treated in terms of log-linear models (see Section 2.1.8 below and in particular Sec. 4.3 of Bishop, Fienberg and Holland, 1975).

Summary quantities such as the SMR (*standardized mortality ratio*, the ratio of observed to expected deaths) can be calculated (see, for example, Hill, 1977, Chap. 17). Although it may be misleading to attempt to summarize the mortality or morbidity of a community in a single figure, the SMR can be used in maps of mortality and perhaps analysed further using techniques like multiple regression, as in Pocock *et al.* (1980).

A general problem with qualitative data concerns continuity corrections. For example, it is often recommended that Yates' correction (Section 1.3.12) be used for all 2×2 contingency tables. There has been much discussion about when to use Yates' correction (see, for example, Liddell, 1976), and this discussion is continuing with no definite conclusion. Other corrections have been proposed (for a discussion see Haber, 1980). However, if one is trying to prove the positive and wishes to be conservative in a statistical test (as in Section 1.3.12) it is best to use Yates' correction (recognizing that it may well overcorrect), whereas if the probability of a type II error is of major concern (as in Section 1.4.3) then it is simpler not to use Yates' correction.

Another approach to an analysis of proportions is to calculate the odds (e.g. number of successes per failure) in different circumstances and then to compare these odds. Using the example from Sections 1.3.10 and 1.3.12, the odds of recovery under treatment A are 34:11 and the odds for treatment B are 64:6. The *odds ratio* is therefore estimated by

$$o = \frac{34/11}{64/6} = \frac{34 \times 6}{64 \times 11} = 0.290.$$

In other words, if we take 'number of successes per failure' as our criterion, then treatment A performs only 0.290 times as well as treatment B.

As often happens when several variables are multiplied together, the analysis can be made much simpler by taking logs:

$$L = \log_e(o) = \log(34/11) - \log(64/6)$$
$$= \log(34) + \log(6) - \log(64) - \log(11) = -1.239.$$

We might add 0.5 to all the counts as a continuity correction and to avoid the chance of dividing by zero or calculating $\log(0)$ (although, as with Yates' correction, there has been much discussion over the advisability of this). Thus,

$$o' = (34.5/11.5)/(64.5/6.5) = 0.302,$$
$$L' = \log_e(o) = -1.196.$$

An estimate of the standard error of L' is given by

$$\text{s.e.}(L') = \sqrt{\frac{1}{34.5} + \frac{1}{6.5} + \frac{1}{64.5} + \frac{1}{11.5}} = 0.534,$$

which can be used to form rough confidence limits for the odds ratio. However, more sophisticated methods are better (see, for example, Fleiss, 1981, Sec. 5.6, and Breslow, 1981).

The expression $\log(34/11) = [\log(34) - \log(11)]$ is the *logit* or *logistic transform* of the recovery rate for treatment A, and L is the *logistic difference* between A and B [see II, §11.10]. Cox (1970) shows how the logistic transform of binary data can be used as the response variable in regression (see Gilbert *et al.*, 1975, for a medical example). Logistic regression is very useful for analysing dose-response curves (see, for example, Brown and Hu, 1980, and the book by Ashton, 1972). Breslow and Day (1980) give a clear and detailed description of logistic regression, particularly as applied to case-control studies.

Section 2.1.5 mentioned how weighted regression can be used to fit general linear models. Unfortunately this can be a poor method for the regression of logits (unless the model is simple and the data extensive), because of the difficulties involved in modelling observed frequencies near zero or one. The *maximum likelihood* method of logistic regression is generally better, even though we need computer programs (Section 2.4.2). Logistic regression can be mathematically involved and should always be handled with care (see, for example, Gordon, 1974, and Greenland, 1979) [see VI, §§11.1.2 and 11.1.8].

The odds ratio has the advantage that we can use it to compare or combine results from several independent studies, including case-control studies (see Section 1.4.3 and, for example, Mantel and Haenszel, 1959, Miller, 1980, and Cox and Snell, 1981, Example V). Advantages and disadvantages of the odds ratio are described in Fleiss (1981, Chap. 6); analysis is often easiest in terms of odds ratios even if the results have to be transformed to some other criterion measure for presentation. The odds ratio can also be generalized to variables with more than two possible values (see, for example, Agresti, 1980).

Another criterion for comparing the two groups is the *relative risk*, the ratio of the proportions of subjects in each group for whom the event of interest occurs. Thus the risk of death under treatment A relative to treatment B is

$$r = \frac{11/45}{6/70} = 2.85.$$

Compare this with the odds ratio of death,

$$o = \frac{11/34}{6/64} = 3.45 \, (= 1/0.290).$$

Although the relative risk has a nice simple interpretation it is not convenient mathematically, and cannot be estimated at all from a case-control study (see, for example, Anderson *et al.*, 1980, Sec. 4.5.2). However, for a rare event, the relative risk and the odds ratio will be nearly equal. For example, if treatment A had a failure rate of 11/450 and treatment B of 6/700 (i.e. around 1 or 2 per cent rather than 10 or 20 per cent), then the relative risk would be 2.85 and the odds ratio $(11/439)/(6/694) = 2.90$.

The odds ratio is related to the logit transform of a proportion, $\log_e[p/(1-p)]$. Other useful transformations for proportions are the *arcsine transformation*, $\sin^{-1}\sqrt{p}$, which is the variance-stabilizing transformation for the binomial distribution [see VI, §2.7.2(c)], and the *probit* transformation [see VI, §6.6], which is related to the cumulative frequency distribution of the standard Normal distribution (and hence to the Normal scores mentioned in Section 1.3.14 of Chapter 1).

The probit transformation also has been widely used in analysing dose-response curves (see Finney, 1971). If individuals had a threshold dose below which they never responded but above which they always responded, and this threshold were Normally distributed in the population, then probit analysis would be appropriate. If the threshold followed a *logistic distribution* (which has slightly heavier tails than the Normal distribution [see II, §11.10]), then logit analysis (i.e. logistic regression) would be appropriate. This idea of a sharp threshold is obviously unrealistic but may help interpretation.

The logit, probit and arcsine transformations are discussed in, for example, Armitage (1971); in practice all three transformations usually give very similar results. Tukey (1977) calls logit $(p)/2$ the folded log or *flog* and he also considers the folded square root or *froot*, $\sqrt{2p} - \sqrt{2(1-p)}$. The transformations $\sqrt{p}$ and $\sqrt{1-p}$ are also useful in analysis of residuals (see Cox, 1970, Sec. 6.6).

Transformations for proportions can be applied more generally to data that fall between two limits; e.g. the arcsine transformation has been found useful in analysing measurements using *visual analogue scales* (see Aitken, 1969).

2.1.8 Further details on categorical data

The use of chi-square tests in contingency tables has been covered but they do not necessarily extract the maximum information from the data in tables larger than 2×2. There are situations where one or both of the variables are ordered categories (ordinal level data); however, chi-square is independent of any reordering of rows or columns in a contingency table.

One way to deal with a $2 \times n$ table where the n categories are in a logical order is to use the so-called '*chi-square for trend*' [see VI, §7.1]. This involves partitioning the value of chi-square and its associated degrees of freedom into two components. One component with 1 d.f. assesses the amount of trend, the other with $(n-2)$ d.f. is additional to the trend. This requires assignment of values to the n categories and they are generally given linear values, e.g. $-1, 0, +1$. This has the difficulty that such linearity in the categories is not generally justified: if it were, then the data could be regarded as interval and analysed with, say, a t test. A further difficulty is that the larger the value of n, the more often individual columns have low totals leading to cells with low values for the expected frequency, so invalidating the use of chi-square in some circumstances [see VI,

§7.3]. Combining categories allows chi-square to be computed, but loses some of the available information.

A solution to both of these problems is to use a non-parametric correlation coefficient which deals with the general $m \times n$ case as well, where both m and n categories are ordered. *Kendall's coefficient of correlation, tau*, is particularly recommended for the analysis of $2 \times n$ or $m \times n$ contingency tables where m and n are both ordered (see, for example, Everitt, 1977). Kendall's coefficient is able to deal with values where there are many ties (in the context of a contingency table, cells with more than one value in them) in an extremely efficient way. Spearman's correlation coefficient (rho) is not as efficient as Kendall's in dealing with ties so is not quite as useful in this case.

Another approach to ordinal data is *ridit analysis*, in which each category is given a score based on the observed cumulative frequency distribution (see, for example, Fleiss, 1981, Sec. 9.4). Ridit analysis is equivalent to methods based on ranks, such as the Mann–Whitney–Wilcoxon test (Section 1.3.8) and Spearman's rho. There is currently much research on building models for ordinal data, often based on sequences or tables of odds ratios (see, for example, McCullagh, 1980).

There have been considerable improvements in the analysis of contingency tables in recent years. The most important of these is to be able to analyse *multiway contingency tables* [see VI, §11.4.3]. For example, suppose the outcome of some trial is positive or negative and we are interested in whether the two different treatments we are dealing with have a consistent effect in males and females. There are circumstances in which we cannot analyse such data simply using 2×2 contingency tables, but need to analyse the $2 \times 2 \times 2$ contingency table.

In recent years it has been shown that a technique called *log-linear models* [see VI, §11.1] provides extremely useful additional insight into multiway tables. The basic idea is that independence means we can multiply probabilities together [see II, §3.5]; thus in Section 1.3.10 we estimated the proportion of patients surviving under treatment A to be given by the proportion of patients receiving treatment A (45/115) times the proportion of patients surviving (98/115), and we checked for independence of treatment and survival by comparing the observed proportions with the expected proportions. Since the log transformation turns multiplication into addition, independence can equally well be investigated by expressing logarithms of probabilities as **sums** of other log probabilities, and we can build models and check their goodness of fit in a similar way to analysis of variance. There is no space here to pursue this subject in great depth but the reader is referred for an elementary introduction to the book by Fienberg (1977). Everitt (1977), Cox (1970) and Bishop, Fienberg and Holland (1975) are references which will take the interested reader further.

There are computer programs which can assist with the analysis of this type of data. In particular the program BMDP3F available in the BMDP series (see Section 2.4.2) deserves mention as being easy to use and producing output which

Table 2.1.9 Cross-tabulation of pregnancy outcome with other variables.

Age	Smoker	OC use before pregnancy	Outcome		Abnormal, %
			Normal	Abnormal	
29	No	Yes	1,051	210	16.7
		No	1,014	178	14.9
	Yes	Yes	204	58	22.1
		No	330	67	16.9
30–34	No	Yes	582	144	19.8
		No	489	85	14.8
	Yes	Yes	125	31	19.9
		No	180	42	18.9
35 +	No	Yes	158	53	25.1
		No	119	31	20.7
	Yes	Yes	35	20	36.4
		No	35	10	22.2

is comprehensible. BMDP4F in the 1983 BMDP series provides even more facilities.

To illustrate log-linear models for contingency tables we have adapted and simplified data from Alberman *et al.* (1980), which should be consulted for definitive conclusions. The problem is to determine whether the outcome of pregnancies is altered by previous use of oral contraceptives (OC). It is well known that adverse outcomes are more likely in older women and in smokers, and it is also known that the use of OC is associated with smoking and differs in different age groups. Hence any association of OC with adverse outcome could be accentuated or even caused by association with smoking or reduced by the fact that OC use is (or at least was in the data studied) less frequent in older women.

The basic data are shown in Table 2.1.9. There are six two-way tables which could be examined (known as two-way *marginal tables*) when looking for associations between any combination of two of the four variables; e.g. Table 2.1.10 shows the marginal table relating outcome with OC before pregnancy. However, these two-way tables may be misleading in view of all the inter-relationships mentioned above, so we proceed to fit various models.

We can denote O = outcome, S = smoking, A = age and P = pill (previous OC use), and then, for example, the interaction between outcome and previous OC use can be written OP. The log-linear model which provides a parsimonious good fit involves OS, OA, OP, PA and PS, giving a likelihood ratio χ^2 of 8.54 with 11 d.f., p = 0.66. If OP is deleted from the model then χ^2 becomes 18.7 with 12 d.f.

Table 2.1.10 Two-way marginal table of pregnancy outcome and pill use.

| | | Outcome | | |
		Normal	Abnormal	Abnormal, %
OC before	Yes	2,155	516	19.3
pregnancy	No	2,167	413	16.0

$$\chi^2 = 9.88, \ P = 0.002$$

(corresponding to $P = 0.096$); thus the difference due to OP is 10.16 with 1 d.f. ($P = 0.0014$). This confirms the result suggested by the marginal table and shows that even allowing for the other associations (OS, OA, PA, PS) there is still an effect associated with OC use.

2.2 MULTIVARIATE ANALYSIS [see VI, Chapter 16]

Multivariate analysis (MVA) is appropriate when we have several response variables. MVA is complicated, but graphical analysis, transformations and assumptions like Normality help (Section 2.2.1). Transformations **between** variables may be useful (Section 2.2.2).

MVA can be used for discrimination and diagnosis (Section 2.2.3), and many other techniques are available (Section 2.2.4). For the theory of MVA we need *matrix algebra* [see I, §6.2]; in practice we need computer programs (Section 2.4.2)

2.2.1 Introduction to Multivariate Analysis

Often we are interested in several variables, each variable having some random variation. Rather than look at each variable in isolation, we can use techniques of *multivariate analysis* to investigate the variation in all the variables simultaneously. Models based on *contingency tables* (Section 2.1.8) can be used if the variables are *qualitative*, as in Bishop, Fienberg and Holland (1975); in this chapter we look at *numerical* variables. For example, if we have measured the serum concentrations of various lipoproteins in a large number of subjects we may want to know how these concentrations vary with each other and with sex, age and weight, and how the relationships differ for different diseases.

A frequently used notation is that we have p variables $X_1, X_2, \ldots, X_p$ for each of n subjects; our data may be thought of as a 'swarm' of n points in p-dimensional space (Cooley and Lohnes, 1971), with points close together representing subjects with similar characteristics. It may also be useful to think of the data as p points in n-dimensional space, each point in this case representing the n values of a particular variable [see I, §5.2].

Classical multivariate analysis is largely based on the *multivariate Normal*

(*MVN*) *distribution* in which each variable has a normal distribution whatever the values of the other variables [see II, § 13.4]. We can combine all values of some of the variables and just look at the distribution of the remaining variables; this is called a *marginal distribution* [see II, § 13.1.2]. All the marginal distributions of an MVN distribution are also multivariate Normal [see II, § 13.4.4].

The data may be inspected by plotting scatter diagrams of two of the variables *conditionally* on the values of other variables (e.g. high density cholesterol versus all other cholesterol for male controls between 55 and 60 years old in a given weight range) and we can see whether transforming the original variables (e.g. taking logs of concentrations) will make the assumption of multivariate Normality more reasonable. For a Multivariate Normal distribution the points in all such scatter diagrams should lie roughly in an ellipse [see II § 13.1.1]. Books such as Gnanadesikan (1977) and Barnett (1981) give many examples of multivariate graphical methods.

Analysis of a multivariate Normal distribution takes into account the means, variances and covariances of the variables, all depending on the scales of measurement. It is clearly unreasonable that our interpretation of the cholesterol levels should depend on whether we recorded the concentrations in millimoles per hundred cubic centimetres or in some other units, and perhaps even on whether weight was recorded in kilograms or grams. A useful first step, by which we give equal importance to each variable, is *standardization*. For each variable we subtract the mean and then divide by the standard deviation: each variable then has variance 1 and the covariance between the two variables is simply their correlation [see II, § 11.4.3]. Standardized values are sometimes called *z-scores*.

If the variables **do** come from a multivariate Normal distribution then the matrix **R** of correlations between all pairs of variables [see II, § 13.3.1], together with the means and variances of the individual variables, are sufficient statistics (Section 1.2.8) and therefore contain **all** the information we can get from the data.

Multivariate data are almost always analysed using standard computer programs, both because the arithmetic is tedious and because we usually want to try several different transformations and look at many different plots to get a feel for the data before carrying out any formal analysis. Examples using these computer programs and explanations of their output can be found in the relevant computer manuals; see Section 2.4.2 for more details.

2.2.2 Principal Components Analysis [see VI, § § 16.3 and 17.2]

To simplify both the interpretation and presentation of data we want to have as few variables as possible. For example, if we have measured a response at several times after a stimulus for different subjects we will want to find a combination of these measurements to summarize the overall response or if we have measured hormone levels we may want some simple representation of hormone imbalance.

Principal components analysis is a method of doing this. The first principal component is the linear combination of the variables that exhibits most variation (hence leaving as little variation as possible unexplained). Subsequent principal components similarly account for as much remaining variation as possible. Mathematically, principal components are the directions of rotated axes in our p-dimensional representation of the data (Section 2.2.1).

As an extreme example, suppose we have measured left and right foot lengths (X_1 and X_2) and left and right hand spans (X_3 and X_4) on a large number of people. Most of the variation between sets of four measurements will be due to the differences in overall stature between subjects, so the first principal component will have positive coefficients for X_1, X_2, X_3 and X_4. The second principal component will probably have positive coefficients for X_1 and X_2 but negative for X_3 and X_4 (or vice versa), since much of the remaining variation is due to some people having relatively large hands and others having relatively large feet. The two remaining principal components should be far less important and may represent differences between left-handed and right-handed people or between different occupations, or just measurement error.

The data in Table 2.2.1 summarize measurements of hormone levels for thirty post-menopausal women. Even with the assumption of multivariate Normality we need fourteen parameters (four means, four standard deviations and six correlations) to present data for four variables. We can try to simplify this by finding the principal components.

Here it seems clear from the correlation matrix **R** that all four variables are positively correlated with each other, but we can use *Bartlett's* test [see VI, §5.10], described, for example, in Cooley and Lohnes (1971), to see whether the correlation matrix is significantly different from the identity matrix (in other words, whether there are any inter-correlations). The test statistic is

$$\chi^2 = -[(n-1) - (2p+5)/6] \log_e(|\mathbf{R}|),$$

Table 2.2.1 Summary of hormone levels of thirty subjects.

Variable	Mean	Variance	s.d.
$X_1(\log_{10}$ oestradiol)	1.040	0.029	0.170
$X_2(\log_{10}$ oestrogen)	1.437	0.037	0.193
$X_3(\log_{10}$ androstenedione)	2.568	0.053	0.230
$X_4(\log_{10}$ testosterone)	2.282	0.059	0.243

$$\text{Correlation matrix } \mathbf{R} = \begin{array}{c} \\ X_1 \\ X_2 \\ X_3 \\ X_4 \end{array} \begin{pmatrix} X_1 & X_2 & X_3 & X_4 \\ 1 & 0.446 & 0.262 & 0.201 \\ 0.446 & 1 & 0.372 & 0.524 \\ 0.262 & 0.375 & 1 & 0.762 \\ 0.201 & 0.524 & 0.762 & 1 \end{pmatrix}$$

where $|\mathbf{R}|$ means the determinant of $\mathbf{R}$ [see I, §6.8]. Here the value is

$$\chi^2 = -[29 - 13/6]\log_e(0.232) = 39,$$

which, if the null hypothesis ('no correlation') were true, would come from approximately a χ^2 distribution on $p(p-1)/2 = 6$ degrees of freedom. The value 39 is highly significant, and we can investigate the inter-relationships between X_1, X_2, X_3 and X_4 by using matrix algebra (or a computer!) to find the principal components. In mathematical terms, we want the *eigenvalues* and *eigenvectors* of $\mathbf{R}$ [see I, §7.1]. The eigenvectors give the principal components and the eigenvalues (which must add up to four, the sum of the diagonal terms of $\mathbf{R}$ [see I, (7.3.6)]) indicate the importance of the corresponding eigenvectors. Bartlett's test can also be used to help us decide how many principal components to extract.

In our example the largest eigenvalue is found to be 2.32 with the corresponding eigenvector (0.363, 0.502, 0.542, 0.567). The second largest eigenvalue is 0.95 with the corresponding eigenvector (0.762, 0.324, -0.398, -0.395). The sizes of the eigenvalues mean that the first principal component represents a proportion $2.32/4 = 0.58$ of the total variation, and the first two together account for a proportion $(2.32 + 0.95)/4$ or 0.82 of the total variation.

The values of x_1, x_2, x_3 and x_4 can be transformed to give *scores* in the direction of the principal components. For example, if $x_1 = 1.279$, $x_2 = 1.447$, $x_3 = 2.444$ and $x_4 = 2.155$ then the corresponding z-scores are (from Table 2.2.1)

$$z_1 = \frac{1.279 - 1.040}{0.170} = 1.41, \qquad z_2 = \frac{1.447 - 1.437}{0.193} = 0.05,$$

$$z_3 = \frac{2.444 - 2.568}{0.230} = -0.54, \qquad z_4 = \frac{2.155 - 2.282}{0.243} = -0.52,$$

and the scores corresponding to the first two principal components are

$$y_1 = 0.363\,z_1 + 0.502\,z_2 + 0.542\,z_3 + 0.567\,z_4 = -0.05,$$
$$y_2 = 0.762\,z_1 + 0.324\,z_2 - 0.398\,z_3 - 0.395\,z_4 = 1.51.$$

We can plot y_1 against y_2 giving a scatter diagram illustrating 82 per cent of the variation between subjects, and can then inspect this scatter diagram for patterns or anomalies. Similarly, we may find it useful to look at half-Normal plots of y_1 and of y_2. Half-Normal plots (Section 1.3.14) can be generalized to give *gamma probability plots* and other plots for multivariate data (see Wilk and Gnanadesikan, 1968, and Gnanadesikan, 1977).

Principal components analysis could also be used on the variance/covariance matrix [see II, §9.6.5] rather than on the correlation matrix, since the variables here are all in the same units of log concentration and all the variances and covariances are comparable. However, analysis of the correlation matrix is generally more meaningful.

2.2.3 Discriminant Analysis [see VI, §16.6]

Discriminant analysis is a technique which has considerable appeal in medicine when we may want to use several variables to help us distinguish between individuals, each of whom falls into one of two or more groups. To take a simple example, in using biochemical tests to classify patients into one of two diagnostic categories, no single test may provide the maximum information, but using results from several tests considerably improves the quality of such classification. The measurement of success of classification can be looked at in terms of the numbers of false positive and false negative misclassifications.

Classical discriminant analysis maximizes the separation between two groups of individuals by using a linear function of a set of variables. It can also be applied to three or more groups, but we shall only consider the problem of separation into two groups. We must initially have a series of individuals (the *training set*) on whom the relevant variables have been measured and for whom we know the classification with certainty. Finding the *linear discriminant function* is then equivalent to multiple regression using group membership as a dummy variable (0 = subject is a member of group A, 1 = subject is a member of group B). Some of the techniques mentioned in Section 2.1.5 have analogues in discriminant analysis; e.g. stepwise discriminant analysis may be appropriate since the emphasis here is on arriving at a correct classification, rather than on trying to obtain an easily interpretable model.

We can subsequently compute the function for as yet unclassified individuals on whom all the relevant variables have been measured (the *test set*). The classification is then made using a discriminant score. This has potential in making most use of readily available information and reducing the necessity for unpleasant, expensive or dangerous diagnostic tests. It has been used in a variety of medical situations, a simple one being that of adding to the information provided by alpha-feto-protein in the diagnosis of neural tube defects (Pettit, King and Evans, 1980).

It is important to realize that there are certain assumptions made about the distribution of the variables which are used in the discriminant function, in particular the scatter must be similar within each group. Any interpretation of results usually also involves the assumption of multivariate Normality [see II, §13.4], which is not as frequent an occurrence in real life as it is in statistics books. The remarks made in earlier sections on testing the assumption of a Gaussian distribution and on the use of transformations and plotting of residuals are all of particular relevance in any preparatory work before doing a discriminant analysis.

A major problem of using a discriminant function is that we will obviously overestimate its success rate if we try to validate it on the same group of patients as was originally used for computing the function itself. The ideal way to avoid this is to have a set of patients for whom the classification has not yet been made: the discriminant function can be used to classify them and when the classification becomes truly known then we can assess the success of the discriminant function in an unbiased way.

However, there is a more practical method known as the *jack-knife* for reducing the classification bias. This involves computing the discriminant function using all the cases except one and using the computed function to classify that case. Then the same thing is done for the next case, and so on, computing the discriminant function as many times as there are cases, each time using all cases except one. This is not as difficult as it sounds with modern computer programs, and leads to a much less biased classification success rate. A computer program that is particularly recommended for this is the program BMDP7M in the BMD series mentioned in Section 2.4.2.

The jack-knife is an important general technique for reducing bias and for estimating precision (see, for example, Mosteller and Tukey, 1977, Chap. 8). When used as here to indicate predictive ability it is an example of *cross-validation* (Stone, 1974).

Discriminant analysis is particularly applicable as an aid to diagnosis, and the Bayes theorem [see VI, §15.2] may be used where the prior probabilities of a particular diagnosis are known; the program BMDP7M mentioned above is able to utilize this in making classifications. There are many different modifications of classical discriminant analysis and several other approaches to discrimination are possible; e.g. logistic regression (Section 2.1.7) may be particularly appropriate if we are trying to build an underlying model. Crandon *et al.* (1980), following on from Clayton, Anderson and McNicol (1976), illustrate logistic discrimination. For further discussion of possible approaches see Titterington *et al.* (1981) and Chapter 3 in this Guidebook.

2.2.4 Other Multivariate Techniques

This section gives a brief indication of when we might use other methods to analyse multivariate data. Robertson *et al.* (1980) give nice examples of various techniques and other examples may be found in, for example, Dixon *et al.* (1981) and Mardia, Kent and Bibby (1979).

Factor analysis [see VI, §16.4] is similar to principal components analysis, but involves the hypothesis that the inter-relationships between all p variables can be explained by fewer than p underlying factors. In principal components analysis we just want to remove the correlations between the variables, but in factor analysis we hope to interpret these inter-correlations by expressing each variable as a linear combination of the factor values, plus residual effects linked with that variable alone.

Once the number of underlying factors has been decided, the factors can be transformed to suggest different plausible models. For example, if one factor represents overall hormone concentration and a second represents the relative levels of male and female sex hormones (see the example in Section 2.2.2), we might want to transform these factors so that one represents male hormone concentrations and the other represents female hormone concentrations. Each factor would then give a high weight to some variables and a low (or zero) weight to others, possibly simplifying the interpretation (or possibly not—see Garside and Roth, 1978).

Factor analysis is mainly used in psychology, to study the existence and nature of qualities like 'social conformity' and 'authoritarianism'. An example of other possible uses is given in Buckatzch and Doll (1952).

Canonical correlations [see VI, §16.5] indicate how one group of variables is related to another group. For example, if we have a set of histological measurements indicating the severity of disease and another set of variables measuring possible risk factors, we can use canonical correlation analysis to produce *canonical variates* X_1 (a linear combination of the risk variables) and X_2 (a linear combination of the histological measurements) in such a way that the correlation between X_1 and X_2 is as high as possible. A scatter diagram of X_1 against X_2 helps to show the extent of the relationship between the two sets, and we may be able to interpret the relationship by seeing which variables contribute most to X_1 and which to X_2.

In a similar way to principal components analysis, we can continue finding more canonical variates to investigate any further relationship between the sets of variables. Canonical correlation analysis can also be generalized to study more than two sets.

Canonical correlation can be thought of as a generalization of ordinary correlation (where each set contains just one variable) and of multiple correlation (where one set has just one variable). For example, if X and Y are variables with a non-linear relationship, then the canonical correlation between the sets $\{(y - \bar{y})$ and $(y - \bar{y})^2\}$ on the one hand and $\{(x - \bar{x})$ and $(x - \bar{x})^2\}$ on the other may be better than ordinary correlation as a numerical assessment of the strength of relationship between X and Y.

Discriminant analysis (Section 2.2.3) may also be seen as a special case of canonical correlation, using a set of dummy variables to indicate group membership.

Multivariate analysis of variance (*MANOVA*) is a natural generalization of ANOVA; one or more of the variables (e.g. sex or treatment) can be used to classify the subjects and we then look for systematic differences between the values of other variables from one category to another.

In ANOVA we assume equal variances in each group, and similarly in MANOVA we assume equal variances and covariances. For example, if we use MANOVA to investigate how arterial pO_2 and pCO_2 vary between different groups of subjects and we plot scatter diagrams of pO_2 against pCO_2 for each group, we would hope that the shapes of the plots are similar (and elliptical), but that the *centroids* (mean pO_2 and mean pCO_2 for each group) are different. Some transformation may help.

Other aspects of MANOVA are similar to ANOVA. For example, *Wilk's lambda* statistic is a ratio of the determinants of two variance/covariance matrices and provides a generalization of the F test. Similarly, *Hotelling's T^2* statistic can be used to test whether centroids are different from one another, but it is not clear how sensitive this test is to non-Normality or to unequal covariance matrices. After carrying out the MANOVA we could look at the variations **within** a category by analysing the pooled residual variance/covariance matrix (perhaps by principal components analysis or canonical correlations, as appropriate) (see, for example, Efron, 1980b).

Cluster analysis is the name for a wide variety of exploratory techniques to divide the subjects into *clusters* (groups of similar subjects). For example, if we have data on a large number of species of bacteria, we may want to define clusters of similar species. Unfortunately there are many plausible approaches, even when we have found an appropriate measure of 'similarity'; we may get radically different results depending on whether we feel it more important to assign two dissimilar species to different clusters or to assign two similar species to the same cluster. This problem is similar to the trade-off between the probabilities of committing type I and type II errors. Cluster analysis is reviewed in Cormack (1971) and Everitt (1974, 1979), an example of its possible use in medicine being in Lewis (1980).

Multi-dimensional scaling [see VI, §17.12] is related to cluster analysis in that we form an $n \times n$ matrix of similarities between subjects, and try to express these similarities by representing the n subjects as points in k-dimensional space, with the distance between two subjects indicating how dissimilar they are. If k is 2, we can plot the points in a scatter diagram and similar subjects will be plotted close together; if k is 1 then we have managed to order the subjects in some way as in Healy and Goldstein (1976).

Cluster analysis and multi-dimensional scaling can also be used to interpret a $p \times p$ matrix of similarities between **variables** (e.g. the matrix of correlations as for principal components analysis or rank correlations).

2.3 SURVIVAL ANALYSIS

This section discusses the particular problems of survival analysis, where we are interested in 'time to death'. If we wish to compare the lengths of time people survive after receiving one of two possible treatments, then we might try to use the techniques of Section 1.3 such as t tests or the Wilcoxon rank sum test. These approaches are perfectly valid when we know all the times, but in practice we rarely do know them completely. We know the survival times of those who have died, but in most analyses of recent data there are some people who are still alive, some who have been lost to follow-up after a certain length of time and some who have died from a cause quite independent of the disease for which they have been treated.

One approach to dealing with survival times that are for one reason or another incomplete (known as *censored* observations [see VI, §6.7.1]) is to compare the proportions of patients surviving (say) five years in each of the two groups. This itself has problems in that the calculation of the proportion surviving is subject to ambiguity. Patients who at the time of analysis could not have had five years of follow-up must be excluded whether alive or not since if we include those who have died but not those who are alive at the last follow-up the proportion dying will be biased upwards. A similar problem exists for those who could have had more than five years follow-up but are censored observations of less than five years (e.g. they were lost to follow-up several years ago), because excluding them will lead to a similar bias. More sophisticated methods of analysis are clearly necessary; some of these (life tables, the log-rank test and Cox's method) are mentioned below. Further details and examples may be found in, for example, Kalbfleisch and Prentice (1980) or Miller (1981).

One method of dealing with survival times is to use the *clinical life table* [see I, §15.2]. This allows the calculation of an actuarial survival curve which is very much less subject to bias (see, for example, Colton, 1974, Chap. 9). Greenwood (1926) gave a method for computing the standard error of the proportion surviving in such a table but this standard error is very unreliable in the presence of large amounts of censoring.

The *log-rank test* is a generalization of the Mantel and Haenszel (1959) method for analysis of contingency tables. It is most suited to data which are already in categories, such as treatment group or pre-/post-menopause. Continuous data (such as age or similar possible risk factors) must be recast as categories in order to use the method. The data are divided into separate strata and the numbers of deaths observed and expected in each treatment category are calculated within each stratum; the difference between observed and expected number of deaths is then pooled across strata to give an overall χ^2 test of significance. This method emphasizes significance testing but it is possible to obtain approximate interval estimates. The Peto *et al.* (1976, 1977) papers provide a very clear exposition of both the analysis and also the prerequisites in terms of the design of studies of survival. Further statistical details are given in Peto and Peto (1972). A very useful computer program is available for simulating clinical trials which are intended to use this method of analysis (see Jones, 1979).

The *hazard function* is an important concept for understanding the modern approaches to survival analysis [see II, §§10.1.1 and 21.6]. It is expressed as the instantaneous probability of dying in a time interval conditional upon having survived to the beginning of that time interval. There are many *parametric methods* of analysis of survival curves which make assumptions about the form of the hazard function, e.g. if the hazard function is a constant then the survival curve is simply an exponential decay. These methods tend to have limited relevance in the medical field because the hazard function may have a very nonregular form.

Cox's model (see Cox, 1972) for analysis of survival curves makes no assumptions about the underlying form of the hazard function, but it does assume that the hazard functions for the groups under study all have the **same** (unknown) shape, the actual hazard differing only by a multiplicative factor for each group. This gives rise to the other term describing this method—the *proportional hazards model*. These multiplicative factors are then analysed by methods akin to multiple regression, so all the assumptions and ramifications of multiple regression (Section 2.1.5) should be borne in mind when using the method. The literature of statistics since 1972 has had many papers studying this model and extensions to it. A few major studies have used it to analyse clinical trials and a few have used it for retrospective studies. Cox's method is most suitable where the explanatory variables are continuous interval (or ratio) scale data, but it is able to deal with categorical data in the same way as does multiple regression by the use of dummy variables.

The result of the Cox analysis gives regression coefficients with asymptotic standard errors which may be used for interval estimation (Section 1.3.11) as well as significance testing. A conditional log likelihood is also obtained so that a form of likelihood ratio testing may also be applied.

The use of residuals from Cox's model is given by Kay (1977), and fitted survival curves may be plotted for the underlying hazard function and thus for any particular group by using the appropriate regression coefficient as a proportional hazard (see Breslow, 1975, and Evans, 1978).

Survival analysis can also be used in many other situations where there is a binary outcome variable (see Section 2.1.7) and which involve long-term observation of the individuals until the 'death' occurs. As an example the methods have been used with success to study the 'survival' of fillings in teeth (or of teeth themselves), where the 'death' is replacement of the filling or extraction of the tooth (Gray, 1976). Many other situations are amenable to this analysis, such as the occurrence or non-occurrence of pregnancy or of morbid events: myocardial infarction, cerebrovascular accidents, relapse of a cancer patient, etc.

Note that in these more general applications the event of interest may occur several times for any one individual, but methods of analysis have only been well developed for the first event. The problem of *multivariate failure times*, i.e. multiple occurrences of similar events or of several different events (*competing risks*) is currently under study; for further details see Kalbfleisch and Prentice (1980, Chap. 7). The literature on *point processes*, e.g. Cox and Isham (1980), is of relevance here.

2.4 COMPUTATION

We have reviewed ways that statistical theory can help us interpret medical results, but to use statistics in practice we must also have some acquaintance with numerical analysis (Section 2.4.1), computers (Section 2.4.2) and common sense (Section 2.4.3).

2.4.1 Statistical Calculation

Obviously all statistical calculations assume that the data accurately represent what they are meant to; this is rather optimistic (Feinstein, 1977a) and the data should at least be 'screened' for errors, as described by Wermuth and Cochran (1979).

Even if the data are correct, the formulae used for theoretical development may not be appropriate for calculation, and some methods are more accurate than others. Formulae using $\sum(x - \bar{x})^2$ are more reliable than those using $\sum x^2 - n(\bar{x})^2$, even though they are algebraically equivalent. For example, suppose X has mean 10 and standard deviation 1. Then the first formula is obtained after subtracting values which typically differ by 10 per cent, but the second subtracts terms differing by only 1 per cent. Consequently, errors in rounding off [see III, §1.3] affect $\sum x^2 - n(\bar{x})^2$ much more than $\sum(x - \bar{x})^2$. Subtracting $\bar{x}$ from each observation is called *correcting for the mean*.

Similarly, if we want to use polynomial regression [see III, §6.1.3, and VI, §8.2.5] to relate Y (incidence of some disease) to X (year $= 1970, 1971, \ldots, 1980$) then if we are using a method that does not automatically correct for the means, we should recode X as $0, 1, \ldots, 10$, or still better as $-5, -4, \ldots, +5$. Simpler numbers also leave less scope for human error. This idea can be extended to give 'orthogonal polynomials' [see III, §6.3] or to correct for the means of X^2, X^4, etc.

Techniques for minimizing such errors come under *numerical analysis*, which is a major field of study in its own right. The problems are usually greater with small computers, particularly microcomputers where the number of digits allowed for internal working in the computer tends to be smaller. For this reason and for other technical reasons associated with the mechanisms for doing arithmetic in a computer, the same program may give slightly different results on different makes of computer.

Many statistical techniques, particularly those in multivariate analysis that invert matrices or calculate eigenvalues [see III, §§4.4 and 4.5], have numerical problems if variables are highly correlated [see III, §6.1.5]. Consequently, if X_1 and X_2 are variables with very similar values we may do better to transform the variables to $Y_1 = (X_1 + X_2)$ and $Y_2 = (X_1 - X_2)$, which will not be so highly correlated. An advantage of analysis based on principal components is that the transformed variables are uncorrelated, so if the principal components have been found accurately we may not need quite such numerical accuracy in further analysis.

It is important to keep intermediate results to a high accuracy and not round off until the end of the calculations. When we calculate $(1.447 - 1.437)/0.193 = 0.05$ we need up to four significant figures and three decimal places on the left-hand side to calculate the right-hand side to one significant figure or two decimal places. Similarly, if $x = 100$ is a typical value to insert in the equation $y = mx + c$ then m should be recorded to two more decimal places than c.

Remember in particular that some quantities such as the mean may be known to greater accuracy than the original values. For example, the mean $\bar{x}_A$ in Section 1.3.6 of Chapter 1 is actually 1.4875, not 1.49, so we could reduce round-off errors by using the more accurate value.

2.4.2 Computer programs

Many calculators now have options to calculate means and variances, and some statistical calculators can carry out simple linear regression or perform χ^2 tests. However, if we have a large volume of data, if we want to try several methods of analysis on the same data set or if we want to use techniques involving complicated arithmetic, we normally use a computer.

Currently the most common scientific computer language is FORTRAN, and many *statistical algorithms* (formal steps to carry out statistical analysis) are given as FORTRAN routines. The journal *Applied Statistics* has an algorithms supplement giving reliable methods of analysis. Other journals and some books also contain appropriate computer programs: for example, Cooley and Lohnes (1971) have routines for *multivariate analysis*, Nijenhuis and Wilf (1978) have *combinatorial* routines that can be used for randomization or non-parametric statistics and Velleman and Hoaglin (1981) have routines for *exploratory data analysis* (both in FORTRAN and in BASIC). Recently more specifically medical computer programs have been published: Breslow and Day (1980) have many routines for analysing case-control studies (particularly using *logistic regression*) and Kalbfleisch and Prentice (1980) cover several topics in *survival analysis*. Unfortunately, published programs occasionally suffer from printing errors which may be difficult to detect and which render the programs incorrect.

A very reliable source of algorithms is the **NAG library**. This is a library of algorithms covering a variety of tasks including many of great use in statistics. They are available in both FORTRAN and ALGOL (another common computer programming language) and are distributed by the Numerical Algorithms Group (NAG), Banbury Road, Oxford, England.

There are many other computer programming languages. One in particular, APL, is worth mentioning as being very elegant and ideal for statistical work (see Anscombe, 1981), but rather daunting for anyone not mathematically minded.

If necessary, published routines may be translated to other computer languages like BASIC for use on small desk-top computers. Most makes of desk-top computer have associated user groups to exchange programs. An advantage of personal computers is that they can be used *interactively* (we can quickly try several different approaches depending on previous analysis) but with many larger computers we must wait hours before seeing any results. Personal computers are subject in some cases to the problems of numerical inaccuracy mentioned in Section 2.4.1 above.

Larger computer centres have many statistical packages for data analysis.

These packages are usually collections of FORTRAN routines and are frequently modified to offer more facilities and improve existing algorithms, so the relative merits of the different packages may vary from year to year and from computer to computer. Currently (1984) the following packages are very often used:

(a) **SPSS** (the Statistical Package for the Social Sciences) (see Nie, 1983) is the most widely available package and is useful for analysing surveys and other large data sets. The statistical options available are those like regression, cross-tabulation (contingency tables), discriminant analysis and factor analysis which are much used in psychology and the social sciences. Each variable can be given a name (e.g. SEX, WEIGHT, DRUG) and particular variable values can also be labelled (e.g. MALE, FEMALE) so the computer printout is easy to interpret without having to remember that 'variable 14 = 2' means 'sex is female'. All the information on the description and labelling of variables can be saved together with the data on a *binary file* in the computer for efficient storage and processing. SPSS also allows us to distinguish between various types of missing data (e.g. between 'the question was not asked' and 'a meaningless answer was received') and it is particularly easy to remove some of the data or to combine different categories. SPSS has very good facilities for creating new variables by transformation or combination of other variables, and for defining groupings of values for a variable. SPSS instructions and the SPSS manual are fairly easy for a casual user to follow.

(b) **BMDP** (the Biomedical Computer Package) by Dixon *et al.* (1983) is generally more statistically sophisticated than SPSS and is more oriented towards medical applications. For example, the package includes simple probability plots, analysis of variance with repeated measures, various techniques for estimating missing values in multivariate analysis, logistic regression, log-linear models for contingency tables and survival analysis (including Cox's model in BMDP-83). BMDP can save data and data descriptions in the same way as SPSS. Its output, together with the manual, is generally comprehensible. The BMDP manual also gives more indication of the statistical theory and the assumptions underlying each option, and is worth reading by anyone interested in statistical computing. Technical reports from the Health Sciences Computing facility at the University of California, Los Angeles (the authors of BMDP), provide theory and annotated output relevant to the programs themselves.

(c) **GENSTAT** (see Alvey *et al.*, 1977) is a more mathematical package than either SPSS or BMDP; various data structures and operations are defined in a formal 'language'. GENSTAT is particularly useful for complicated analysis of variance and covariance since it uses a general method for fitting ANOVA models and can easily handle random effects and missing data. GENSTAT also offers several recently developed techniques in multivariate analysis and can be used to fit general linear models (see GLIM below). Its output is more difficult to interpret than SPSS or BMDP but it has great flexibility and new methods of analysis can be obtained using its matrix handling facilities.

(d) **GLIM** (General Linear Interactive Modelling) (see Baker and Nelder, 1978) is a very powerful program to fit general linear models to data. It requires considerable statistical expertise and familiarity with the notation but can solve many apparently different problems within the one framework. GLIM can be used, for example, for probit analysis in biological assay, to fit log-linear models to categorical data, to fit Cox's model in survival analysis or in a case where preliminary ANOVA suggests that one transformation simplifies interpretation (e.g. by removing interactions), but a different transformation seems appropriate from the residuals. Its current versions, GLIM-3, is about to be enhanced by a new version to be called GLIM-4/PRISM which will include some graphics facilities. The present version of GLIM tends to be difficult if not impossible to use with extremely large data sets, but the new version may improve on this.

(e) **SAS** (Statistical Analysis System) (see Ray, 1982) is extremely comprehensive but has until recently only been available on IBM-compatible computers. It originated from North Carolina State University and is marketed by the SAS Institute with offices in Europe as well as North America. It has a very wide coverage of statistical facilities with good algorithms (very necessary for IBM computers with their word size and architecture). It is fairly easy to use and includes matrix manipulation facilities (as does GENSTAT) which enable new methods to be programmed. It has a direct interface with BMDP which has some facilities not available in SAS (including reading BMDP binary files). SAS/GRAPH is a further package with colour graphic output including special statistical features. It also has a powerful report-writing facility for formating output of results as the user wants. SAS has comprehensive manuals and a very good library of supplemental procedures covering techniques not yet in the main SAS package.

(f) **SIR** (Scientific Information Retrieval) (see Robinson *et al.*, 1980) is not really a statistical package but is for handling databases. It is worth mentioning here partly because the problems of storing and organizing data in any large study are very considerable. SIR can create data files with all the labelling of variables and their values for future reading by either SPSS or BMDP. It is particularly useful for hierarchical data (variable amounts of data on each individual in the study) which are not as easily handled by the other major packages.

(g) **MINITAB** (see Ryan, Joiner and Ryan, 1976) is a development of a fairly simple program designed to be used interactively and is particularly effective for teaching statistics. It is implemented on many small computers and its latest release contains many of the features found in the larger packages. It also contains some of the robust techniques mentioned in Section 1.2.7 and simple plotting of data, including 'box and whisker' diagrams.

Many other packages are available; if you have a choice of computer programs, look at examples using each to decide which you prefer.

Computers are also often used for *simulation* [see II, §5.6]; it can be very instructive to create an artificial set of data and then compare different methods of analysis (e.g. Riggs, Guarneiri and Addelman 1978, and Rubin, 1979). Another special use is *numerical approximation*; many functions cannot be calculated exactly and approximations must be used (e.g. to tabulate probability levels for test statistics). Abramowitz and Stegun (1970) give several useful approximations [see III, Chapter 6].

2.4.3 Uses and abuses of computers

Computers have taken a great deal of the drudgery out of statistical calculation, and many of the techniques mentioned in this chapter are only practical because of the availability of computer programs. Some researchers use the computer as a giant black box into which they put all their data and their question (or many questions) and expect a *P*-value to be regurgitated for entry in the blank space(s) in their paper. This may be valid, but is clearly dangerous (see 'fishing expeditions' below) and is not using the computer to its full potential. What are the areas where computers are particularly useful?

(a) Uses of computers

(i) *Large amounts of data.* By 'large' we mean the product of cases and variables (the number of individual data items) is greater than 500. As soon as the amount of data becomes large the probability of mistakes being made in calculation of simple statistics, even by the obsessionally careful, becomes considerable.

(ii) *Complex calculations.* Long calculation can arise both from statistical analysis (particularly multivariate methods) and from using mathematical models or simulation. Even where, say, five variables have been measured the computation of the ten correlation and regression coefficients becomes tedious and prone to error on a hand calculator because of the repeated entry of data. In most cases there are good package programs that will provide the correct answers if the data are correct. The methods involving iterative calculation (such as maximum likelihood in many instances) are particularly suited to computers because by their nature computers are good at iterative calculations provided the algorithms used are efficient.

(iii) *Data screening.* Section 2.4.1 emphasized the necessity of checking for errors in the data. Computers can be used to assist in this process of data screening, and at the very least the minimum and maximum should be examined for each variable. The kurtosis (see Section 1.1.4) is a sensitive indicator of gross errors in a single variable: a kurtosis of greater than 3 is very rare in genuine data but values of 10 or more are not unknown where there are data errors giving rise to extreme values (very high, very low or both together). It would be unusual to compute the kurtosis for descriptive purposes but there are several computer programs which will do this routinely.

Data checking can become much more sophisticated, examining pairs or sets of variables where apparently reasonable values for a single variable seem less reasonable when taken in context. Cook's distance has been referred to in Section 1.3.14 of Chapter 1 and a program that computes this and draws attention to data points which may be extreme is BMDP-9R. The fact that a data point is an extreme value does not necessarily mean that it is an error, and external objective criteria must be used to decide on its rejection. Alternatively, the computer may let us use the more robust methods mentioned in Section 1.2.7.

v) *Plotting.* Modern computers are able to plot graphs as easily as to calculate equations. Special purpose plotters are available which can plot in several colours on paper, on a television-like screen or directly onto microfilm or microfiche. Elementary plots are particularly useful for data screening, and the plotting of residuals in a variety of manners is to be recommended, as in Section 1.3.14.

v) *Exploring the data.* Computers have great potential for allowing the researcher to 'listen to what the data is trying to say'. The general approach is to allow for the known sources of variation and to see if what is then left has any pattern; there should be none if the known sources of variation are the only ones measured which do affect the data. This approach, followed by Tukey and others, has its own problems but may well lead to more careful thought and can generate interesting hypotheses and insights. Daniel and Wood (1980) illustrate the use of computers in finding successive possible explanations for patterns in the data.

) *Abuses of computers*

i) *'Fishing expeditions'.* When there are no well-defined questions posed by the researcher the computer offers the potential for asking very many questions but then selecting only those with significant '*P*-values'. It could well be that all these are statistically significant only by chance and any conclusions that are drawn assuming these to be valid tests of hypotheses may be totally wrong. If they are used to generate hypotheses which are then tested using *other* data then the approach is valid. In the jargon of Tukey, it is not possible to regard all interesting findings from an exploratory data analysis as candidates for confirmatory data analysis using the same data.

(ii) *Lack of scepticism.* The scepticism towards *P*-values in the above paragraph should be extended to a scepticism regarding both the data and the computer programs being used. There is a tendency for investigators to be mesmerized by computer-produced results and to lose all common sense. The process of entering data from which the computer can produce results may take some time, but it is hazardous to omit checking the data in order to meet the publishing deadline on a paper.

The computer may be programmed incorrectly, generally in regard to the actual data being analysed rather than in the methods of calculation. For example, the location of the data in particular columns of a punched card might be misspecified or the fact that blanks or '99' are to be regarded as missing data for age in years might have been forgotten. The well-known statistical packages do have occasional errors in them but these are very rare compared to the errors in data description or task description. Even rarer, though by no means impossible, are errors in the calculations carried out by the computer. Vigilance is needed at all times!

(iii) *Remoteness of investigator.* The investigator who does everything by hand is closer both to the data and to the methods of analysis than is the computer user. Everyone should do by hand at least one simple analysis of the type being done on a computer, and sophisticated methods should not be used unless the investigator can give to a colleague a clear explanation of what is being done in comprehensible terms. The computer should be used to give many plots of the basic data so that the distributions of individual variables and the simple relationships in the data are familiar.

(iv) *Abdication of responsibility.* Where statistical significance is taken as the sole arbiter of significance the clinician has abdicated responsibility for deciding what is important. A clinical trial could show that a difference in lowering of blood pressure between two drugs of 0.1 mm Hg is *statistically* significant, but it is the practical or clinical significance which should be remembered.

(v) *Complexity.* Computers have allowed the highly sophisticated methods of statistics to be applied in almost any set of data. There is a tendency for these methods to be used simply for the sake of it, whereas simplicity is to be preferred. It is refreshing to find eminent statisticians reminding readers of this, such as Cox and Snell (1981).

J. E. H. S.
S. J. W. E.

REFERENCES

References are flagged with a T if they are difficult matters of technical detail. Those flagged with an * contain further discussions of detail which are written for a more general audience.

Abramowitz, M., and Stegun, I. A. (Eds) (1970). *Handbook of Mathematical Functions*, Dover, New York. T

Abramson, J. H. (1979). *Survey Methods in Community Medicine*, 2nd ed., Churchill Livingstone, Edinburgh.

Agresti, A. (1980). Generalized odds ratios for ordinal data, *Biometrics*, **36**, 59–67. T

Aitken, R. C. B. (1969). A growing edge of measurement of feelings, *Proc. Royal Soc. Med.*, **62**, 989–996.

Alberman, E., Pharoah, P., Chamberlain, G., Roman, E., and Evans, S. (1980). Outcome of pregnancies following the use of oral contraceptives, *Int. J. Epidem.*, **9**, 207–213.

Alvey, N. G., Banfield, C. F., Baxter, R. I., Gower, J. C., Krzanowski, W. J., Lane, P. W., Leech, K. P., Nelder, J. A., Payne, R. W., Phelps, M. K., Rogers, C. E., Ross, G. J. S., Simpson, H. R., Todd, A. D., Wedderburn, R. W. N., and Wilkinson G. N. (1977). *GENSTAT, A General Statistical Program*, The Statistics Department, Rothamsted Experimental Station.

Anderson, S., Auquier, A., Hauck, W. W., Oakes, D., Vandaele, W., and Weisberg, H. I. (1980). *Statistical Methods for Comparative Studies*, Wiley, New York.

Anscombe, F. J. (1961). Examination of residuals, *Proc. fourth Berkeley Symposium on Maths, Statistics and Probability*, **1**, 1–36. T

Anscombe, F. J. (1981). *Computing in Statistical Science through APL*, Springer-Verlag, New York.

Anscombe, F. J., and Tukey, J. W. (1963). The examination and analysis of residuals, *Technometrics*, **5**, 141–160.*

Armitage, P. (1971). *Statistical Methods in Medical Research*, Blackwell, Oxford.

Armitage, P. (1975). *Sequential Medical Trials*, Blackwell, Oxford.

Armitage, P., and Gehan, E. A. (1974). Statistical methods for the identification and use of prognostic factors, *International Journal of Cancer*, **13**, 16–36.

Armitage, P., and Hills, M. (1982). The two-period cross-over trial, *The Statistician*, **31**, 119–131.

Ashton, W. D. (1972). *The Logit Transformation*, Statistical monographs and courses no. 32, Griffin, London.

Baker, R. J., and Nelder, J. A. (1978). The GLIM System Release 3, Numerical Algorithms Group, Oxford. T

Barker, N., Hews, R. J., Huitson, A., and Poloniecki, J. (1982). The two-period cross-over trial, *BIAS*, **9**, 67–128.

Barnett, V. (Ed.) (1981). *Interpreting Multivariate Data*, Wiley, New York.

Barnett, V. (1982). *Comparative Statistical Inference*, 2nd ed., Wiley, New York.

Berkson, J. (1946). Limitations of the application of fourfold table analysis to hospital data, *Biometrics*, **2**, 47–53.

Bishop, Y. M. M., Fienberg, S. E. and Holland, P. W. (1975). *Discrete Multivariate Analysis: Theory and Practice*, MIT Press, Cambridge, Massachusetts. T*

Box, G. E. P. (1954). Some theorems on quadratic forms applied in the study of analysis of variance problems, I. Effect of inequality of variance in the one-way classification, *Annals of Math. Stats.*, **25**, 290–302. T

Box, G. E. P. (1980). Sampling and Bayes' inference in scientific modelling and robustness, *J. Royal Stat. Soc. A*, **143**, 383–430. *

Box, G. E. P., and Cox, D. R. (1964). An analysis of transformations, *J. Royal Statist. Soc. B*, **26**, 211–252. *

Box, G. E. P., and Tiao, G. C. (1973). *Bayesian Inference in Statistical Analysis*, Addison–Wesley, Reading, Massachusetts. *

Breslow, N. E. (1975). Analysis of survival data under the proportional hazards model, *Int. Stat. Rev.*, **43**, 45–58.

Breslow, N. E. (1981). Odds ratio estimators when the data are sparse, *Biometrika*, **68**, 73–84.

Breslow, N. E., and Day, N. E. (1980). *Statistical Methods in Cancer Research*, Vol. 1—*The Analysis of Case-Control Studies*, IARC Scientific Publications no. 32, Lyon.

Brown, B. W., and Hu, M. S. (1980). Setting dose levels for the treatment of testicular cancer, in *Biostatistics Casebook*, pp. 123–152, Wiley, New York.

Buckatzch, J., and Doll, R. (1952). An experimental factor analysis of cancer mortality in England and Wales 1921–30, *Journal of Hygiene*, **50**, 384–393.

Burch, P. R. J. (1978). Smoking and lung cancer: the problem of inferring cause, *J. Royal Statist. Soc. A*, **141**, 437–477.

Burkhardt, R., and Kienle, G. (1978). Controlled clinical trials and medical ethics, *Lancet*, **ii**, 1356–1359.

Byar, D. P., Simon, R. M., Friedewald, W. T., Schlesselman, J. J., DeMets, D. L., Ellenberg, J. H., Gail, M. H., and Ware, J. H. (1976). Randomized clinical trials, perspectives on some new ideas, *New England J. Med.*, **295**, 74–80.

Canadian Cooperative Study Group (1978). A randomized trial of aspirin and sulfinpyrazone in threatened stroke, *New England J. Med.*, **299**, 53–59.

Cancer Research Campaign Working Party (1980). Trials and tribulations: thoughts on the organisation of multicentre clinical studies, *Brit. Med. J.*, **281**, 918–920.

Chalmers, T. C. (1975). Randomization of the first patient, *Medical Clinics of North America*, **59**, 1035–1038.

Clayton, J. K., Anderson, J. A., and McNicol, G. P. (1976). Preoperative prediction of postoperative deep vein thrombosis, *Brit. Med. J.*, **ii**, 910–912.

Cochran, W. G., and Cox, G. M. (1957). *Experimental Designs*, 2nd ed., Wiley, New York.

Colquhoun, D. (1971). *Lectures on Biostatistics*, Oxford University Press, Oxford.

Colton, T. (1974). *Statistics in Medicine*, Little, Brown and Company, Boston, Massachusetts.

Conover, W. F. (1980). *Practical Nonparametric Statistics*, Wiley, New York.

Cooley, W. W., and Lohnes, P. R. (1971). *Multivariate Data Analysis*, Wiley, New York.

Cormack, R. M. (1971). A review of classification (with discussion), *J. Royal Statist. Soc. A*, **134**, 321–367. T

Cornish-Bowden, A., and Eisenthal, R. (1974). Statistical considerations in the estimation of enzyme kinetic parameters by the direct linear plot and other methods, *Biochem. J.*, **139**, 721–730. *

Cox, A., Rutter, M., Yule, B., and Quinton, D. (1977). Bias resulting from missing information: some epidemiological findings, *Br. J. Prev. & Social Medicine*, **31**, 131–136.

Cox, D. R. (1958). *Planning of Experiments*, Wiley, New York.

Cox, D. R. (1970). *Analysis of Binary Data*, Chapman and Hall, London.

Cox, D. R. (1972). Regression models and life tables, *J. Royal Statist. Soc. B*, **34**, 187–220. *

Cox, D. R., and Isham, V. (1980). *Point Processes*, Chapman and Hall, London. *

Cox, D. R. and Snell, E. J. (1981). *Applied Statistics, Principles and Examples*, Chapman and Hall, London.

Crandon, A. J., Peel, K. R., Anderson, J. A., Thompson, V., and McNicol, G. P. (1980). Prophylaxis of pre-operative deep vein thrombosis: selective use of low-dose heparin in high-risk patients, *Brit. Med. J.*, **281**, 345–347.

Daniel, C., and Wood, F. S. (1980). *Fitting Equations to Data*, 2nd ed., Wiley, New York.

Darby, S. C., and Fearn, T. (1979). The Chatham blood pressure study. An application of Bayesian growth curve models to a longitudinal study of blood pressure in children, *Int. J. Epidem.*, **8**, 15–21.

Dawid, A. P., and Skene, A. M. (1979). Maximum likelihood estimation of observer error-rates using the EM algorithm, *Appl. Statist.*, **28**, 20–28.

Diem, K., Lentner, C., and Seldnip, J. (Eds) (1982). *Documenta Geigy Scientific Tables, Volume II: Statistics*, Ciba-Geigy, Ltd, Basle.

Dixon, W. J., Brown, M. B., Engelman, L., Frane, J. W., Hill, M. A., Jennrich, R. I., and Toporek, J. D. (1981). *BMDP Statistical Software*, University of California Press, Berkeley.

Draper, N. R., and Smith, H. (1981). *Applied Regression Analysis*, 2nd ed., Wiley, New York.

Edwards, A. W. F. (1972). *Likelihood*, Cambridge University Press, Cambridge.

Efron, B. (1979). Bootstrap methods; another look at the jackknife, *Ann. Statist.*, **7**, 1–26. T

Efron, B. (1980a). Randomizing and balancing a complicated sequential experiment, in *Biostatistics Casebook*, pp. 19–30, Wiley, New York.

Efron, B. (1980b). Which of two measurements is better?, in *Biostatistics Casebook*, pp. 153–170, Wiley, New York. *

Efron, B. (1981). Nonparametric estimates of standard error and confidence intervals, *Canadian J. Statistics*, **9**, 139–172. T

Ellenberg, J. H. and Nelson, K. B. (1980). Sample selection and the natural history of disease, *J. Amer. Med. Assoc.*, **243**, 1337–1340.

Evans, S. J. W. (1978). *Survival in Oral Cancer*, MSc thesis, University of London.

Everitt, B. S. (1974). *Cluster Analysis*, Heinemann Educational Books, London.

Everitt, B. S. (1977). *The Analysis of Contingency Tables*, Chapman and Hall, London.

Everitt, B. S. (1979). Unresolved problems in cluster analysis, *Biometrics*, **35**, 169–181. *

Feinstein, A. R. (1977a). Clinical biostatistics XLI. Hard science, soft data and the challenges of choosing clinical variables in research, *Clin. Pharmacol. Ther.*, **22**, 485–498.

Feinstein, A. R. (1977b). *Clinical Biostatistics*, C. V. Mosby Company, St Louis.

Fienberg, S. E. (1977). *The analysis of Cross-Classified Categorical Data*, MIT Press, Cambridge, Massachusetts.

Finney, D. J. (1971). *Probit Analysis*, 3rd ed., Cambridge University Press, Cambridge.

Fisher, R. A., and Yates, F. (1963). *Statistical Tables for Biological, Agricultural and Medical Research*, 6th ed., Oliver & Boyd, Edinburgh.

Fleiss, J. L. (1981). *Statistical Methods for Rates and Proportions*, 2nd ed., Wiley, New York.

Freiman, J. A., Chalmers, T. C., Smith, H., and Kuebler, R. R. (1978). The importance of beta, the type II error and sample size in the design and interpretation of the randomized control trial, *New England J. Med.*, **299**, 690–694.

Friedman, L. M., Furberg, C. D., DeMets, D. L. (1981). *Fundamentals of Clinical Trials*, John Wright, PSG Inc., Boston.

Garside, R. F., and Roth, M. (1978). Multivariate statistical methods and problems of classification in psychiatry, *Br. J. Psychiatry*, **133**, 53–67.

Gehan, F. A., and Freireich, E. J. (1974). Non-randomized controls in cancer clinical trials, *New England J. Med.*, **290**, 198–203.

George, S. L. (1980). Sequential clinical trials in cancer research, *Cancer Treatment Reports*, **64**, 393–397.

Gilbert, J. P., Meier, P., Rumke, C. L., Saracci, R., Zelen, M., White, C., Armitage, P., Schneider, B., Holford, T., and Ricketts, H. T. (1975). Report of the committee for the assessment of biometric aspects of controlled trials of hypoglycaemic agents, *J. Amer. Med. Assoc.*, **231**, 583–608.

Gnanadesikan, R. (1977). *Methods for Statistical Data Analysis of Multivariate Observations*, Wiley, New York.

Gordon, T. (1974). Hazards in the use of the logistic function with special reference to data from prospective cardiovascular studies, *J. Chron. Dis.*, **27**, 97–102. T

Gore, S. M., and Altman, D. G. (1982). *Statistics in Practice*, British Medical Association, London.

Gray, J. (1976). *Community Dentistry*, MSc thesis, University of London.

Greenland, S. (1979). Limitations of the logistic analysis of epidemiological data, *Amer. J. Epidem.*, **110**, 693–698.

Greenwood, M. (1926). The natural duration of cancer, *Report on Public Health and Medical Subjects, HMSO, London*, **33**, 1–26.

Haber, M. (1980). A comparison of some continuity corrections for the chi-squared test on 2×2 tables, *J. Amer. Statist. Assoc.*, **75**(371), 510–515. T

Hayden, G. F., Kramer, M. S., and Horwitz, R. I. (1982). The case-control study. A practical review for the clinician, *J. Amer. Med. Assoc.*, **247**, 326–331.

Healy, M. J. R. (1968). The disciplining of medical data, *Brit. Med. Bull.*, **24**, 210–214.

Healy, M. J. R., and Goldstein, H. (1976). An approach to the scaling of categorized attitudes, *Biometrika*, **63**, 219–229. T

Hill, A. B. (1962). *Statistical Methods in Clinical and Preventative Medicine*, Livingstone, Edinburgh.

Hill, A. B. (1963). *Medical Ethics and Controlled Trials, Brit. Med. J.*, **1**, 1043–1049.

Hill, A. B. (1977). *A Short Textbook of Medical Statistics*, Hodder and Stoughton, London.

Hills, M., and Armitage, P. (1979). The two-period cross-over clinical trial, *Br. J. Clin. Pharmacol.*, **8**, 7–20.

Hocking, R. R. (1976). The analysis and selection of variables in linear regression, *Biometrics*, **32**, 1–49. *

Hollander, M., and Wolfe, D. A. (1973). *Nonparametric Statistical Methods*, Wiley, New York.

Horwitz, R. I. (1979). Selected annotated bibliography of case-control studies, *J. Chron. Dis.*, **32**, supplement.

Huber, P. J. (1981). *Robust Statistics*, Wiley, New York. T

Hulley, S. B., Rosenman, R. H., Bawol, R. D., and Brand, R. J. (1980). Epidemiology as a guide to clinical decisions. The association between triglyceride and coronary heart disease, *New England J. Med.*, **302**, 1383–1389 (+ letters, **303**, 1060–1062).

John, J. A., and Quenouille, M. H. (1977). *Experiments: Design and Analysis*, 2nd ed., Griffin, London.

Jones, D. (1979). Computer simulation as a tool for clinical trial design, *Int. J. Biomed. Computing*, **10**, 145–150.

Joossens, J. V., and Brems-Heyns, E. (1975). High power polynomial regression for the study of distance, velocity and acceleration of growth, *Growth*, **39**, 535–551.

Kalbfleisch, J. D., and Prentice, R. L. (1980). *The Statistical Analysis of Failure Time Data*, Wiley, New York.

Kay, R. (1977). Proportional hazard regression models and the analysis of censored survival data, *Appl. Statist.*, **26**, 227–237.

Kershner, R. P., and Federer, W. T. (1981). Two-treatment crossover designs for estimating a variety of effects, *J. Amer. Statist. Soc.*, **76**, 612–619. T

Largo, R. H., Gasser, T. H., Prader, A., Stuetzle, W., and Huber, P. J. (1978). Analysis of the adolescent growth spurt using smoothing spline functions, *Annals of Human Biology*, **5**, 421–434.

Leaper, D. J., Horrocks, J. C., Staniland, J. R., and De Dombal, F. T. (1972). Computer-assisted diagnosis of abdominal pain using 'estimates' provided by clinicians, *Brit. Med. J.*, **4**, 350–354.

Lewis, M. S. (1980). Spatial clustering in childhood leukaemia, *J. Chronic Dis.*, **33**, 703–712.

Liddell, D. (1976). Practical tests of 2×2 contingency tables, *Statistician*, **25**, 295–304. *

Lindley, D. V. (1965). *Introduction to Probability and Statistics*. Part 2: *Inference*, Cambridge University Press, Cambridge.

McCullagh, P. (1980). Regression models for ordinal data, *J. Royal Statist. Soc. B*, **42**, 109–142. T

McGill, R., Tukey, J. W., and Larsen, W. A. (1978). Variations of box plots, *Amer. Statistician*, **32**, 12–16.

McPherson, K., Healy, M. J. R., Flynn, F. V., Piper, K. A. J., and Garcia-Webb, P. (1978). The effect of age, sex and other factors on blood chemistry in health, *Clin. Chim. Acta*, **84**, 373–397.

Mantel, N., and Haenszel, W. (1959). Statistical aspects of analysis of data from retrospective studies, *J. Nat. Cancer Inst.*, **22**, 719–748.

Mardia, K. V., Kent, J. T., and Bibby, J. M. (1979). *Multivariate Analysis*, Academic Press, New York. *

Maritz, J. S. (1981). *Distribution-Free Statistical Methods*, Chapman and Hall, London. *

Meier, P. (1975). Statistics and medical experimentation, *Biometrics*, **31**, 511–529.

Miller, R. G. (1980). Combining 2×2 contingency tables, in *Biostatistics Casebook*, pp. 73–83, Wiley, New York.

Miller, R. G. (1981). *Survival Analysis*, Wiley, New York.

Miller, R. G., Efron, B., Brown, B. M., and Moses, L. E. (1980). *Biostatistics Casebook*, Wiley, New York.

Mitchell, D. M., Collins, J. V., and Morley, J. (1980). An evaluation of cusum analysis in asthma, *Br. J. Dis. Chest*, **74**, 169–174.

Mosteller, F., and Tukey, J. W. (1977). *Data Analysis and Regression*, Addison-Wesley, Reading, Massachusetts.

Nelder, J. A., and Wedderburn, R. W. M. (1972). Generalized linear models, *J. Royal Statist. Soc. A*, **135**, 370–384. T

Nie, N.H. (Ed.) (1983). SPSS-X User Guide, McGraw-Hill, New York.

Nijenhuis, A., and Wilf, H. S. (1978). *Combinatorial Algorithms*, 2nd ed., Academic Press, New York. T

Pauker, S. G., and Kassirer, J. P. (1980). The threshold approach to clinical decision making, *New England J. Med.*, **302**, 1109–1117.

Pearson, E. S., and Hartley, H. O. (Eds) (1970). *Biometrika Tables for Statisticians*, Vol I, 3rd ed., Griffin, London.

Peterson, A. V., and Fisher, L. D. (1980). Teaching the principles of clinical trials, design and management, *Biometrics*, **36**, 687–697.

Peto, R. (1979). The British way of death, *New Scientist*, **83**, 649–651.

Peto, R., and Peto, J. (1972). Asymptotically efficient rank invariant test procedures (with discussion), *J. Royal Statist. Soc. A*, **135**, 185–206. T

Peto, R., Pike, M. C., Armitage, P., Breslow, N. E., Cox, D. R., Howard, S. V., Mantel, N., McPherson, K., Peto, J., and Smith, P. G. (1976). Design and analysis of randomized clinical trials requiring prolonged observation of the patient (I), *Br. J. Cancer*, **34**, 585–611.

Peto, R., Pike, M. C., Armitage, P., Breslow, N. E., Cox, D. R., Howard, S. V., Mantel, N., McPherson, K., Peto, J., and Smith, P. G. (1977). Design and analysis of randomized clinical trials requiring prolonged observation of the patient (II), *Br. J. Cancer*, **35**, 1–39.

Pettit, B. R., King, G. S., and Evans, S. (1980). The potential of multivariate discriminant analysis in the antenatal detection of neural tube defects, *Clin. Chim. Acta*, **102**, 191–198.

Phillips, D. S. (1978). *Basic Statistics for Health Science Students*, Freeman, San Francisco.

Pike, M. C., and Morrow, R. H. (1970). Statistical analysis of patient-control studies in epidemiology. Factor under investigation an all-or-none variable, *Br. J. Prev. & Soc. Med.*, **24**, 42–44.

Pocock, S. J. (1978). Size of cancer clinical trials and stopping rules, *Br. J. Cancer*, **38**, 757–766 (+ letters **40**, 171–172).

Pocock, S. J. (1982). Statistical aspects of clinical trial design, *Statistician*, **31**, 1–17.

Pocock, S. J. (1983). *Clinical Trials*, Wiley, Chischester.

Pocock, S. J., Shaper, A. J., Cook, D. G., Packham, R. F., Lacey, R. F., Powell, P., and Russell, P. F. (1980). British regional heart study: geographic variations in cardiovascular mortality, and the role of water quality, *Brit. Med. J.*, **280**, 1243–1249.

Prentice, R. L., and Marek, P. (1979). A qualitative discrepancy between censored data rank tests, *Biometrics*, **35**, 861–867. T

Randles, R. H., and Wolfe, D. A. (1979). *Introduction to the Theory of Nonparametric Statistics*, Wiley, New York. T

Ray, A. A. (Ed.) (1982). *SAS User's Guide*, SAS Inst. Inc., Cary. N. Carolina.

Riggs, D. S., Guarnieri, J. A., and Addelman, S. (1978). Fitting straight lines when both variables are subject to error, *Life Sciences*, **22**, 1305–1360. *

Roberts, R. S., Spitz, W. O., Delmore, T., and Sackett, D. L. (1978). An empirical demonstration of Berkson's bias, *J. Chronic Diseases*, **31**, 119.

Robertson, E. A., Van Steirtegham, A. C., Byrkit, J. E., and Young, D. S. (1980). Biochemical individuality and the recognition of personal profiles with a computer, *Clin. Chem.*, **26**, 30–36.

Robinson, B. N., Anderson, G. D., Cohen, E., Gazdzic, W. F., Karpel, L. C., Miller, A. H., and Stein, J. R. (1980). *SIR Scientific Information Retrieval Users Manual*, version 2, SIR Inc., Evanston, Illinois.

Rosa, A. A., Fryd, D. S., and Kjellstrand, C. M. (1980). Dialysis symptoms and stabilization in long-term dialysis. Practical applications of the CUSUM plot, *Arch. Intern. Med.*, **140**, 804–807.

Rubin, D. B. (1979). Using multivariate matched sampling and regression adjustment to control bias in observational studies, *J. Amer. Statist. Assoc.*, **74**, 318–328. *

Ryan, T. A., Joiner, B. L., and Ryan, B. F. (1976). *MINITAB Student Handbook*, Duxbury Press, North Scituate, Massachusetts.

Sackett, D. L. (1979). Bias in analytical research, *J. Chron. Dis.*, **32**, 51–63.

Schwartz, D., Flamant, R., and Lellouch, J. (1980). *Clinical Trials*, Academic Press, New York.

Siegel, S. (1956). *Nonparametric Statistics for the Behavioural Sciences*, McGraw-Hill Kogakusha, Tokyo.

Simon, R. (1977). Adaptive treatment assignment methods and clinical trials, *Biometrics*, **33**, 743–749. T

Snedecor, G. W., and Cochran, W. G. (1980). *Statistical Methods*, 7th ed., Iowa State University Press, Ames, Iowa.

Spiegelhalter, D. J., and Smith, A. F. M. (1981). Decision analysis and clinical decisions, in *Perspectives in Medical Statistics* (Eds J. F. Bithell and R. Coppi), Academic Press, London.

Stone, M. (1974). Cross-validatory choice and assessment of statistical predictions, *J. Royal Statist. Soc. B*, **36**, 111–147. T

Titterington, D. M., Murray, G. D., Murray, L. S., Spiegelhalter, D. J., Skene, A. M., Habbema, J. D. F., and Gelpke, G. J. (1981). Comparison of discrimination techniques applied to a complex set of head injured patients, *J. Royal Statist. Soc. A*, **144**, 145–175. T

Tukey, J. W. (1977). *Exploratory Data Analysis*, Addison-Wesley, Reading, Massachusetts.

Velleman, P. F., and Hoaglin, D. C. (1981). *Applications, Basics and Computing of Exploratory Data Analysis*, Duxbury Press, Boston, Massachusetts.

Wade, A., and Wingate, D. (1980). Use of pentagastrin test as a combined teaching and research project for medical students, *Lancet*, **ii**, 516–519.

Wald, A. (1950). *Statistical Decision Functions*, Wiley, New York.

Wallenstein, S., Zucker, C. L., and Fleiss, J. L. (1980). Some statistical methods useful in circulation research, *Circulation Research*, **47**, 1–9.

Wermuth, N., and Cochran, W. G. (1979). Detecting systematic errors in multi-clinic observational data, *Biometrics*, **35**, 683–686.

Westgard, J. O., and Hunt, M. R. (1973). Use and interpretation of common statistical tests in method-comparison studies, *Clin. Chem*, **19**, 49–57.

Wilk, M. B., and Gnanadesikan, R. (1968). Probability plotting methods for the analysis of data, *Biometrika*, **55**, 1–17.

Winer, B. J. (1971). *Statistical Principles in Experimental Design*, 2nd ed., McGraw-Hill, Kogakusha, Tokyo.

Wold, S. (1974). Spline functions in data analysis, *Technometrics*, **16**, 1–11.

Zelen, M. (1979). A new design for randomized clinical trials, *New England J. Med.*, **300**, 1242–1245.

3

Formal Approaches to the Analysis of Clinical Decisions

3.1 INTRODUCTION

3.1.1 A place for mathematics

Traditionally, the major decisions of treatment and patient care have been the responsibility of the trained medical practitioner. The manner in which the physician reached his decision was rarely, if ever, questioned, nor was the quality of his decision-making monitored in any objective or scientific way. Indeed, the expression, 'the art of clinical medicine', is still used frequently to describe the abilities of those entrusted with the care of the health of others. However, it has long been recognized that the quality of clinical decision-making depends in part on the physician's knowledge and experience and that clinical decision-making, in common with all forms of management, is not immune to errors of judgement. Thus, over the past twenty-five years, medical research has begun to devote more attention to the general problems of decision-making in a clinical environment. In particular, attention has been focused on methods of data-processing and decision-making developed initially for business and scientific applications, and these can now be shown to have a useful role in clinical medicine.

Above all, this research has been motivated by a desire to improve the quality of patient care. However, there have been other major changes in medicine during this period which have influenced the way in which research has proceeded. Changes in medical technology have been dramatic. Many new investigative tests are now available but some carry a high cost in monetary terms. Others can cause the patient considerable discomfort. The clinician must now decide which expensive tests are really necessary, balancing the needs of the individual patient with a desire to preserve limited resources for future use. Such decisions are particularly acute when the clinician is working within a State-funded health service. Once such a test has been carried out, the clinician is obliged to make effective use of the information gained. Computers are now a recognized tool of management and provide an efficient means of accessing patient records and processing data. With the advent of the microcomputer, information-handling technology can be used at the bedside in a way which was not previously possible. Finally, there is a steadily increasing demand for automated or formal systems which can 'advise' junior or paramedical personnel in circumstances where difficult clinical decisions must be taken without the aid of expert advice.

This chapter describes some of the findings of recent research, highlighting the various roles which have been found for mathematical ideas. The discussion focuses on three related topics. The first is a group of mathematical ideas, which need to be understood by all persons responsible for clinical decision-making. In the second we survey mathematical methods which can assist decision-making by improving the accuracy of diagnosis. Finally, we look briefly at the mathematical aspects of some related issues likely to be encountered by a research team setting up a formal system for diagnosis [see VI, Chapter 19].

It is worth emphasizing that, in restricting our discussion to mathematical ideas, we will not be commenting in any detail on a number of issues which would be included in a full description of the impact of formal procedures in clinical decision-making. In particular, we will not be discussing the use of computers and database management systems *per se*, although numerous studies have already shown that such systems can improve the quality of clinical decision-making simply by making relevant information more easily accessible. Also, we shall not discuss the question of acceptability of formal systems, although this again is an important issue. Leaving aside the performance characteristics of a formal system, acceptability is determined in part by the manner in which the system is implemented and in part by the attitudes of the clinicians involved. A system which is easy to use is clearly more acceptable than one which forces medically trained personnel to adopt inconvenient working practices or which requires that the user understands complicated computer protocols. A system which is designed to assist the physician rather than replace him will be viewed more favourably. The solution to problems of acceptability lies in appropriately packaging the system and in educating the user. Thus, complicated mathematical ideas need not be avoided simply to make the system more acceptable. Currently there are very few formal procedures for clinical decision-making in routine use. The main reasons for this are the problems of acceptability and the mediocre performance of many experimental systems due to their use of inappropriate mathematical techniques. It is hoped that this chapter will demonstrate that there exists a substantial body of mathematical theory which has yet to be fully utilized by applied research in this area.

3.1.2 The clinical decision problem

Once a person declares himself to be ill and seeks medical advice, the physician concerned initiates a course of action which he hopes will return his patient to an acceptable state of health. This course of action will be determined by a series of decisions taken during the period the patient remains in his care. Some decisions will be concerned directly with treatment. For example:

Should the patient be treated surgically or with chemotherapy?
What is the appropriate dose of drug for this patient?
How long should treatment be maintained?
Should treatment A be started now or should we do nothing and await developments?

Other decisions are taken during the investigation of the patient's illness:

Is an ultrasound scan of this patient's liver necessary?

Yet others could be called management decisions:

Should this patient suffering from chest pain be admitted to a coronary care unit, a general medical ward or sent home?
Should this patient be informed of his prognosis?

All such decisions are similar. In each case the physician must choose one option from a small set of alternatives, the objective being to 'move' the patient from his present state of health to a preferred state of health. Henceforth we shall refer to these alternatives as 'treatments' although we recognize that we are extending the literal meaning of the word.

Difficulties arise in clinical decision-making because it is often the case that the precise outcome of a particular treatment cannot be predicted with certainty at the time the decision must be taken. Sometimes it is the treatment itself which has unpredictable outcomes. For example, all surgery carries some risk of peri-operative death and many drugs can produce unpleasant side-effects in certain persons. On other occasions, the effect of a treatment cannot be predicted accurately simply because the nature of the patient's illness has not been established with certainty. Any choice among treatments must take these alternative outcomes into account. Note that we shall continue to use the word 'outcome' to describe these uncertain events, even when the uncertainties arise from the diagnostic process.

The relevance of a particular outcome to the choice of treatment is determined in part by the likelihood that the outcome will occur and in part by the ensuing consequences of that outcome for the patient. Consider a situation in which a choice must be made between treating a patient, who has a chronic but stable condition surgically, or doing nothing. Surgery may bring about the patient's death or may lead to a good recovery. The consequences of the alternative outcomes of surgery are very different for the patient but, on determining that the probability of peri-operative death is low, the physician may decide that, on balance, surgery is the preferred treatment. Note that this decision could be reversed if either the probability of death were increased or if the value of successful surgery were diminished to a point where the state of health of the patient following surgery was little better than the state of health before surgery. Similarly, if a decision has to be made between two treatments, the more effective of which might produce side-effects, the final choice depends both on the likelihood of the side-effects occurring and on the unpleasantness of these side-effects as perceived by the patient.

Thus, in its most general form, the clinical decision can be viewed as a considered choice of one treatment from a shortlist of feasible treatments, having due regard for the various outcomes, the likelihood of each outcome and the consequences of each outcome, beneficial or otherwise, for the patient.

In Section 3.2 we describe a mathematical theory for decision-making and show how this theory is relevant to clinical medicine. Our argument is not that all clinical decisions should be determined by a strict application of a mathematical theory. Rather it is that decision theory should be used as a tool of medical research for examining those decisions where correct choice of treatment has always proved difficult and should act as a yardstick against which more pragmatic or *ad hoc* procedures for decision-making can be compared. We will show that the theory provides a means of identifying where further information should be collected in order to clarify awkward decision problems. An awareness of the basic ideas of decision analysis allows the physician to assess his own mechanisms for arriving at clinical decisions. This, in turn, may increase his consistency or perhaps improve his use of those resources which are in short supply.

3.1.3 Diagnosis

The information necessary for a reasoned choice of treatment comes from three distinct sources. One obvious source is the patient. A second is the pool of specialist knowledge acquired by training and from books of reference. Finally, the experienced physician will have some knowledge of an epidemiological nature through his acquaintance with the population of which his patient is a member, and, having faced similar decisions in the past, he will be able to recall relevant case histories. A proportion of the time, the physician summarizes part of this information by pronouncing a diagnosis or perhaps a prognosis. Although a diagnosis does not in itself have any effect on the patient's current state of health, it can be viewed as an 'allocation' of the patient to a particular category which has relevance for future management. We refer to such categories as *disease classes* or simply *diseases*, even though it is quite possible to diagnose a 'broken leg' or even 'abdominal pain meriting immediate admission'. In some circumstances, if the physician is confident that his diagnosis is correct, subsequent decisions regarding treatment may be simplified. Much of the current research into formal procedures for clinical decision-making reflects this thinking and has been concerned solely with improving the accuracy of diagnosis.

It is generally accepted that a simple examination or even a single *lead symptom* is sufficient for the physician to determine a shortlist of diseases, one of which will be the eventual diagnosis. Research has concentrated on improving the accuracy of this final choice. The majority of formal procedures for diagnosis are statistical in nature. Data—signs, symptoms, history and the results of special tests— collected from patients whose diseases have already been confirmed are used to establish the character of each disease group. A new patient is then diagnosed using a statistical calculation which determines how typical the patient's individual pattern of signs and symptoms is of each disease group in turn. This approach emphasizes the information available from case histories and makes limited use of medical knowledge. However, data-based methods for diagnosis tend to be robust procedures and are relatively unaffected by occasional errors incurred when recording the results of a patient examination. Furthermore, the majority of such procedures quantify diagnostic uncertainty using probabilities estimated from the database and thereby avoid problems of subjective judgement and bias.

The problem of allocating an individual to a category on the basis of a fixed set of measurements is not unique to medicine. The general issues are described in both the statistical and engineering literature under the headings of *discriminant analysis* [see VI, §16.6] and *pattern recognition* respectively. Although the primary objective of discriminant analysis is to make maximum use of the information in the database as it pertains to the classification of a new individual, there is no single best procedure for achieving this. In any given application, secondary considerations, such as the number of disease categories, the number of measurements made on each individual, whether the data are measured on discrete or continuous scales and whether or not all the patient records in the database are complete, dictate the form of the discriminant rule which should be used. In medicine, the selection of a mathematical procedure for diagnosis may be subject to even more practical considerations, such as the nature of the computing facilities available at the implementation site. Section 3.3 begins with a description of those discrimination procedures which have already been used extensively for diagnosis. Later sections describe alternative discrimination procedures which have only been used occasionally in medicine but merit further attention.

Statistical rules for diagnosis yield results in one of two forms. A first group yields a simple prediction of the form 'the patient has disease X'. Although such rules appear to give an unambiguous result, they can be misleading in that they do not distinguish definitive diagnoses from those which are subject to uncertainty. A second group of diagnostic rules yields sets of probabilities. For example, where there are three possible diseases, the diagnosis might be reported as 'the probability that the patient has disease X is 0.78, the probability of disease Y is 0.18 and the probability of disease Z is 0.04' [see II, §3.2]. This second form of output is most useful when the diagnosis is to be used for allocating treatment.

3.1.4 Further introductory reading

An excellent introduction to formal reasoning methods in diagnosis is given by Wulff (1976), while the case for mathematical methods in medical decision-making is made by Card and Good (1974). Early books on the topic include a general description of the mathematical aspects of decision-making by Lusted (1968) and two collections of articles edited by Jacquez (1964, 1972). More recently, special issues of the *Journal of the Royal College of Physicians, London* (1975, 1979) and the *New England Journal of Medicine* (1975) have contained numerous articles which give a good indication of the nature of research in this area. See also Bunker, Barnes and Mosteller (1977) and the two conference proceedings edited by de Dombal and Grémy (1976) and Alpèrovitch, de Dombal and Grémy (1979) for further examples.

3.2. DECISION THEORY

3.2.1 A prescription for clinical decision-making

Consider the following simple *decision problem* [see II, §2.3]:

> A physician must choose between two treatments. The patient is known to have one of two diseases but the diagnosis is not certain. A thorough examination of the patient was not able to resolve the diagnostic uncertainty. The best that can be said is that the probability that the patient has disease A is p.

The problem may be represented graphically as in Figure 3.2.1, this structure being known as a *decision tree*. It summarizes all the possibilities foreseen by the decision-maker. In the event, exactly one path through the tree will be realized, this path depending partly on the choice of treatment (X or Y) and partly on the actual disease state (A or B). The various paths depend on treatment–disease combinations and the branches are labelled to indicate these. The probability of each disease is also indicated.

Following convention, a node where a decision has to be made is represented by a square. The paths leading from such a node represent the options or treatments from which a choice must be made. Alternative *outcomes* of treatment—in this case, the alternative diagnoses—are shown emanating from a *chance node* represented by a small circle. It is important to distinguish between a path through the tree and the state of health the patient finds himself in as a result. The latter we shall call a *consequence*. A value u is associated with each consequence, as discussed below.

Decision theory [see VI, Chapter 19] is based on the assumption that, given any two consequences, the decision-maker can either state which consequence he

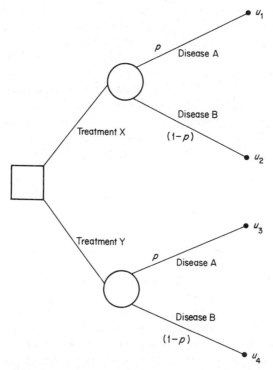

Figure 3.2.1 A simple decision tree. □ indicates a decision node; paths from it represent options. ○ indicates a chance node; possible 'outcomes' are represented with their probabilities of occurrence. p is the probability that the patient has disease A. Each of the four possible combinations of treatment and disease is associated with a 'utility', u.

prefers or he can say that he has no preference, i.e. both consequences have the same value to him. In the latter case the decision-maker is said to be indifferent to the two consequences. Decision theory further assumes that the decision-maker is rational. Simple axiomatic schemes exist which provide a strict definition of rationality (see de Groot, 1970, for example). Much of the essence of these schemes is illustrated by the following transitivity axiom: given any three consequences, if the first is preferred to the second and the second is preferred to the third then the first must be preferred to the third. In no way does the mathematical definition of *rational* transcend the usual intuitive meaning of the word.

Such axioms lead to the conclusion that in any decision problem one can identify a worst or least preferred consequence and a best consequence, and can rank the remaining consequences in strict order of preference. However, simply ranking consequences does not in itself lead to an unambiguous procedure for deciding treatment. The probabilities of the different outcomes have to be taken into account. If specific values could be assigned to each consequence, a natural strategy for decision-making would be to choose that treatment which had the greatest expected consequential value. Here the term 'expected' is used in its statistical sense. The *expected value* associated with a particular treatment is defined to be a weighted sum of the values assigned to the various consequences, the weights being the probabilities of the corresponding outcomes [see II, §8.1]. If values $u_1, \ldots, u_4$ were assigned to the four consequences in the example described above (see Figure 3.2.1), treatment X would be chosen in preference to treatment Y when

$$pu_1 + (1-p)u_2 > pu_3 + (1-p)u_4. \tag{3.2.1}$$

There are, of course, many different choices of the u values consistent with a single preference ranking, some leading to the choice of treatment X and others to the choice of treatment Y. The axiomatic basis of decision theory leads to a well-defined procedure for assigning preference values to consequences which resolves this difficulty. These values are known as *utilities* [see VI, §19.1] and are obtained as follows.

Let the utility of the worst (i.e. least desirable) possible consequence, W, equal zero and let the utility of the best possible consequence, B, equal one. Let C be a consequence with intermediate ranking and consider the hypothetical decision problem represented by Figure 3.2.2. Here one can either choose a path which guarantees consequence C or a path where the outcome is uncertain. For the latter path only two of the possible consequences are considered; either the best consequence, which is postulated to occur with probability q, or the worst consequence, occurring with probability $1 - q$. This hypothetical decision can be

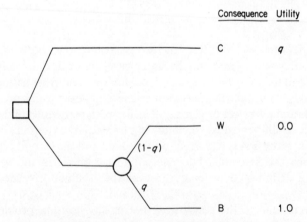

Figure 3.2.2 The hypothetical decision problem used in defining the utility of the consequence C.

viewed as a straight choice between a certain consequence and a simple gamble, and it is clear that the choice depends both on the probability, q, and the decision-maker's willingness to gamble. If q were very close to one then the gamble would almost certainly be preferred, but q close to zero would probably result in the decision-maker choosing the sure consequence. The decision-maker questions himself carefully as to the value of q which would leave him indifferent to the two options. The utility of consequence C is defined to be that value of q.

An example, given by Spiegelhalter (1980), may help to make this method of evaluating consequences more tangible. Consider a situation where you are suddenly blinded by an accident. You are offered the prospect of an operation which can return normal sight but the operation carries some risk of death. Let q be the probability that the operation is a success. What is the smallest value of q that you would be prepared to accept if you were going to have the operation? That value is your personal utility for the state of blindness on a scale where death has utility zero and normal sight (and health) has utility one.

It can be shown that the axioms referred to above imply the following formal prescription for clinical decision-making:

(a) Identify the set of feasible treatments

$t_1, \ldots, t_I$, say.

(b) Identify all the likely outcomes for each treatment

$O_{11}, \ldots, O_{1J_1}, \ldots, O_{I1}, \ldots, O_{IJ_I}$.

(c) Assess the probabilities that each outcome will occur

$p_{11}, \ldots, p_{1J_1}, \ldots, p_{I1}, \ldots, p_{IJ_I}$.

(d) Assess the utility of each consequential state of health

$u_{11}, \ldots, u_{1J_1}, \ldots, u_{I1}, \ldots, u_{IJ_I}$.

(e) Calculate an expected utility for each treatment

$$e_i = \sum_{j=1}^{J_i} p_{ij} u_{ij} \quad i = 1, \ldots, I.$$

(f) Choose that treatment which has the maximum expected utility; i.e. choose t_* where

$$e_* = \max_i \{e_i, i = 1, \ldots, I\}.$$

Good introductions to decision theory are given by Raiffa (1968) and Lindley (1971). A recent text by Weinstein *et al.* (1981) deals specifically with the role of decision analysis in medicine. Krischer (1980), in a bibliography of applications of decision analysis, cites 110 applications to health care.

It is worth emphasizing the essential elements of this prescription. Uncertainty must be quantified using probabilities, consequences of decisions must be valued using utilities and decisions must be determined by selecting that treatment having the highest expected utility. Decision theory is an optimal procedure. No other method of determining treatment can yield a greater *return* to the decision-maker over a long series of decisions, provided that the return associated with each possible consequence is defined in units which truly reflect the decision-maker's personal assessment of worth. It should also be noted that this prescription is sufficiently general to accommodate those decision problems where some of the outcomes of certain treatment choices involve events where further decisions must be made. This feature is best illustrated by example and is discussed further in Section 3.2.2.

Decision-making in the face of uncertainty involves a gamble [see VI, §19.3] and thus it is correct that the final decision should, in part, reflect the decision-maker's propensity to gamble. Applying decision theory in clinical medicine raises a number of interesting questions regarding the identity of the decision-maker. In some situations it is clear that the choice of treatment will only affect the patient and thus it is the patient's utilities which should be used. In other situations, e.g. where a physician must decide which patient will benefit from scarce resources, the issue is more controversial. In practice, the situation is further complicated by the fact that it can be very difficult to assess a utility directly. The patient may have no conception of the possible consequences of certain treatments and the direct assessment of utilities using hypothetical gambles can prove daunting. Practical methods for assessing or approximating utilities are considered in Section 3.3.3. Here, however, we shall assume for the time being that utilities can be obtained and discuss a number of further issues.

Consider again the decision problem described by Figure 3.2.1 and assume that u_1, u_2, u_3 and u_4 are utilities for the four possible outcomes. This decision problem is sufficiently general to illustrate a number of interesting points. It may occasionally happen that the decision-maker prefers consequence 1 to consequence 3 and prefers consequence 2 to consequence 4. In this case the value of p is immaterial. Treatment X is the obvious choice. Although this situation would occur very rarely in the two-treatment, two-disease problem it does suggest a way in which more complicated decision problems might be simplified prior to a detailed evaluation of the probabilities and utilities involved.

In a second extreme case we may know with certainty that the patient has disease A. In these circumstances, it is sufficient to know which of consequence 1 and consequence 3 is preferred. A similar argument may be used when we are almost certain of the patient's disease. When p is close to 1.0, the sides of (3.2.1) are closely approximated by u_1 and u_3 respectively and thus, providing the gains and losses associated with each consequence are not too dissimilar, we may again make the correct decision based simply on our preference for consequence 1 and

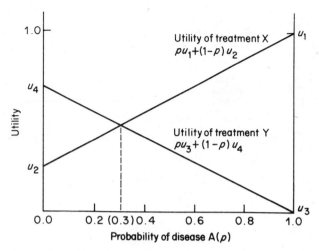

Figure 3.2.3 Sensitivity analysis of the decision depicted in
Figure 3.2.1.

consequence 3. Precise values for the utilities need not be known. This makes explicit the simplifications which arise from accurate diagnosis.

Figure 3.2.3 displays the expected utility of each of the two treatments X and Y. Arbitrary values have been chosen for each of the four utilities, but the expected utilities have been plotted as functions of the probability p. It can be seen that in this case any small error in the assessment of p would be unimportant unless p was near the value 0.3. Thus, a graph of this type can be used to determine whether the decision is sensitive to errors in the assessment of a disease probability. Similarly, for a fixed value of p, the relative height of each line can be recalculated for different choices of any of the utilities and thus the sensitivity of the decision to inaccuracies in utility assessment can be judged. This is a simple example of a general technique known as *sensitivity analysis* which may be applied to all decision problems. The value of such a technique lies in its ability to pinpoint those features of a complicated decision which need greatest attention and those other areas which can be overlooked.

3.2.2 Some illustrative examples

Teather, Emerson and Handley (1974) describe an application of decision theory to the use of heparin therapy in the treatment of deep vein thrombosis. When a doctor sees a patient with myocardial infarction he has to decide whether the patient should be started on anticoagulant therapy as soon as he is admitted to hospital, thereby reducing the risk of a pulmonary embolism, or whether the decision should be delayed until a deep vein thrombosis develops subsequently.

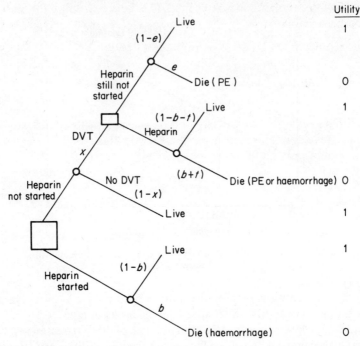

Figure 3.2.4 Decision tree for heparin treatment (from Teather *et al.*, 1974).

The issue is one of balancing the risk of death from pulmonary embolism with the risk of a bleeding complication of heparin.

The decision tree for this problem is given in Figure 3.2.4. Note that the tree includes a description of the supplementary decision which would have to be taken if deep vein thrombosis developed following an initial decision not to start heparin therapy. The decision-maker is faced with several sources of uncertainty and here these are quantified using four probabilities defined as follows:

b = probability of a fatal haemorrhage given heparin
e = probability of a fatal pulmonary embolus (PE) complicating untreated deep vein thrombosis (DVT)
t = probability of a fatal pulmonary embolus complicating heparin-treated deep vein thrombosis
x = probability of deep vein thrombosis developing

The authors ignore the cost of treatment and other non-fatal consequences of treatment and adopt a very simple but adequate utility structure which assigns the value zero to death and one to life. The expected utility of each treatment option can now be calculated. Starting from the right-hand side of the tree, the supplementary decision is considered first. The expected utility for starting a patient on heparin once a deep vein thrombosis starts is $(1 - b - t)$. That is,

$1 - b - t = P(\text{live}|\text{DVT and heparin}) \times \text{utility (live)}$

$\qquad + P(\text{die from PE or haemorrhage}|\text{DVT and heparin})$
$\qquad \times \text{utility (die)}$

$\qquad = (1 - b - t) \times 1.0 + (b + t) \times 0.0.$

If not started on heparin, the expected utility is $(1 - e)$. It follows that, if a patient is not being treated with heparin when a deep vein thrombosis develops, such treatment should only be initiated if $b + t < e$. If we assume, for purposes of illustration, that this condition is satisfied, then we may now consider the primary decision using the reduced tree displayed in Figure 3.2.5.

The expected utility associated with the optimal treatment in the supplementary decision is now assigned to the consequence identified with no heparin initially but deep vein thrombosis subsequently, because the decision-

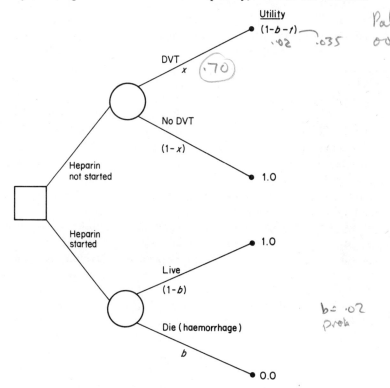

Figure 3.2.5 Collapsed decision tree for heparin treatment. $1 - b - t$ is the expected utility for the supplementary decision to start a patent on heparin once DVT has been diagnosed.

maker has already decided how he would act in these circumstances. Computation of the expected utilities associated with heparin and no heparin on admission leads to the conclusion that heparin should be given if

$$(1 - x) + x(1 - b - t) < 1 - b,$$

i.e. if

$$x > b/(b + t).$$

Teather, Emerson and Handley (1974) then discuss plausible values for the four probabilities and relate these quantities to factors such as patient age, previous history of varicose veins or thromboembolism and smoking habits, before specifying a formal treatment allocation rule. For example, for patients over the age of 70, they estimate that the probability of a fatal bleed given heparin (b) is 0.02 and that the probability of a fatal pulmonary embolism complicating treated deep vein thrombosis (t) is 0.035. Thus, if x, the probability of deep vein thrombosis occurring, is greater than $0.02/(0.02 + 0.35) = 0.36$ then such a patient should be treated with heparin on admission. The authors quote an incidence rate for deep vein thrombosis of 70 per cent in untreated patients aged more than 70 years. Clearly such patients should be treated from admission. A simple sensitivity analysis shows that this decision would not be changed if the probability estimates for b and t were modified slightly.

A second illustration of the use of decision analysis is given by Pauker and Pauker (1977) who are concerned with the use of amniocentesis for the pre-natal diagnosis of genetic disorders. Amniocentesis carries with it a risk of spontaneous abortion. Furthermore, such a test may yield a false-positive result which could lead to the parents requesting an unnecessary abortion. One possible decision tree for this situation is given in Figure 3.2.6, although the authors do extend this description to include other eventualities.

The probabilities associated with spontaneous abortion due to amniocentesis or otherwise, the probability of an affected foetus and the false positive and false negative error rates of the test may depend on individual circumstances, but are generally well known by the clinican responsible for advising the parents. Straightforward calculations can be used to obtain the expected utility of each option as a function of the utilities attached to each consequence. However, it is these utilities which are at the heart of this decision problem; the attitudes of parents to abortion and congenitally handicapped children differ markedly. It is argued that a physician who understands the concepts of decision theory will be able to see whether or not the decision is sensitive to the informal 'utilities' that parents may suggest during consultation and thus better counsel the parents to ensure that the final decision really does reflect their wishes. The authors conclude: 'The decision is sufficiently complex, however, that many couples find it bewildering. Decision analysis provides a systematic means of both com-

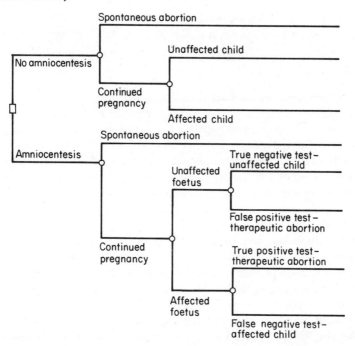

Figure 3.2.6 Decision tree for counselling on prenatal diagnosis of genetic disorders (from Pauker and Pauker, 1977).

municating the issues to the parents and obtaining measures of the relative costs or burdens of the outcomes from them.'

The preceding examples show clearly the insight which one can gain when a clinical decision problem is formulated within the framework of decision theory. In both cases the decision trees are relatively simple but do indicate how sequences of decisions can be incorporated and how the various sources of uncertainty can be exposed. Two further examples may help to reinforce the importance of evaluating the consequences of alternative treatments in a manner which is relevant to the patient. McNeil, Weichselbaum and Pauker (1978) compared the use of surgery versus radiation therapy in the treatment of lung cancer. The former results in an increased five-year survival rate but carries a risk of death within a short time of surgery. Patients interviewed who had operable lung cancer were found to have a variety of attitudes towards surgery and some were quite averse to taking risks involving the possibility of immediate death. The authors argue that radiation therapy would be a more appropriate choice for these patients. Similar attitudes expressed in two letters which appeared in *The Sunday Times* of 6 July 1980 on the subject of surgery in the treatment of breast cancer: 'Nothing prepares one either for the successive annihilating waves of disgust and depression which make life more or less intolerable. The rate of survival may look good in the statistics, but statistics don't count the cost' and 'Given my present knowledge, I would prefer death to the radical operation.'

3.2.3 Assessment of utility

In any practical clinical decision problem, where utilities for different health states are required, there are two separate considerations. First, the various states of health need to be defined. We distinguish between those health states which can be described or indexed by a single clearly defined attribute and those health states which are more complicated and must be described in terms of two or more component attributes. For example, a decision problem may involve a series of alternative treatments which lead to consequences which can be expressed simply in terms of life expectancy. In a slightly more complicated example the consequences could be described in terms of life expectancy with or without a fixed level of disability. Two distinct attributes are involved here. At the most general level, health states could possibly be described in terms of five attributes: life expectancy, level of pain, degree of physical disability, degree of mental disability and a measure of the 'burden' which the patient places on his immediate family.

Where health states are difficult to describe as a function of distinct attributes, it may be possible to proceed with a finite list of health states obtained by identifying a continuum of similar health states as a single quantity. Utilities for this finite set of states could then be assessed directly. For example, Spiegelhalter and Smith (1981) describe a study of the choice of treatment for a severe liver disease. A group of clinicians reduced the continuum of consequences to just six categories:

1. peri-operative death;
2. death within one year, confined to bed;
3. death within one year, mobile but unable to work;
4. death within five years, mobile but unable to work;
5. death within five years, able to work;
6. survival past five years, able to work.

When the question of treatment was considered for any particular patient, the actual consequences envisaged were approximated by health states from this list.

Second, a means of assigning values to consequences is required. The basic procedure involving hypothetical gambles has already been described. Where a consequence is defined in terms of more than one attribute, it is possible to assess utilities for each consequence by considering each attribute separately and then computing aggregate utilities in a way which reflects the relative importance of each attribute. A detailed theoretical discussion of *multiattribute utility theory* is given by Raiffa and Keeney (1976). Examples of the use of multiattribute utilities in clinical decision-making are given by Krischer (1976), who considers the treatment of cleft lip, and Pauker (1976), who discusses the merits of coronary-bypass surgery. Krischer evaluated the alternative outcomes of cleft lip surgery using four attributes: monetary cost, clarity of speech, hearing loss and disfigurement. Pauker, on the other hand, considered just two attributes: length of life and a measure of quality of life.

Hypothetical gambles can also be used to assign utilities to consequences described by a single continuous attribute. Card, Rusinkiewicz and Phillips (1977) describe an experiment to determine the utility of varying degrees of sight. It is assumed that utility for sight can be expressed as an increasing function of visual acuity although there is no reason to expect the relationship to be linear. A sequence of gambles is used to determine the utility of fixed levels of visual acuity and then a curve is fitted through these values. It is recognized that no individual will be totally consistent when presented with a series of gambles and thus revealed utilities are subject to a degree of assessment error. The utility curves obtained are, in essence, curves of best fit to the data available.

Spiegelhalter and Smith (1981) describe similar techniques for summarizing an individual's utility for remaining years of life. Figure 3.2.7 displays the utilities obtained from a 30 year old man when the method of gambles was used to discover how he valued a life expectancy of two and a half, five, ten and twenty years respectively. It was assumed that a life expectancy of forty years had a utility of 1.0. If a smooth curve can be found which passes close to these points then the individual's utility for different life expectancies, x, can be obtained. Spiegelhalter and Smith considered two simple families of curves [see IV, §2.11]:

$$\text{Exponential: } u(x) = \frac{1 - e^{-kx/40}}{1 - e^{-k}},$$

and

$$\text{Logarithmic: } u(x) = \frac{\log(1 + bx/40)}{\log(1 + b)},$$

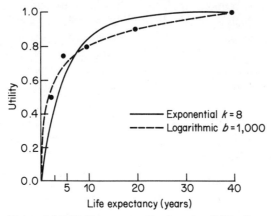

Figure 3.2.7 Utility curves for length of life (from Spiegelhalter and Smith, 1981).

both curves being the graphs of one-parameter functions, the parameters being k and b respectively. The best fitting curves from each family are displayed. The authors point out that the concave nature of these curves reflects risk aversion on the part of the subject and that the degree of curvature is a simple function of the parameter in each case. Thus it may be possible, in situations such as this, to summarize an individual's utility for a continuously varying attribute by a single number.

When it is not possible to elicit utilities from the patient, one approach is to adopt a set of utilities which represent a consensus opinion. Careful thought must be given to the choice of parties to the consensus but, in those circumstances where it is believed that different utilities for a particular consequence simply reflect the difficulties in assessing utilities rather than systematic differences between participants, it is possible to use standard statistical techniques to estimate the 'true' utility [see VI, §19.3.3]. Spiegelhalter and Smith (1981), in their discussion of the treatment of liver disease, provide an example of this approach.

Several studies have suggested alternative ways of evaluating consequences. A survey of methods for valuing health states in the context of health programme evaluation is given by Culyer (1978) and Rosser and Kind (1978). These include the use of *linear analogue scales* where the best and worst consequences are fixed at either end of a 10 cm line and individuals are asked to mark the 'position' of intermediate consequences. Another method is to value a health state in terms of the number of days spent in this state, which is equivalent to one day of good health.

Occasionally *ad hoc* scales for valuing outcomes turn out to be utility scales. Perhaps the most important of these is survival rate. If a particular consequence is 'normal health with probability p' then the utility of this state is simply p, when expressed on a utility scale where certain survival has utility one and certain death has utility zero. Pauker and Kassirer (1975) describe a study of the treatment choices in appendicitis using survival rates. In general, we note that choice of treatment remains unchanged if utilities are subject to simple linear transformations which maintain the order of preference. Thus, scales whose end points are not zero and one may be used provided that the relative positions of intermediate consequences approximate to the utilities of those consequences. However, if non-utility scales are used to value consequences, resulting decisions are not necessarily optimal and may contradict the rationality axioms.

3.3 MATHEMATICAL METHODS FOR DIAGNOSIS

3.3.1 Principles of discriminant analysis

We will now consider mathematical methods which may be used to assign a new patient to one of several disease classes. Although most of the methods to be described can be generalized to several, i.e. five to ten diseases, we shall assume that just two diseases are possible. It is further assumed that the patient has exactly one of the diseases in question and that the incidence rate for each disease is known. That is, we can identify a target population for the diagnostic rule and know the proportions of that population having each disease. In the discussion we need to be able to distinguish between the features of a patient which are potentially quantifiable, e.g. sex or systolic blood pressure, and the values we obtain when these features are actually recorded for a particular patient, such as 'male' and '140 mm Hg'. Here we shall call the former *features* and the latter *indicants*.

Assume that over a period of time a sizable collection of patient records has been gathered from patients now known to have had either of the two diseases, A and B say. Expert opinion has determined a list of features known to be useful in discriminating between A and B. The problem of selecting a best sub-set of features for diagnosis is discussed in Section 3.4.3. For each patient in the database, we have a record of the disease and the indicants corresponding to each feature on the list. In addition, data are available from the new patient but, in this case, only the indicant pattern is known.

In practice, features are assessed on a variety of measurement scales. Some features may be scored as present or absent, while others may be scored using 'none', 'mild', 'moderate' and 'severe' type scales. Yet other features, such as age or biochemical measurements, may be recorded on continuous scales. Many discriminant rules require all features to be measured on the same type of scale, but it is always possible to recode continuous data in a discrete form, albeit with the loss of some information. Therefore, our discussion concentrates on procedures for discrete data. A second complication, which frequently arises in the practical situation, is that some indicants are missing from some of the cases included in the database. For most procedures we shall assume that full data are available, but will indicate when missing data would affect the usefulness of the procedure.

As indicated earlier, discriminant procedures are of two types. Some simply yield a statement of the disease class to which the patient should be assigned. Such procedures are surveyed in Section 3.3.2. Others yield a set of disease probabilities. As we have seen, such probabilities may subsequently be used to describe uncertain aspects of a treatment decision. Even when the sole objective of diagnosis is to classify a patient, a probabilistic diagnosis is still of value. The assignment of a patient to a disease class involves a decision which is equivalent to a decision concerning treatment. The appropriate decision tree for the classification decision, when just two diseases are possible, is given in Figure 3.3.1. The similarity with Figure 3.2.1 is evident. A *classification rule* where one assigns a new patient to the disease class having greatest probability corresponds to the special case where the utility of correct classification is one and the utility of an incorrect classification is zero.

Before proceeding it may be helpful to discuss very briefly some general

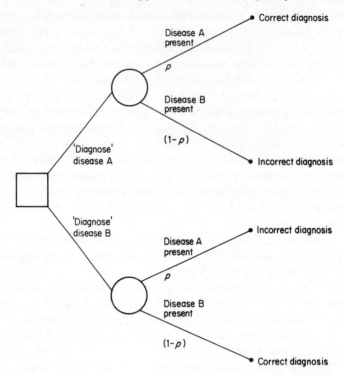

Figure 3.3.1 Decision tree for the classification decision between
two diseases.

statistical ideas which are relevant to discriminant analysis. (Further details and
references are given in Chapter 1 of this book and in Volumes II and VI.)

A probability is a measure of uncertainty attached to a particular event. All
probabilities are conditional probabilities in the sense that a probability is not
meaningful unless a set of 'prevailing conditions' are specified [see II, §3.9]. For
example, the probability that a particular patient has appendicitis cannot be
specified unless we state which group or population of patients is being
considered. The probability of appendicitis may also change on learning that the
patient has abdominal pain and has arrived in a doctor's surgery complaining of
feeling unwell. However, in certain contexts it is convenient to distinguish
between *conditional* and *unconditional probability*. Consider the population of
patients defined as those who arrive at a hospital complaining of chest pain. Then,
with reference to this population, we may consider the 'unconditional' probability that a patient has a broken rib as distinct from the conditional
probability that a patient has angina, given that he has a history of cardiac pain.
We write $P(D_i)$ to indicate the probability that a patient has disease i and
$P(S_1, \ldots, S_k)$ (or $P(\mathbf{S})$) for the probability that a patient has a certain set of

indicants. Conditional probabilities, such as the probability that a patient has disease i given that he has a certain set of indicants, is represented as $P(D_i|S_1,\ldots,S_k)$ or $P(D_i|\mathbf{S})$. The conditional probability $P(S_1,\ldots,S_k|D_i)$, the probability that a patient with disease i will exhibit the indicant pattern $S_1,\ldots,S_k$ is known as the likelihood of $S_1,\ldots,S_k$ given disease i.

In practice, it is rare for any of the probabilities associated with either diseases or indicant patterns to be known exactly. These quantities must be estimated from the data to hand. The simplest approach, the so-called *actuarial* or *full multinomial* method, is to count those patients satisfying certain conditions. Consider a sample of 100 patients drawn from all patients complaining of chest pain. If eight of these patients are found to have broken ribs then 0.08 is one estimate of the probability that the next patient drawn from this population will have a broken rib [see II, §2.3]. This estimate is a reasonable statistical approximation to the true probability of broken ribs in the population in question. However, it is clearly possible to improve the accuracy of this estimate by increasing the sample size. If three of the patients with broken ribs complain of severe pain then an estimate of P(severe pain|broken ribs) is 0.375. However, this estimate is likely to be poor as it is based on data from only eight patients. The problem of very small sample sizes leading to poor estimates of certain probabilities is central to all statistical approaches to diagnosis.

Consider a more realistic situation in which ten features, all of which can be either present or absent, are to the used to discriminate between two diseases. A total of 2^{10} (i.e. 1,024) indicant patterns are possible and thus, to cover all eventualities, 2,048 probabilities of the form $P(D_i|S_1,\ldots,S_{10})$ where $i=1,2$ must be estimated. If all these probabilities were to be estimated directly, an extremely large database would be necessary. Furthermore, it would have to contain numerous representatives of all possible indicant combinations. Such a direct approach is not practicable. The only alternative is to model the relationship between disease probability and indicant complex.

In common with all mathematical modelling, the statistician views the probability that a patient has a particular disease as some function of the features, $X_1,\ldots,X_k$, say, which are to be used for diagnosis. This may be written

$$P(D_i) = f_i(X_1,\ldots,X_k;\theta_1,\ldots,\theta_j). \tag{3.3.1}$$

where the f_i represent prescribed functional forms that depend, in part, on the values assigned to the 'model parameters' $\theta_1, \theta_2,\ldots,\theta_j$. In some circumstances these are known constants in the expression. More generally they are estimated using the database. The precise form of the function $f_i(.)$ is open to considerable choice, although the form will usually reflect a set of assumptions about the relationships between indicant patterns and disease probabilities along with other considerations such as the ease with which the function can be evaluated in practice. In view of the arbitrariness of such models, it is necessary to have a set of criteria whereby discriminants can be compared and the best discriminant selected. This matter is discussed further in Section 3.4.3.

Although $P(D_i|S)$ can be modelled directly, one can also exploit the fact that, by Bayes' theorem [see II, §16.4],

$$P(D_i|S) = P(S|D_i)P(D_i)/P(S). \tag{3.3.2}$$

In words, Bayes' theorem states that the probability of a particular disease given a set of indicants is proportional to the product of the probability of observing the same indicant pattern in a patient known to have disease i and the incidence rate for disease i. The value of this approach lies in the fact that the likelihood $P(S|D_i)$ allows greater scope for modelling. The incidence rates are known and the scaling factor $P(S)$ can be obtained using the partition law of probability [see II, §16.2] once the likelihoods have been estimated. When just two diseases are possible,

$$P(S) = P(S|D_1)P(D_1) + P(S|D_2)P(D_2).$$

For a more general statement of the partition law see Volume II, Theorem 16.2.1. A detailed discussion of the relative merits of both approaches is given by Dawid (1976). In Section 3.3.3 we describe by far the most popular model for the likelihood, the so-called *Bayes' independence model*, and in Section 3.3.4 we consider a number of alternatives. Direct estimation of $P(D_i|S)$ is considered again in Section 3.3.5 and illustrated by the *logistic discriminant*. It is worth emphasizing, in view of the frequency with which Bayes' theorem is mentioned in medical diagnosis, that (3.3.2) is a statement of a standard result of probability theory and this equation should not be confused with the Bayes' independence model.

We conclude this section with a simple example to illustrate how the composition of the database can have a marked effect on estimates of certain disease probabilities. Consider a situation where just one symptom, pain, is to be used to discriminate between two diseases. Cross-tabulating that symptom with the confirmed disease, we might obtain a contingency table [see VI, §§5.4.1, 5.4.2 and 7.5.1] of the form of Table 3.3.1.

If the new patient has mild pain then the probability that he has disease A can be estimated directly from the first column of the table and is 5/7 in this example.

Table 3.3.1

	Pain		
	Mild	Severe	
Disease A	50	10	60
Disease B	20	20	40
	70	30	100

(Artificial data)

Table 3.3.2

	Pain		
	Mild	Severe	
Disease A	50	10	60
Disease B	120	120	240
	170	130	300

(Artificial data)

However, the validity of this probability depends on the numbers of patients in the database with each disease being in the same ratio as the relative incidence of each disease in the population. If, in fact, disease B were four times as likely as disease A and the database reflected this, the equivalent contingency table would be as shown in Table 3.3.2.

The probability that the new case has disease A is now 5/17. If simple actuarial estimates of disease probabilities are to be unbiased, the database must contain cases of each disease in the same proportions as the disease incidence rates. The same comment applies whenever the database is used to yield a direct estimate of a disease probability. Note also that in this example the likelihoods of mild pain in each of the disease groups can be obtained from the rows of either table and are

$$P(\text{mild pain}|\text{disease A}) = 5/6$$

and

$$P(\text{mild pain}|\text{disease B}) = 1/2.$$

No systematic bias is induced into likelihood estimation by the manner in which the database is collected. However, the number of representatives of each disease will have a bearing on the accuracy of probability estimates.

3.3.2 Predictive procedures

The simplest predictive procedure is the clinical algorithm or *flowchart*. The user reaches a decision by tracing a path through the chart. The strength of such systems lies in their simplicity and the fact that they are cheap to implement; a chart or a book of flowcharts can be used to advise in many situations. The weakness of such systems is their strictly deterministic character. If a particular piece of information is misleading or incorrectly recorded, the user could be led down the wrong branch of the flowchart and a totally erroneous diagnosis could result. Where the use of clinical algorithms is reported, it would appear that they have been derived informally by one or more experienced physicians. Diagnosis achieved in this way is similar to the problem of biological identification. Payne and Preece (1980) provide a good survey of the mathematics of this subject and

Mesel *et al.* (1976) give a description of a working system which is used by general practitioners to determine cancer therapy. Essex (1980) combines diagnosis with management in a series of flowcharts designed for use by the 'barefoot doctors' responsible for primary medical care in Tanzania.

The so-called *nearest neighbour models* provide a second class of predictive procedures. When large numbers of features are considered, each case in the database usually displays a unique indicant pattern and it is rare for a new patient to match any of the confirmed cases exactly. The simplest nearest neighbour procedure searches the database for a patient whose indicant pattern is closest to the indicant pattern of the new case and then declares the diagnosis for the new patient to be the same as that for the confirmed case. The biggest problem with this approach is the need to define a measure of 'distance' between cases. This is particularly difficult when the features are measured on a mixture of discrete and continuous scales. Many distance measures are arbitrary although the same problem does arise in statistical *cluster analysis*. The technical issues are discussed by Hartigan (1975) and many other texts on multivariate analysis [see VI, Chapter 17]. The sensitivity of the diagnosis to the peculiarities of individual cases in the database can be avoided to some extent by identifying several nearest neighbours and looking at the proportions of these cases having each disease. A description of nearest neighbour methods for discrete data is given by Hills (1967). Practical applications of nearest neighbour methods have tended to be informal in operation, providing the user with summaries of the patients close to the new patient and leaving the final judgement to the physician. Fries (1972) describes a system used at Stanford University which provides the user with a written report on the prognosis of those patients attending a rheumatology clinic who match a new patient on a certain set of selected indicants. Diagnostic systems based on nearest neighbour ideas require the full data to be available for access at all times. This typically requires a substantial computer system which is seen as a limitation to the approach. In common with cluster analysis, missing data creates added complexity to the meaning of distance between cases.

By far the most widely known predictive procedure is Fisher's *linear discriminant function*. Let $X_1, \ldots, X_k$ be a set of features and let

$$y = a_1 X_1 + a_2 X_2 + \cdots + a_k X_k$$

be a score which can be computed for a patient once his particular indicant pattern is observed. If this score exceeds a threshold the patient is said to have one disease, if not, he has the other. This is the first example of a diagnostic rule where the modelling concept discussed above is evident. Even so, direct estimation of disease probabilities is not attempted. The coefficients $a_1, \ldots, a_k$ and the threshold are the model parameters chosen to maximize the number of correct diagnoses when the rule is applied to the database. For an indication of the manner in which these coefficients are obtained see VI, §16.6. A detailed description is given by Lachenbruch (1975). The statistical literature contains numerous accounts of the properties of the linear discriminant. It can be shown that this method of classification is optimal in the case where the distribution of features in each disease class has a multivariate Normal distribution with a common variance–covariance structure [see II, §13.4] (see Mardia, Kent and Bibby, 1979, Chap. 11). Thus the linear discriminant is best suited to situations where features are measured on continuous scales. When distribution assumptions can be substantiated, it is possible to obtain expected classification error rates. Again, a guide to the literature is given by Lachenbruch. A recent example of the use of the linear discriminant is provided by Ellis and Goldberg (1979) who describe a study where laboratory test data were used to classify patients with hepatobiliary disease into fourteen disease groups. Goldstein and Dillon (1978) discuss the use of the linear discriminant with discrete data. One reason for the popularity of the linear discriminant, apart from its simplicity (note that a new patient can be classified using a simple calculation once the coefficients and threshold are known), was the wide availability of computer programs for calculating the coefficients. However, in medical applications particularly, its use is declining in favour of the logistic discriminant (see Section 3.3.5).

3.3.3 Bayes' independence model

One plausible form for the likelihood of a given indicant pattern is given by the expression

$$P(\mathbf{S}|D_i) = \prod_{j=1}^{k} P(S_j|D_i);$$

i.e. the likelihood of the complete set of k indicants is found by computing the product of the likelihoods of each indicant taken separately. As likelihoods for individual indicants can be estimated from simple tables such as Table 3.3.1, there is, in principle, no upper limit to the number of features which can be considered. Furthermore, neither the estimation of the separate likelihoods nor the calculation of disease probabilities for a new patient is affected by missing data. However, this model is founded on the assumption that all the features used for diagnosis are conditionally independent of each other [see II, §§3.5 and 6.5]. Conditional independence is a notoriously elusive concept but may be illustrated as follows. Consider two indicants or features, S_1 and S_2, say, and disease D. S_1 and S_2 are conditionally independent, given D, if

$$P(S_1 S_2|D) = P(S_1|D)P(S_2|D).$$

Note that we have to say what the conditioning is *on*. Extending this a stage further, consider two features, pain severity and age, and two diseases A and B. We say that pain severity and age are conditionally independent if and only if, separately for those patients having disease A and those having disease B, the probability that a patient will suffer severe pain does not depend on his/her age.

Table 3.3.3 Data consistent with the assumption that age
and pain are *conditionally* independent, given disease.

		Disease A		Disease B	
	Age, years	< 40	≥ 40	< 40	≥ 40
Pain	Mild	40	10	8	20
	Severe	10	3	12	30

(Artificial data)

Table 3.3.4 Data contradicting the assumption that age
and pain are conditionally independent, given disease.

		Disease A		Disease B	
	Age, years	< 40	≥ 40	< 40	≥ 40
Pain	Mild	30	20	20	30
	Severe	2	28	28	2

This is not the same as saying pain and age are independent in the target population as a whole (i.e. in this case those having A or B). Tables 3.3.3 and 3.3.4 illustrate how the conditional independence property may be checked using the database. In each case a three-way contingency table is displayed. In the first of these tables neither of the 2×2 sub-tables defined by the different diseases shows any sign that pain and age are related. A simple chi-squared test for independence in each sub-table would indicate that there are no grounds for rejecting the independence hypothesis [see Section 1.3.10 and VI, §7.5]. In Table 3.3.4, however, the frequencies indicate that severe pain is positively associated with age in disease A but negatively associated with age in disease B. Here is a clear example of two features which are not conditionally independent.

For each of these two sets of data we now form the two-way table obtained by pooling the frequencies from each disease group. These are displayed in Tables 3.3.5 and 3.3.6 respectively. This allows an assessment of the degree of association between the two features in the population as a whole. In Table 3.3.5 we have clear evidence that pain and age are related unconditionally even though they were conditionally independent. In Table 3.3.6 pain and age are clearly independent unconditionally even though these same data indicated that these features were not conditionally independent. Unconditional independence of two symptoms [see II, §3.5] does not imply conditional independence and neither does the reverse hold.

In practice, the operational simplicity of Bayes' theorem has made this procedure for diagnosis very popular. A recent review article (Sadegh-Zadeh,

Table 3.3.5 Contingency table formed by ignoring disease state in Table 3.3.3. Data contradicts the assumption that pain and age are independent unconditionally.

		Age, years < 40	≥ 40
Pain	Mild	48	30
	Severe	22	33

Table 3.3.6 Contingency table formed by ignoring disease state in Table 3.3.4. Data now supports the assumption that pain and age are independent unconditionally.

		Age, years < 40	≥ 40
Pain	Mild	50	50
	Severe	30	30

1980) lists 362 papers describing diagnosis, published prior to 1978, which refer to Bayes' theorem. The majority of these articles describe applications of the Bayes' independence model. Unfortunately, few of the articles pay more than lip service to the conditional independence assumption and frequently assume that it is unconditional independence which is necessary. Failure to ensure that the features being used are conditionally independent effectively means that the same diagnostic information is used twice or even more often. The result is that the disease probabilities obtained tend to give a false impression of certainty.

For examples of effective use of the independence model the reader is referred to an account of automated diagnosis of the cause of abdominal pain by de Dombal *et al.* (1972) and to an example of computer-aided prognosis in severe head injury described by Jennett *et al.* (1976). Both authors have subsequently published numerous papers which describe various aspects of these studies. For comment on the estimation of the likelihoods for each feature see Titterington *et al.* (1981). Hilden and Bjerregaard (1976) suggest ways in which the independence model can be adapted when the conditional independence assumption is not strictly appropriate. A continuous feature can be incorporated in the independence model either by replacing the continuous scale by a discrete scale or by assuming that the feature has a particular probability density.

Recent experience indicates that diagnostic procedures which make use of the conditional independence assumption can be very powerful, but specific applications require an extensive investigation of the inter-relationships among the important features. Some appreciation of statistical methods for the analysis of discrete data is necessary.

3.3.4 Other methods for modelling feature likelihoods

A variety of alternative models for feature likelihoods have been proposed which are appropriate when inter-relationships between features are known to be present. Although they are widely varying in nature they all share the common property that they do not rely on the conditional independence assumption. For this reason, they deserve greater attention in medical applications than they are receiving at present. When the number of features is less than five or six, *log-linear models* may be used [see VI, Chapter 11]. A detailed description of the theory of log-linear models is given by Bishop, Fienberg and Holland (1975); see also Section 2.1.8 of this Guidebook. The method is very flexible and it is possible to incorporate features measured on both continuous and discrete scales. The essence of this approach is that the statistician has the capability of investigating every possible pair-wise and higher order relationship. The resulting model thus reflects the true pattern of relationships between disease and features rather than reflecting assumptions about these relationships. The penalty for this degree of sophistication is the upper limit on the number of features which can be included in the model. This limit is determined by problems of tractability which arise when the models are being fitted and a need for larger and larger databases as the number of features is increased. Missing data causes no additional complexity but can lead to a considerable increase in the amount of statistical analysis necessary when specifying the discriminant. Early computational problems have now largely been overcome with the wide availability of computer packages for fitting log-linear models. See the discussion in Chapter 2, Section 2.4.

Modelling strategies which are intermediate between the independence model and the log-linear model include the *Lancaster models* and the *Bahadur expansion*. For a description of these models see, for example, Goldstein and Dillon (1978) and Moore (1973).

Latent class models represent and provide yet another means of calculating disease class probabilities without having to invoke the assumption that the features are independent within disease classes. Here, the strategy is to cluster the data into groups so that, as far as possible, the features are independent within the groups. These groups are the latent classes. By noting which cases in the database are assigned to which latent class, we can determine how typical each latent class is of each disease class. The diagnosis of a new patient is effected by first using the Bayes' independence model to assign the patient to a latent class and then determining disease probabilities using the partition law [see II, Theorem 16.2.1]. See Fielding (1977) for the general theory of latent class analysis and Skene (1978) for details of how this model can be used for diagnosis. Latent

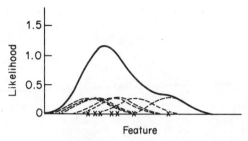

Figure 3.3.2 Kernel estimate of the likelihood
of a single continuous feature.

class models have two useful properties. They can be extended to include features measured on both discrete and continuous scales and their operation is unaffected by missing data either in the database or in the indicant complex collected from the patient to be diagnosed.

The final group of procedures to be considered here are those known as *kernel-based procedures*. These procedures are essentially non-parametric in nature; the basic idea is illustrated by Figure 3.3.2 which displays a kernel estimate for the likelihood of one disease as a function of one continuous feature. The likelihood, or probability density as it is here, is a 'mountain' created by summing the effects of small 'mountains' placed over each of the values of the features that have actually been observed. Figure 3.3.3 considers two diseases and a single feature and indicates how likelihoods h_1 and h_2 can be calculated for a new patient. Even when just two features are considered, quite complicated likelihood surfaces can arise. The nature of these surfaces also depends to a large

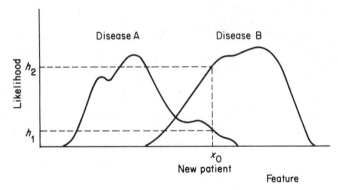

Figure 3.3.3 Calculation of disease probabilities using kernel based estimates of likelihoods.
$P(\text{disease A}|\text{feature} = x_0) = h_1 P(A)/(h_1 P(A) + h_2 P(B))$,
$P(\text{disease B}|\text{feature} = x_0) = h_2 P(B)/(h_1 P(A) + h_2 P(B))$,

where $P(A)$ and $P(B)$ are disease incidence rates.

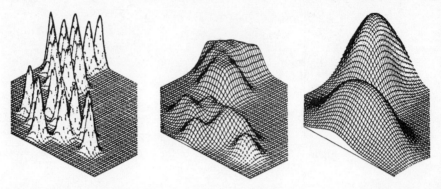

Figure 3.3.4 A bivariate likelihood surface for different choices of component kernels (from Meisel, 1972).

extent on the shape adopted for the 'component mountains', as Figure 3.3.4 indicates. Kernel methods, though intuitively appealing, involve extensive computation as the number of features is increased and missing data creates further difficulties. Meisel (1972), Breiman, Meisel and Purcell (1977) and Habbema, Hermans and Remme (1978) provide further details of kernel methods for continuous features. See also a comparison of continuous kernel methods with Fisher's linear discriminant, described by Hermans and Habbema (1975). Analogous methods for discrete data have been proposed. These are described by Aitchison and Aitken (1976), Murray and Titterington (1978) and Titterington (1980). An example of the use of discrete kernel methods in medicine is given by Titterington *et al.* (1981).

3.3.5 Logistic discrimination

The logistic discriminant model takes the form

$$\log\left[\frac{P(D_i)}{1 - P(D_i)}\right] = a_0 + a_1 X_1 + \cdots + a_k X_k, \tag{3.3.3}$$

i.e. the model, an extension of the linear discriminant, is founded on the assumption that the log of the odds in favour of disease *i* can be expressed as a linear combination of the features. Once suitable values have been found for the coefficients $a_0, \ldots, a_k$, the right-hand side of (3.3.3) can be evaluated for any given indicant pattern **S**. If the resulting score is *y*, say, an estimate of the probability of $P(D_i|\mathbf{S})$ is given by

$$P(D_i|\mathbf{S}) = \frac{e^y}{1 + e^y}.$$

This method of discrimination is described by Day and Kerridge (1967) for two diseases; the method is extended to several diseases by Anderson (1972).

Anderson (1975) describes a further extension, the quadratic logistic model. As the logistic model estimates $P(D_i|S)$ directly, it is necessary to introduce a correction term when the composition of the database does not reflect disease incidence in the population being considered. Anderson (1972) considers this problem further.

Despite its unusual form, this model is very general and includes other popular models as special cases. For examples of the use of the logistic discriminant in medicine see Clayton, Anderson and McNicol (1976), Titterington *et al.* (1981) and Spiegelhalter (1982).

3.3.6 Use of artificial intelligence

A number of attempts to develop formal procedures for diagnosis have avoided the use of statistical procedures and employed ideas of *artificial* or *machine-based intelligence*. Diagnosis is achieved using computer programs which access a large database of logical rules designed to summarize the relevant medical knowledge and reflect clinical experience. It is argued that by following orthodox lines of reasoning, such programs result in a better handling of rarely seen conditions. The emphasis is very much on the logical manipulation of medical knowledge and no large-scale processing of patient records is attempted. Such an approach has obvious advantages when the number of diseases under consideration is large and useful classifications follow in a logical manner from certain patterns of symptoms.

Perhaps the most widely known of these systems is the MYCIN system (Shortliffe, 1976) which was designed to assist physicians in the selection of antibiotics for patients with infections. A review of progress in this area is given by Shortliffe, Buchanan and Feigenbaum (1979). Artificial intelligence research has concentrated on a number of related topics: the interpretation of natural language, the representation in a database of natural language-based knowledge, algorithms for deductively searching a database to resolve a problem and the man–machine interface all have an application in medical decision-making. However, medical diagnosis presents special problems for logical systems due to the non-specific nature of many features. To date, artificial intelligence systems have tended to employ *ad hoc* scoring systems to represent uncertainty but as yet no consistent method of incorporating diagnostic uncertainty into such systems has been devised. The limited success of early data-based systems has lead to a situation where research workers in artificial intelligence have tended to avoid the use of probabilistic models. This separation is unfortunate. The most profitable direction for future research in clinical decision-making is almost certainly the embedding of specific systems which make use of probabilistic models and the general principles of decision theory within wider information processing systems. For an excellent discussion of the strengths and shortcomings of both statistical and knowledge-based approaches, see Spiegelhalter and Knill-Jones (1984).

3.4 OTHER RELATED TOPICS

3.4.1 Developing a diagnostic rule

The development of a formal procedure for diagnosis is a complex process. Following initial decisions determining the target population for the procedure, the nature of the eventual users and the range of diseases to be considered, a list of features is drawn up containing all those signs, symptoms, etc., which might possibly be useful for discriminating between the diseases. Appropriate measurement scales must be chosen. For some features the scale may be obvious but, more often, it is necessary to choose between discrete and continuous scales or determine the number and character of the distinct responses possible on a discrete scale. For example, a patient's age could be recorded in years or decades. Pain levels could be scored as absent or present, or on the four-point scale— 'none', 'mild', 'moderate', 'severe'. In different circumstances, the four-point scale 'none', 'moderate', 'severe', 'very severe' might be an even better choice. In each case a balance must be struck between the use of an extensive scale which may enhance the discriminating power of the feature and a simple scale which minimizes the chances of measurement error.

An understanding of the effects of measurement error and the way in which it can be controlled is central to the development of formal decision procedures. Good and Card (1971), in an important discussion, describe how the discriminatory power of features can be seriously degraded by errors of measurement. We reproduce their simplest example to illustrate the problem. Consider a binary feature being used to discriminate between two diseases, D_1 and D_2. Assume that when the feature is elicited without error it is known to be of reasonable discriminatory power. Specifically, assume that the likelihood of the feature being present in patients with D_1 is 0.80 while the likelihood of the same feature being present in patients with D_2 is only 0.10. In this case the errors of observation can be of two types. The observer may say that the feature is absent when it is actually present or he/she may record the presence of the feature when it is really absent. The probabilities that each of these types of error occurs are indicated by α and β, which are known as the false negative and false positive error rates respectively [see §1.3.3]. Good and Card propose the use of a measure of discriminatory power known as *expected weight of evidence* and then investigate how this measure is degraded as either α or β is increased. Considering the simplest case where α equals β, the percentage information loss is given in Figure 3.4.1 as a function of $\alpha + \beta$.

The startling fact revealed by this graph is that when α and β are as small as 0.05 there is a loss of expected weight of evidence of 25 per cent and when α and β are 0.15 the loss rises to nearly 60 per cent, rendering the feature almost worthless for diagnosis. The authors derive similar results for measurement errors associated

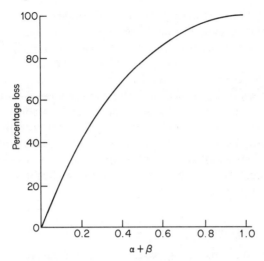

Figure 3.4.1 Percentage loss of expected weight of evidence as a function of $\alpha + \beta$ (assuming indicant likelihoods as stated in the text). (from Good and Card, 1971).

with polychotomous discrete features and features measured on continuous scales.

Measurement error can have several causes. Some features are inherently difficult to assess. For example, even experienced physicians can disagree on whether a patient's liver is palpable or not. On the other hand, disagreement between observers as to whether a patient's level of pain is mild or moderate can be minimized by careful definition of precisely what is meant by mild and moderate in this setting. Measurement error may be a function of the clinician's experience. Thus a popular strategy, when establishing measurement scales prior to initial data collection, is to choose rather more extensive scales than are perhaps necessary, in the knowledge that these scales can be collapsed at a later stage when it can be shown that this does not significantly degrade the discriminant. One then ensures that those clinicians contributing cases to the database understand clearly the meanings of each scale and perhaps, also, one conducts a pilot study to assess the degree of measurement error. In Section 3.4.2 we review methods for quantifying the degree of observer agreement and indicate how the consistency and bias of individual observers can be estimated.

Once the database is available, a period of extensive data analysis and experimentation follows to determine which of the many features in the original list should be incorporated into the final discriminant, the most appropriate form for that discriminant and whether the original or simpler measurement scales should be used. Initially a feature might be considered because it has traditionally been recognized as a valuable source of information to determine diagnosis. However, it may be eventually excluded from consideration either because it has a low discriminatory power for the specific diseases in question or because it is of limited usefulness, given that other features have already been included. In traditional methods of diagnosis there is a high degree of redundancy in the information collected. Such redundancy is unnecessary in formal systems where the information provided by single features is exploited more fully. Some features may be very useful in certain rare circumstances but useless for the majority of cases; others may be discarded once it is confirmed that the scale of measurement necessary for the feature to be of value will lead to significant measurement error by the eventual users.

3.4.2 Measuring observer error

The extent to which a particular feature attracts measurement error can be assessed by a study in which several different observers independently measure the feature on a common set of patients. When the feature is measured on a continuous scale one would not expect complete agreement between observers. Rather, it is to be hoped that the variation between observers within patients is small compared with the variation in measurements obtained across patients. Standard statistical methods exist for determining the sizes of such variation. The reader is referred to the discussion of analysis of variance models in Chapter 2 and a review of alternative methods by Landis and Koch (1975a).

When a feature is measured on a discrete scale, some agreement between observers is to be expected. In fact, even two observers making no attempt to record a feature correctly would still agree occasionally by chance alone. The extent to which chance agreements arise depends in turn on the relative frequencies with which the possible values of the feature occur. Consider the two contingency tables displayed in Table 3.4.1. Each represents the pattern of agreements and disagreements obtained when two observers independently measured two binary features on 100 patients. In each case there were eighty-two agreements. However, the first feature was equally likely to be present or absent in an individual patient and thus, in this case, one would have expected fifty agreements by chance alone. (Consider the expected number of agreements if two fair coins were tossed simultaneously 100 times.) The second feature was known to be present in 90 per cent of the population from which the sample was drawn and thus eighty-two agreements are expected by chance alone (eighty-one 'present, present' agreements and one 'absent, absent' agreement—i.e. $82 = 100 \times (0.9 \times 0.9 + 0.1 \times 0.1)$). In the first case there is considerable evidence of agreement; in the second there is no evidence of agreement at all.

In assessing observer agreement on discrete scales, correction must be made for chance agreement. The most popular statistic for measuring such agreement is

Table 3.4.1 Observed agreements for two observers and two binary features.

Feature 1

		Observer 1	
		Present	Absent
Observer 2	Present	41	9
	Absent	9	41

Total = 100

Feature 2

		Observer 1	
		Present	Absent
Observer 2	Present	81	9
	Absent	9	81

Total = 100

the *Kappa statistic,* defined as

$$K = \frac{\text{number of observed agreements} - \text{number of expected agreements}}{\text{number of trials} - \text{number of expected agreements}}$$

Kappa takes the value zero when there is chance agreement only and the value one when agreement is perfect. Further properties of this statistic are described by Landis and Koch (1975b). The definition is sufficiently flexible to accommodate polychotomous scales and agreement between more than two observers. Furthermore, it is possible to carry out a range of hypothesis tests using the statistic.

Theodossi *et al.* (1980) described a large study which makes extensive use of the Kappa statistic. Liver biopsies are used routinely in the diagnosis of hepatobiliary disease. The study investigated the extent of agreement between six histopathologists who were asked to score twenty-seven features normally requested for diagnosis on a four-point scale on each of sixty biopsies. For eight of the features there was no evidence of anything other than chance agreement among the participants.

For discrete features, when interest focuses on the ability of the observer rather than on inherent properties of the feature or the measurement scale, it is possible to use data from the same type of study to estimate a set of error rates for each observer. An error rate is a probability—the probability that a particular observer will record a value *i* for the feature when the true value is *j*. Inspection of error rates can identify the consistent observer or the observer who may be interpreting a scale differently from his colleagues. Details of the estimation procedure are given by Dawid and Skene (1979) and an example of the use of error rates is provided by Wilson *et al.* (1980).

3.4.3 Measuring the performance of diagnostic systems

There are two quite distinct aspects to the measurement of performance. First and foremost is the ability of the system to *separate* patients into their correct disease groups. However, it must be reiterated that diagnosis almost always leads to a decision regarding treatment and, when certain diagnosis is not possible, it is the probability of each disease which must be incorporated into the decision problem. Thus a good diagnostic system should also yield disease probabilities which are reliable. If it is calculated that a patient with a certain indicant set has a certain disease with a probability of, say, 0.9 then the system is *reliable* if 90 per cent of all patients with that indicant set are found to have the disease in question. Titterington *et al.* (1981) give the following two examples to show that a balance must be struck between separation and reliability. If, in the case of two diseases, a rule always assigns the probability of 0.51 to the correct disease, then the separation is perfect but the probabilities are clearly unrealistic. On the other hand, if the rule ignores all features and simply assigns disease probabilities equal to the incidence rates, then the probabilities are certainly reliable but of little value. An extensive review of these issues together with many methods of measuring both separation and reliability is given in a series of papers by Habbema, Hilden and Bjerregaard (1978, 1981), Habbema and Hilden (1981) and Hilden, Habbema and Bjerregaard (1978a, 1978b).

Any assessment of performance requires a set of test data, where the true disease for each patient is known. These data should be distinct from the training data and represent a random sample from the eventual target population for the system. As we have indicated, the majority of diagnostic systems contain parameters estimated using the training data. Such systems are in a sense optimal for the training data. Using the training data as test data thus leads to optimistic measures of performance for the system. In practice, data are expensive to collect and there is a natural tendency to include as much data in the training set as possible in order to obtain the best possible rule. One possibility for assessment is to use the jack-knife or 'leaving one out' method of assessment. The rule is developed using all the data available with the exception of that from one patient. The disease probabilities for this patient are computed and then the whole process is repeated for each patient in turn. Assessment bias is reduced but the computation costs are usually high.

The simplest way to assess separation is to construct classification matrices. Each case in the test dataset is classified according to some simple criteria; usually it is assigned to a disease class having highest probability. From this, conditional probabilities of the form P (diagnosed D_i|truth is D_j) can be estimated and confidence intervals for these estimates obtained (see Section 1.3.11). Competing procedures can thus be compared using these error rates. However, this approach is unsatisfactory as no single measure of performance is available (except perhaps the number of cases correctly classified) and the relative seriousness of various errors of diagnosis or the near misses are not taken into account.

A simple modification of this approach is to classify only those patients where the largest disease probability exceeds a particular threshold. Here, the number of unclassified cases is a further measure of system performance. The merit of this measure is that it mirrors one possible way of using a formal system which would appear to have been largely ignored to date. A formal system can easily be used as a screening device, to be operated by junior staff or para-medical personnel, to identify those cases where the diagnosis is unambiguous from the cases which need referral to a more competent authority.

Clearly, a system provides good separation when computed probabilities for the true disease are consistently near one and other disease probabilities are near zero. A wide range of scoring functions have been proposed to quantify this phenomenon. One possibility, the so-called *logarithmic score*, is obtained by calculating the log of the probability assigned to the true disease for each case in the test dataset and averaging this value over all cases. Alternatively, one can calculate a *quadratic score* for each patient and average these. If there are k diseases possible and the true disease for a particular patient is disease 1, say, then the quadratic score for this patient is

$$(1 - p_1)^2 + \sum_{j=2}^{k} p_j^2,$$

where p_i is the probability produced by the rule for the ith disease. Note that the logarithmic score only uses the probability calculated for the correct disease class while the quadratic score incorporates the probabilities for all disease classes.

None of the preceding methods takes the relative seriousness of the different types of error into account. Earlier, it was pointed out that the allocation of a patient to a disease class on the basis of a set of disease probabilities was in fact a decision problem which could easily be expressed within the framework of decision theory. Here, the utilities attached to each consequence are the gains or losses associated with each correct or incorrect classification. It follows, therefore, that the method of assessing separation which is theoretically most sound is to evaluate these utilities with reference to the situation where the diagnostic rule will eventually be used and choose that decision rule which yields the highest average gain.

Assessment of reliability is more difficult. Ideally one should obtain a large number of patients for each indicant set and then see how the proportions having each disease agreed with the disease probabilities given by competing procedures.

Clearly this is not possible, although an approximate measure of reliability can be obtained by identifying groups of patients in the test dataset having sets of disease probabilities which are similar and observing the proportions of each group who have each disease. Titterington *et al.* (1981) and Spiegelhalter (1982) describe this approach in detail for the case where there are three disease classes. Alternative measures of reliability are given by Hilden, Habbema and Bjerregaard (1978a).

Distinguishing between separation and reliability allows a further comment on the popularity and general performance characteristics of the Bayes' independence model for diagnosis. In those applications where many features are incorporated into this rule it is almost certain that the conditional independence assumption will be violated and, as a result, the reliability of the rule is likely to be poor. The rule will tend to be optimistic, suggesting greater separation than is in fact the case. However, it may well be that, because many features have been included, the true separation is better than that achievable with competing rules which have an upper limit on the number of features which can be included. This, allied to the rule's simplicity, may account for its popularity and for its successful applications. It is worth noting that violating the assumptions of the independence model will have less impact when the discriminant is being used to identify certain diagnoses than when the model is being used to calculate disease probabilities needed for the resolution of a difficult decision regarding treatment.

In conclusion, we note that the various methods available for comparing the performance of diagnostic rules can be used to compare discriminants based on different assumptions and distinct models, as well as to compare very similar discriminants which differ only in the inclusion or exclusion of a particular subset of features or in the choice of measurement scales for certain features. There is no optimal method for determining the best rule for diagnosis. One can only proceed by extensive experimentation backed by sound medical judgement and an understanding of the strengths and limitations of the many statistical procedures which are available.

A.S.

REFERENCES

Aitchison, J., and Aitken, C. G. G. (1976). Multivariate binary discrimination by the kernel method, *Biometrika*, **63**, 413–420.

Alpèrovitch, A., de Dombal, F. T., and Grémy, F. (Eds) (1979). *Evaluation of Efficacy of Medical Action*, North-Holland, Amsterdam.

Anderson, J. A. (1972). Separate sample logistic discrimination, *Biometrika*, **59**, 19–36.

Anderson, J. A. (1975). Quadratic logistic discrimination, *Biometrika*, **62**, 149–154.

Bishop, Y. M. M., Fienberg, S. E., and Holland, P. W. (1975). *Discrete Multivariate Analysis: Theory and Practice*, MIT Press, Cambridge, Massachusetts.

Breiman, L., Meisel, W., and Purcell, E. (1977). Variable kernel estimates of multivariate densities, *Technometrics*, **19**, 135–144.

Bunker, J. P., Barnes, B. A., and Mosteller, F. (1977). *Costs, Risks and Benefits of Surgery*, Oxford University Press, New York.

Card, W. I., and Good, I. J. (1974). A logical analysis of medicine in *Companion to Medical Studies* (Eds R. Passmore and J. S. Robson), Vol. 3, Chapter 60, Blackwell, Edinburgh.

Card, W. I., Rusinkiewicz, M., and Phillips, C. I. (1977). Utility estimation of a set of states of health, *Meth. Inform. Med.*, **16**, 168–175.

Clayton, J. K., Anderson, J. A., and McNicol, G. P. (1976). Preoperative prediction of postoperative deep vein thrombosis, *Brit. Med. J.*, **2**, 910–912.

Culyer, A. J. (1978). Need, value and health state measurement, in *Economic Aspects of Health Services* (Eds A. Culyer and R. G. Wright), pp. 9–31, Martin Robertson, London.

Dawid, A. P. (1976). Properties of diagnostic data distributions. *Biometrics*, **32**, 647–658.

Dawid, A. P., and Skene, A. M. (1979). Maximum likelihood estimation of observer error rates using the EM algorithm. *Appl. Statist.*, **28**, 20–28.

Day, N. E., and Kerridge, D. F. (1967). A general maximum likelihood discriminant, *Biometrics*, **23**, 313–323.

de Dombal, F. T., and Grémy, F. (Eds) (1976). *Decision Making and Medical Care: Can Information Science Help?*, North-Holland, Amsterdam.

de Dombal, F. T., Horrocks, J. C., Staniland, J. R., and Guillou, P. J. (1972). Pattern recognition: a comparison of the performance of clinicians and non-clinicians with a note on the performance of a computer-based system, *Meth. Inform. Med.*, **11**, 32–37.

de Groot, M. (1970). *Optimal Statistical Decisions*, Addison-Wesley, New York.

Ellis, G., and Goldberg, D. M. (1979). Discriminant function analysis applied to laboratory tests in patients with hepatobiliary disease, *Comput. Biomed. Res.*, **12**, 483–501.

Essex, B. J. (1980). *Diagnostic Pathways in Clinical Medicine*, Churchill Livingstone, Edinburgh.

Fielding, A. (1977). Latent structure analysis, in *Exploring Data Structures* (Eds C. A. O'Muircheartaigh and C. P. Payne), pp. 125–157, Wiley, New York.

Fries, J. F. (1972). Time-oriented patient records and a computer databank, *J. Amer. Med. Assoc.*, **222**, 1536–1542.

Goldstein, M., and Dillon, W. R. (1978). *Discrete Discriminant Analysis*, Wiley, New York.

Good, I. J., and Card, W. I. (1971). The diagnostic process with special reference to errors, *Meth. Inform. Med.*, **10**, 176–188.

Habbema, J. D. F., Hermans, J., and Remme, J. (1978). Variable kernel density in discriminant analysis, in *COMPSTAT* 1978 (Eds L. C. A Corsten and J. Hermans), pp. 178–185, Physica Verlag, Vienna.

Habbema, J. D. F., and Hilden, J. (1981). The measurement of performance in probabilistic diagnosis—IV. Utility considerations in therapeutics and prognostics, *Meth. Inform. Med.*, **20**, 80–96.

Habbema, J. D. F., Hilden, J., and Bjerregaard, B. (1978). The measurement of performance in probabilistic diagnosis—I. The problem, descriptive tools, and measures based on classification matrices, *Meth. Inform. Med.*, **17**, 217–226.

Habbema, J. D. F., Hilden, J., Bjerregaard, B. (1981). The measurement of performance in probabilistic diagnosis—V. General recommendations, *Meth. Inform. Med.*, **20**, 97–100.

Hartigan, J. (1975). *Clustering Algorithms*, Wiley, New York.

Hermans, J., and Habbema, J. D. F. (1975). Comparison of five methods to estimate posterior probabilities. *E.V.D. in Med. und Biol.*, **6**, 14–19.

Hilden, J., and Bjerregaard, B. (1976). Computer-aided diagnosis and the atypical case, in *Decision Making and Medical Care: Can Information Science Help?* (Eds. F. T. de Dombal and F. Gremy), pp. 365–378, North-Holland, Amsterdam.

Hilden, J., Habbema, J. D. F., and Bjerregaard, B. (1978a). The measurement of performance in probabilistic diagnosis—II. Trustworthiness of the exact values of the diagnostic probabilities, *Meth. Inform. Med.*, **17**, 227–237.

Hilden, J., Habbema, J. D. F., and Bjerregaard, B. (1978b). The measurement of performance in probabilistic diagnosis—III. Methods based on continuous functions of the diagnostic probabilities, *Meth. Inform. Med.*, **17**, 238–246.

Hills, M. (1967). Discrimination and allocation with discrete data, *Appl. Statist.*, **16**, 237–250.

Jacquez, J. A. (Ed.) (1964). *The Diagnostic Process*, Michigan University Press, Ann Arbor.

Jacquez, J. A. (Ed.) (1972). *Computer Diagnosis and Diagnostic Methods*, C. C. Thomas, Springfield, Illinois.

Jennett, B., Teasdale, G., Braakman, R., Minderhoud, J., and Knill-Jones, R. (1976). Predicting outcome in individual patients after severe head injury, *Lancet*, i, 1031–1034.

Journal of the Royal College of Physicians, London (1975), **9**, 191–269. Special issue on statistical methods for clinical decision-making.

Journal of the Royal College of Physicians, London (1979), **13**, no. 4. Special issue devoted to the conference on clinical decision-making: Picking the Best Test, held at the Royal College of Physicians, June 1979.

Krischer, J. P. (1976). The utility structure of a medical decision-making problem, *Oper. Res.*, **24**, 951–972.

Krischer, J. P. (1980). An annotated bibliography of decision analytic applications to health care, *Oper. Res.*, **28**, 97–113.

Lachenbruch, P. A. (1975). *Discriminant Analysis*, Macmillan, New York.

Landis, J. R., and Koch, G. G. (1975a). Review of statistical methods in the analysis of data arising from observer reliability studies (Part I), *Statist. Neerland.*, **29**, 101–123.

Landis, J. R., and Koch, G. G. (1975b). Review of statistical methods in the analysis of data arising from observer reliability studies (Part II), *Statist. Neerland.*, **29**, 151–161.

Lindley, D. V. (1971). *Making Decisions*, Wiley, London.

Lusted, L. B. (1968). *Introduction to Medical Decision Making*, Thomas, Springfield, Illinois.

McNeil, B. J., Weichselbaum, R., and Pauker, S. G. (1978). Fallacy of the five-year survival in lung cancer, *New England J. Med.*, **299**, 1397–1401.

Mardia, K. V., Kent, J. T., and Bibby, J. M. (1979). *Multivariate Analysis*, Academic Press, London.

Meisel, W. S. (1972). *Computer Oriented Approaches to Pattern Recognition*, Academic Press, New York.

Mesel, E., Wirtschafter, D. D., Carpenter, J. T., et al. (1976). Clinical algorithms for cancer chemotherapy—systems for community-based consultant-extenders and oncology centers, *Meth. Inform. Med.*, **15**, 168–173.

Moore, D. H. (1973). Evaluation of five discrimination procedures for binary variables, *J. Amer. Statist. Assoc.*, **68**, 399–404.

Murray, G. D., and Titterington, D. M. (1978). Estimation problems with data from a mixture, *Appl. Statist.*, **27**, 325–334.

New England Journal of Medicine (1975), **293**, 211–244. Issue on decision-making in health care.

Pauker, S. G. (1976). Coronary artery surgery: the use of decision analysis, *Ann. Intern. Med.*, **85**, 8–18.

Pauker, S. G., and Kassirer, J. P. (1975). Therapeutic decision making: a cost-benefit analysis, *New England J. Med.*, **293**, 299–234.

Pauker, S. P., and Pauker, S. G. (1977). Prenatal diagnosis: a directive approach to genetic counselling using decision analysis, *Yale J. Biol. Med.*, **50**, 275–289.

Payne, R. W., and Preece, D. A. (1980). Identification keys and diagnostic tables: a review, *J. Roy. Statist. Soc. A*, **143**, 253–292.

Raiffa, H. (1968). *Decision Analysis: Introductory Lectures on Choices under Uncertainty*, Addison-Wesley, Reading, Massachusetts.

Raiffa, H., and Keeney, R. L. (1976). *Decisions with Multiple Objectives: Preferences and Trade-offs*, Wiley, New York.

Rosser, R., and Kind, P. (1978). A scale of valuations of states of illness: is there a social consensus?, *Int. J. Epidemiol.*, **7**, 347–358.

Sadegh-Zadeh, K. (1980). Baysian diagnostics: a bibliography, *Metamedicine*, **1**, 107–124.

Shortliffe, E. H. (1976). *Computer Based Medical Consultations: MYCIN*, Elsevier/North-Holland, New York.

Shortliffe, E. H., Buchanan, B. G., and Feigenbaum, E. A. (1979). Knowledge engineering for medical decision making: a review of computer-based clinical decision aids, *Proc. IEEE*, **67**, 1207–1224.

Skene, A. M. (1978). Discrimination using latent structure models, in *COMPSTAT 1978* (Eds L. C. A. Corsten and J. Hermans), pp. 199–204, Physica Verlag, Vienna.

Spiegelhalter, D. J. (1980). *Quantifying the Value of Medical Treatment*, Presented to the British Association for the Advancement of Science Annual Meeting, Salford, September 1980.

Spiegelhalter, D. J. (1982). Statistical aids in clinical decision-making, *The Statistician*, **31**, 19–36.

Spiegelhalter, D. J., and Knill-Jones, R. P. (1984). Statistical and knowledge-based approaches to clinical decision-support systems with an application in gastroenterology. *J. Roy. Statist. Soc. A*, **147**, (To appear).

Spiegelhalter, D. J., and Smith, A. F. M. (1981). Decision analysis and clinical decisions, in *Perspectives in medical statistics* (Eds J. F. Bithell and R. Coppi), Academic Press, London.

Teather, D., Emerson, P. A., and Handley, A. J. (1974). Decision theory applied to the treatment of deep vein thrombosis, *Meth. Inform Med.*, **13**(2), 92–97.

Theodossi, A., Skene, A. M., Portmann, B., Knill-Jones, R. P., Patrick, R. S., Tate, R. A., Kealey, W., Jarvis, K. J., O'Brian, D. J., and Williams, R. (1980). Observer variation in assessment of liver biopsies including analysis by Kappa statistics, *Gastroenterology*, **79**, 232–241.

Titterington, D. M. (1980). A comparative study of kernel-based density estimates for categorical data, *Technometrics*, **22**, 259–268.

Titterington, D. M., Murray, G. D., Murray, L. S., Spiegelhalter, D. J., Skene, A. M., Habbema, J. D. F., and Gelpke, G. J. (1981). Comparison of discrimination techniques applied to a complex set of head injured patients, *J. Roy. Statist. Soc. A.*, **144**, 145–175.

Weinstein, M. C., Fineberg, H. V., Elstein, A. S., Frazier, H. S., Neuhauser, D., Neutra, R. R., and McNeil, B. J. (1981). *Clinical Decision Analysis*, W. B. Saunders, Philadelphia.

Wilson, M. E., Williams N. B., Baskett, P. J. F., Bennett, J. A., and Skene, A. M. (1980). Assessment of fitness for surgical procedures and the variability of anaesthetists' judgments, *Brit. Med. J.*, **1**, 509–512.

Wulff, H. R. (1976). *Rational Diagnosis and Treatment*, Blackwell Scientific Publications, Oxford.

Mathematical Methods in Medicine
Edited by D. Ingram & R. F. Bloch
© 1984 John Wiley & Sons Ltd.

4

Statistical Methods in Human Genetics and Immunology

The material in this chapter falls into two parts. Sections 4.1, 4.2 and 4.3 cover statistical methods used in the study of genetic data in populations. Sections 4.4 and 4.5 are concerned with methods for testing genetic hypotheses in the study of disease. The emphasis of the chapter as a whole is on applications in human immunology and the genetic analysis of disease. A brief glossary of terms is included at the end of the chapter to assist the general reader.

4.1 INTRODUCTION TO POPULATION GENETICS

Population genetics usually involves the quantitative investigation of the distribution of known genetic markers (see Section 1.2) [see II, §§4.3 and 10.1]. The population studied might be a racial or ethnic group, a genetically isolated group (isolate) or even a group of individuals affected by some clinical disorder. For several reasons, populations are studied to estimate the distribution of alleles and genotypes of as many markers as possible. First of all, the relationship between genotype and allele frequencies **within** a population demonstrates whether or not there is ongoing selection or mutation with respect to the gene of interest. In the second place, comparisons of gene and genotype frequencies of various races, ethnic groups, isolates or diseased populations are interesting, in their own right, as a means of providing unambiguous measures of the genetic difference between the groups being studied. Furthermore, if one makes appropriate adjustment for other factors which might cause genetic differences, such as drift and consanguinity, one can estimate the effects of selection and mutation. Finally, the joint distribution [see II, §§6.1.1 and 13.1.1] of the alleles of genetic markers known to be on the same chromosome is of interest because such an association may indicate linkage disequilibrium which, in turn, might indicate selective advantage of a haplotype or selective advantage of some unknown locus very close to one or both of the loci being investigated.

In Sections 4.1, 4.2 and 4.3 we consider the theory of the distribution of alleles and genotypes which is used in population studies. We begin with the expected distribution of genes and genotypes when there is no selection, mutation or inbreeding, and then indicate how one would expect these factors to influence the genotypic distribution. We will indicate methods for determining through a sample whether or not there is evidence of departures from the expected distribution within a population. We then consider methods for comparing the distribution of a genetic marker in two samples obtained from different populations and for summarizing quantitatively differences observed at several genetic markers. To compare healthy populations, a quantity called *genetic distance* is often computed. Comparing diseased individuals with normal individuals is often done through computation of *relative risk*. Finally, we indicate how one can test for *linkage disequilibrium* between two markers and provide methods for quantitating such disequilibria and for estimating the haplotype frequencies.

Population genetics involves many issues and many quantitative methods other than those we include here. Indeed, whole texts have been written in this area (Cavalli-Sforza and Bodmer, 1971; Li, 1976). In this chapter we have addressed ourselves only to those issues which have to date been of importance in the population genetics of human immunology. Many of the methods we consider have been used and may continue to be used in the study of human diseases.

4.2 THE HARDY–WEINBERG THEOREM

The Hardy–Weinberg theorem (Hardy, 1908; Weinberg, 1908) states that if we have a genetic locus 'A' with two alleles (A_1 and A_2) then the frequency of the genotypes A_1A_1, A_1A_2 and A_2A_2 after one generation of random mating will be an explicit function of the population frequencies of the alleles. Specifically, after one generation of random mating the genotype frequencies will be as given in Box 4.2.1 [see II, §2.2]. The interesting features of this theorem are that it is true

---

Box 4.2.1 The Hardy–Weinberg theorem

Consider a locus having two alleles A_1 and A_2.

Let   the relative frequency of $A_1 = p_1$,

      the relative frequency of $A_2 = p_2$,

      where $p_1 + p_2 = 1$.

Then, after one generation of random mating, the relative frequencies of the genotypes are as given below:

Genotype	Relative frequency	
A_1A_1	p_1^2	
A_1A_2	$2p_1p_2$	(4.2.1)
A_2A_2	p_2^2	

regardless of the initial distribution of the three genotypes and that if there is random mating and no selection or mutation, the relative frequencies of the alleles A_1 and A_2 will not change. The latter can easily be demonstrated by noting that the relative frequency of A_1 after one generation of random mating, p_1^*, is

$$p_1^* = (p_1^2 \times 1) + 2p_1p_2(1/2) = p_1(p_1 + p_2) = p_1.$$

A final point is that one can extend the Hardy–Weinberg theorem to a situation in which there are k alleles $A_1, A_2, \ldots, A_k$, each with frequency $p_i (i = 1, 2, \ldots, k)$. After one generation of random mating with no selection or mutation, the frequencies of the genotypes are as given in Box 4.2.2.

Box 4.2.2 The Hardy–Weinberg theorem generalized to a locus with k alleles

The alleles are $A_1, A_2, \ldots, A_k$ each with population relative frequency of p_1, $p_2, \ldots, p_k$, respectively.

Then after one generation of random mating the relative frequencies of the genotypes $A_1A_1, A_1A_2, \ldots, A_kA_k$ are

$$\begin{aligned}
&p_i^2 &&\text{for } A_iA_i, \text{ where } i = 1, 2, \ldots, k, \\
&2p_ip_j &&\text{for } A_iA_j, \text{ where } i = 1, 2, \ldots, k; j = i + 1, \ldots, k.
\end{aligned} \qquad (4.2.2)$$

4.2.1 Application of the Hardy–Weinberg theorem: Estimates of gene frequency

For situations in which we have a recessive allele, A_2, the homozygote, A_1A_1, and the heterozygote, A_1A_2, are indistinguishable and allele frequency can not be estimated by direct gene counting. The Hardy–Weinberg theorem might then be applied to estimate the allele frequency. Examples of recessive alleles are the alleles for as yet undefined antigens in the histocompatibility system. These are 'recessive' in the sense that individuals who are homozygous for a known allele may be indistinguishable from individuals who are heterozygous for the known allele and one that is not yet defined. This has been found relevant to histocompatibility studies of races other than Caucasians (Ward, 1975; Ward and Biegel, 1976; Ruderman and Ward, 1977), and of certain population isolates where a large proportion of the population has alleles for as yet undefined specificities (Ferreira, Ward and Amos, 1975).

On applying the Hardy–Weinberg theorem, we can see that the gene frequencies are a function of the phenotype frequencies. These relationships, given in Box 4.2.3, can be used to obtain estimates of genotype frequencies. A procedure for estimating phenotype and genotype frequencies is given in Box 4.2.4 [see VI, §2.1.3.1]. Haldane (1956) has shown that use of (4.2.7) gives a biased underestimate; thus 4.2.8) is often used. However, other methods have been suggested (Haldane, 1956b; Li, 1976; Huether and Murphy, 1980) for obtaining

Box 4.2.3 Gene frequency as a function of phenotype frequency under Hardy–Weinberg equilibrium

Consider a locus with k dominant (or codominant) alleles $A_1, A_2, \ldots, A_k$ and u recessive or unknown alleles $x_1, x_2, \ldots, x_u$ ($u = 0, 1, \ldots$).

Let p_i denote the frequency of allele $A_i (i = 1, 2, \ldots, k)$,

$\quad q$ denote the total of the u frequencies of alleles $x_1, x_2, \ldots, x_u$,

$\quad f_i$ denote the relative frequency of phenotypes indicating the presence of allele $A_i (i = 1, 2, \ldots, k)$.

and b denote the relative frequency of individuals who are not positive for any of the codominant alleles and, thus, have only alleles $x_1, x_2, \ldots, x_u$.

Then, under the Hardy–Weinberg theorem,

$$p_i = 1 - \sqrt{1 - f_i}, \tag{4.2.3}$$

$$q = \sqrt{b}. \tag{4.2.4}$$

We also have, with or without Hardy–Weinberg equilibrium,

$$q = 1 - \sum_{i=1}^{k} p_i. \tag{4.2.5}$$

Box 4.2.4 Estimates of allele frequencies from phenotype frequencies

Let O_i be the number of individuals in a sample of N individuals indicating presence of a dominant or codominant allele $A_i (i = 1, 2, \ldots, k)$,

$$\hat{f}_i = \frac{O_i}{N},$$

$\quad O_b$ be the number of individuals in a sample of N who do not indicate the presence of any of the codominant alleles $A_1, A_2, \ldots, A_k$,

and $\quad \hat{b} = \dfrac{O_b}{N}.$

Then $\hat{f}_i$ and $\hat{b}$ estimate f_i and b given in Box 4.2.3 and we estimate the frequency of dominant alleles $A_1, A_2, \ldots, A_k$ under Hardy–Weinberg equilibrium as

$$\hat{p}_i = 1 - \sqrt{1 - \hat{f}_i}. \tag{4.2.6}$$

An estimate of q is

$$\hat{q} = \sqrt{\hat{b}}. \tag{4.2.7}$$

Alternatively, we can estimate the frequency of unknown alleles by $\hat{q}$, where

$$\hat{q} = 1 - \sum_{i=1}^{k} \hat{p}_i. \tag{4.2.8}$$

Example 4.2.1 Estimation of gene frequencies using the observed phenotype frequencies and assuming that the genotypic distribution is in Hardy–Weinberg equilibrium

A sample of $N = 68$ individuals from the Old Order Amish (Ward *et al.*, 1972)

HLA-A allele	(i)	Number of individuals indicating presence of allele (O_i)	Estimated phenotype frequency (f_i)	Estimated gene frequency $(\hat{p}_i)$ (4.2.6)
A1	1	23	0.338	0.186
A2	2	32	0.470	0.272
A3	3	27	0.397	0.223
A9	4	8	0.118	0.061
A10	5	1	0.015	0.008
A11	6	19	0.279	0.151[*]
A19	7	0	0.000	0.000
A28	8	1	0.015	0.008
Undefined	b1	0	0.000	0.091[a]

[a] Equation (4.2.8).

unbiased estimates [see VI, §3.3.2]. Example 4.2.1 applies the results presented in Boxes 4.2.1 to 4.2.4 to estimate frequencies of alleles for HLA-A locus antigens. These alleles are all codominant. However, at the time the study was done several antigens were undefined and thus (4.2.8) is used to estimate the total frequency of the alleles for these antigens.

4.2.2 Detecting departures from Hardy–Weinberg equilibrium

The observation of departures from Hardy–Weinberg equilibrium in a population might be due to mutation or selection. However, observed departures might also result from other factors such as sampling variation (see Section 1.1.1), inbreeding, assortative mating and genetic drift. To obtain some idea of whether departures observed in a sample reflect real departures in the population rather than sampling variability, one usually does a chi-squared test (Section 1.3.9) of goodness of fit [see VI, Chapter 7]. The number of degrees of freedom for such a test is equal to the number of distinguishable genotypes minus the number of alleles.

In Box 4.2.5 we present a procedure for testing the goodness of fit of observed data to the results expected under the hypothesis of Hardy–Weinberg equilibrium. The first step is to obtain maximum likelihood estimates [see VI, Chapter 6] of the allele frequencies. This is best done by selecting a random sample of

---

Box 4.2.5 Estimating allele frequency by gene counting and tests for goodness of fit to Hardy–Weinberg equilibrium

We have k dominant (or codominant) alleles $A_1, A_2, \ldots, A_k$, and u recessive or unknown alleles $x_1, x_2, \ldots, x_u$.

(a) To obtain the maximum likelihood estimates of allele frequency through gene counting in a sample of N individuals:

Let O_{ii} denote the frequency of individuals who are known to be homozygous $A_i A_i (i = 1, 2, \ldots, k)$,

O_{xx} denote the frequency of individuals who do not have any of the alleles $A_i (i = 1, 2, \ldots, k)$,

O_{ij} denote the number of individuals who are heterozygous for A_i and A_j,

and O_{ix} denote the number of individuals having A_i and some recessive (or undefined) allele.

Then the maximum likelihood estimates of the frequency of $A_i (i = 1, 2, \ldots, k)$ and the total frequency of the alleles $x_i (i = 1, 2, \ldots, u)$ are, by gene counting,

$$\hat{p}_i = \frac{\sum\limits_{i=1}^{k} O_{ii} + \frac{1}{2} \sum\limits_{j=1}^{i-1} O_{ji} + \frac{1}{2} \sum\limits_{j=i+1}^{k} O_{ij} + \frac{1}{2} O_{ix}}{N} \qquad (4.2.9)$$

and

$$\hat{q} = \frac{O_{xx} + \frac{1}{2} \sum\limits_{i=1}^{k} O_{ix}}{N} \qquad (4.2.10)$$

(b) To test for goodness of fit to Hardy–Weinberg equilibrium we compute:

$$E_{ij} = 2\hat{p}_i \hat{p}_j N \qquad (i \neq j; i = 1, 2, \ldots, k-1; j = i+1, \ldots, k), \qquad (4.2.11)$$

$$E_{ix} = 2\hat{p}_i \hat{q} N \qquad (i = 1, 2, \ldots, k), \qquad (4.2.12)$$

$$E_{ii} = \hat{p}_i^2 N \qquad (i = 1, 2, \ldots, k), \qquad (4.2.13)$$

$$E_{xx} = \hat{q}^2 N, \qquad (4.2.14)$$

$$X_{ij}^2 = \frac{(O_{ij} - E_{ij})^2}{E_{ij}} \qquad (i = 1, 2, \ldots, k, x; j = i, i+1, \ldots, k, x), \qquad (4.2.15)$$

and

$$X^2 = \sum_{i=1}^{k} \sum_{j=i}^{k} X_{ij}^2 + \sum_{i=1}^{k} X_{ix}^2 + X_{xx}^2 \qquad (4.2.16)$$

(c) X^2 of (4.2.16) follows a chi-squared distribution with the number of degrees of freedom given by

$$\text{d.f.} = \frac{(k+r+1)(k+r)}{2} - (k+r), \tag{4.2.17}$$

where $r = 1$ if there are unknown or recessive alleles and 0 otherwise. We conclude that we do have evidence of departure from Hardy–Weinberg equilibrium in our sample at the α level of significance [see VI, §§5.2.1(f) and 5.2.1(h)] if X^2 is greater than the $1 - \alpha$ percentile of the chi-square distribution with this number of degrees of freedom.

(d) If there are recessive or unknown alleles and we do not know whether an individual who indicates only allele A_i is $A_i A_i$ or $A_i x_i$ (see Box 4.2.3), then our first approximations to the maximum likelihood estimates (MLE) of $p_i (i = 1, 2, \ldots, k)$ and q are obtained by (4.2.6) and (4.2.7). We then use a method cited by Cavalli-Sforza and Bodmer, originally proposed by Bernstein (1930), and set

$$D = 1 - \sum_{i=1}^{k} \hat{p}_i - \hat{q}. \tag{4.2.18}$$

Our estimates of p_i and q are then

$$\hat{p}_i^* = \hat{p}_i(1 + D/2) \qquad (i = 1, 2, 3, \ldots, k), \tag{4.2.19}$$

and

$$\hat{q}^* = \left(\hat{q} + \frac{D}{2} \right)\left(1 + \frac{D}{2} \right). \tag{4.2.20}$$

We can reapply (4.2.18) through (4.2.20) and obtain better approximations to the MLE of p_i and q (i.e. $\hat{p}_i^{**}$ and $\hat{q}^{**}$).

(e) In these cases, individuals who are positive for exactly one codominant allele $(O_{i \cdot})$ are not homozygous $A_i A_i$ (thus $O_{i \cdot} = O_{ii} + O_{ix}$) and we compute

$$E_{i \cdot} = \hat{p}_i^{*2} + 2\hat{p}_i^* \hat{q}^* \qquad (i = 1, 2, \ldots, k), \tag{4.2.21}$$

instead of E_{ii} and E_{ix} of (4.2.16), and X^2 follows the chi-square distribution with

$$\text{d.f.} = (\text{number of distinguishable genotypes} - 1) - k. \tag{4.2.22}$$

individuals of known genotype. Allele frequency estimates may then be obtained through gene counting as indicated in Box 4.2.5. These estimates are used with the equations of Box 4.2.2 to obtain the genotype frequencies which would be expected under Hardy–Weinberg equilibrium (as given in equations

4.2.11 to 4.2.13). Computation of the chi-squared statistic, to test the difference between observed and expected frequencies, is then quite straightforward.

For situations in which gene counting cannot be done, initial estimates of allele frequencies can be obtained using the methods outlined in Box 4.2.4. Following this, one might use an iterative scheme, first proposed by Bernstein (1930) and since presented in several standard textbooks on human genetics (e.g. Cavalli-Sforza and Bodmer, 1971), to obtain approximate maximum likelihood estimates of gene frequency under Hardy–Weinberg equilibrium. This scheme is outlined in equations (4.2.18) through (4.2.20). Alternatively, one might use a likelihood maximizing procedure (Kaplan and Elston, 1972) to obtain maximum likelihood estimates of the allele frequencies under Hardy–Weinberg equilibrium. The number of degrees of freedom is computed using (4.2.17) if we estimate gene frequencies by gene counting, and (4.2.22) otherwise. Note that a sufficient number of distinguishable genotypes is necessary to ensure that there is at least one degree of freedom for the chi-squared test statistic. In Example 4.2.2 we show how this method has been used to test the departure of the HLA-Bw4 and Bw6 genotypes from Hardy–Weinberg equilibrium using data obtained by van Rood and van Leeuwen (1965).

Example 4.2.2 Testing goodness of fit to Hardy–Weinberg equilibrium of HLA-Bw4, Bw6 genotypes in a sample of 347 individuals
Bw4 and Bw6 are codominant alleles (at the time these data were observed by van Rood and van Leeuwen, 1965, they were called 4a and 4b respectively).

Phenotype (genotype)	O_{ij}	Number observed	Number expected
Bw4 + Bw6 + (Bw4 Bw6)	O_{12}	175	164.3
Bw4 + Bw6 − (Bw4 Bw4)	O_{11}	46	51.4
Bw4 − Bw6 + (Bw6 Bw6)	O_{22}	126	131.2
		347	

(a) By gene counting, (4.2.9), the allele frequencies of Bw4 and Bw6 (p_1 and p_2) are estimated to be

$$\hat{p}_1 = \frac{46 + \frac{1}{2}(175)}{347} = 0.385, ^-$$

$$\hat{p}_2 = \frac{126 + \frac{1}{2}(175)}{347} = 0.615.$$

(b) Thus by (4.2.11) the expected frequency of Bw4 + Bw6 + is

$$E_{12} = 2\hat{p}_1\hat{p}_2 \times 347 = 2 \times 0.385 \times 0.615 \times 347 = 164.3.$$

Similarly, the expected frequency of the Bw4 Bw4 genotype is from (4.2.13)

$$E_{11} = \hat{p}_1^2 = 0.385^2 \times 347 = 51.4$$

and, for the Bw6 Bw6 genotype,

$$E_{22} = \hat{p}_2^2 = 0.615^2 \times 347 = 131.2.$$

(c) The number of degrees of freedom is (using (4.2.17) with $r = 0$)

$$\text{d.f.} = \frac{3 \times 2}{2} - 2 = 1.$$

(d) Finally, using (4.2.16), $X^2 = 1.48$ and thus $P > 0.2$. This we accept the null hypothesis and conclude that we have a good fit to Hardy–Weinberg equilibrium.

4.2.3 Some effects of inbreeding on the genotypic distribution

On observing statistically significant departures from Hardy–Weinberg equilibrium in a sample, it is desirable to know to what extent these departures are due to selection and to what extent they are due to non-selective factors such as inbreeding and drift. To do this we need to consider (a) how inbreeding alone affects the genotypic distribution, (b) how selection might affect the genotypic distribution and (c) how the combination of selection and inbreeding affects the genotypic distribution.

Inbreeding has the direct effect on the genotypic distribution of increasing the frequency of individuals homozygous for each allele. Individuals can be homozygous only if their parents have an allele in common. This could occur by chance alone when individuals are not inbred. However, in an inbred individual the probability is increased by the chance that both parents share an allele which has been transmitted from their common ancestor. It turns out that the probability of this homozygosity by descent depends on how closely an individual's parents are related to each other. For this reason inbreeding is measured for an individual in terms of a quantity called the *inbreeding coefficient* which is the probability of homozygosity by descent. The level of inbreeding in a population is, in turn, expressed in terms of the *mean inbreeding coefficient*.

The value of the inbreeding coefficient is known and tabulated for the more common types of inbreeding (i.e. offspring of individuals who are either first, second or third cousins) (Falconer, 1960). However, particularly in an isolate, the parents of an inbred individual can be related in several ways (e.g. they might be second cousins through both the maternal and paternal sides of the family). For these situations there are methods of sequentially computing the coefficient for each generation (Cruden, 1949) and computer analysis of pedigrees can be used to calculate inbreeding coefficients directly (Mange, 1964). Using these methods a mean inbreeding coefficient of about 0.03 has been observed with Amish pedigrees (McKusick, 1978).

The effects of inbreeding on the distribution of genotypes in a population with probability of homozygosity by descent, F, has been given by Cavalli-Sforza and Bodmer (1971) for a situation where there are two alleles. In Box 4.2.6 this has been generalized for the case of k alleles. It is obvious that, as the level of inbreeding increases, the relative frequency of homozygotes with respect to each allele will increase. However, Cavalli-Sforza and Bodmer (1971) call attention to the result of Li and Horvitz (1953) which indicates that one would probably need an enormous sample in order to observe a statistically significant departure from Hardy–Weinberg equilibrium if inbreeding alone was responsible for the departure. Specifically, in a population with mean inbreeding coefficient F, the expected number of individuals required to detect a departure from Hardy–Weinberg equilibrium at a locus with two alleles at the 0.05 level of significance is $3.84/F^2$ [see VI, Table 5.2.1]. In general, for a locus with k alleles we need the quantity N_k as given in Box 4.2.7. Since most human isolates studied have $F < 0.05$ (Cavalli-Sforza and Bodmer, 1971), we would need at least 1,500 people to detect a departure from Hardy–Weinberg equilibrium at a two-allele locus. Thus, we might conclude that any departure from Hardy–Weinberg equilibrium observed in samples of less than 1,000 individuals must be due to other factors in addition to inbreeding.

Box 4.2.6 The effect of inbreeding on the genotypic distribution

Let p_i be the frequency of allele $A_i (i = 1, 2, \ldots, k)$, and F be the mean level of inbreeding.

Then, after one generation, we have the following genotype frequencies:

for $A_i A_i$ $p_i^2 + F p_i(1 - p_i)$, where $i = 1, 2, \ldots, k$,

for $A_i A_j$ $2 p_i p_j (1 - F)$, where $i = 1, 2, \ldots, k - 1; j = i + 1, i + 2, \ldots, k$.

$$(4.2.23)$$

Box 4.2.7 The expected number of individuals required to detect departures from Hardy–Weinberg equilibrium in a population with inbreeding

Let k be the number of alleles,

  F be the mean inbreeding coefficient,

and G be the number of distinguishable genotypes.

$\chi^2_{G-k, 1-\alpha}$ denotes the $(1 - \alpha)$ percentile of the chi-square distribution with $G - k$ degrees of freedom.

Then, to detect a departure from Hardy–Weinberg equilibrium in a population with mean inbreeding coefficient F at the locus with k alleles, the expected sample size is

$$N_k = \chi^2_{G-k, 1-\alpha}/F^2.$$

$$(4.2.24)$$

4.2.4 Some effects of selection and mutation on the genotypic distribution

We now consider selection in favour of the homozygous genotype and selection in favour of the heterozygous genotype. As a first example, we consider a locus with a single deleterious allele, **B**. The disadvantage to individuals with genotypes involving **B** is expressed in terms of their *fitness* relative to individuals not having **B**, where fitness is the ability of an individual to live and reproduce. Thus all genotypes homozygous or heterozygous for alleles other than **B** are denoted **AA** and the fitness of each of these genotypes is set at one. The fitness of the genotype **BB** is set at $1 - s$ (where $0 < s < 1$) and the *dominance* of **B** is represented by the quantity h in defining the fitness of **AB** to be $1 - hs$ $(0 < h < 1)$. Thus if **B** is completely recessive, h is zero, and the fitness of **AB** is the same as that of **AA**. This is all summarized in Box 4.2.8 where we give the model and the genotype frequencies with and without inbreeding.

The loss of individuals due to selection is frequently referred to as *genetic load*. By comparing the values of genetic load with and without inbreeding, we see that load with inbreeding differs from load without inbreeding by a quantity which is

---

Box 4.2.8 Genotype frequencies with a single deleterious allele— mutational load (from Cavalli-Sforza and Bodmer, 1971)

Let p be the frequency of allele **A**,

     $q = 1 - p$,

     $1 - s$ be the fitness of **BB**$(0 < s < 1)$,

     $1 - hs$ be the fitness of **AB**$(0 < h < 1)$,

and F be the coefficient of inbreeding.

The genotype frequencies are then:

		Genotype frequency	
Genotype	Fitness	No inbreeding after selection	Inbreeding after selection
AA	1	p^2	$p^2 + pqF$
AB	$1 - hs$	$2pq(1 - hs)$	$2pq(1 - F)(1 - hs)$
BB	$1 - s$	$q^2(1 - s)$	$(q^2 + pqF)(1 - s)$
Total		$1 - sq^2 - 2pqhs$	$1 - sq^2 - 2pqhs$ $- sq(1 - 2ph - q)F$
Load		$2pqhs + sq^2$	$(2pqsh + sq^2)$ $+ sq(1 - 2ph - q)F$

proportional to the inbreeding coefficient F. For this reason one is more likely to see the effects of selection in an inbred isolate than in a large, randomly mating population. This linear relationship has led to the use of mortality data at various levels of inbreeding to compute the mutational load (Schull and Neel, 1970). The best-fitting line of the form $-\log(\text{mortality}) = A + BF$ is obtained and the estimated lethal equivalents in the population lie between A and $A + B$, since F lies between 0 and 1.

In a population with a deleterious allele **B**, we will observe fewer individuals homozygous for the allele in each generation (see Box 4.2.8). Hence the relative frequency, q, of this allele will decrease. Since there is also the possibility of mutation from **A** to **B** with probability μ, the ultimate lower bound on the gene frequencies will be a function of the *mutation rate* and the *selection coefficients* (μ and s). In Box 4.2.9 we give the equilibrium frequencies of a deleterious allele for situations in which it is recessive and for situations in which it is dominant. The equilibrium frequencies of phenotypes are also given for each case. These latter frequencies are obtained on application of the Hardy–Weinberg theorem and are frequently used to estimate the mutation rate or the selection coefficient. The relationship between the equilibrium gene frequency of a deleterious allele for cases of partial dominance ($h > 0$), derived by Kimura (1961), is given in Box 4.2.9.

In Example 4.2.3 we indicate how the equations of Box 4.2.9 have been used to

---

Box 4.2.9 Equilibrium frequency of a deleterious allele and its associated phenotypes (from Cavalli-Sforza and Bodmer, 1971)

Let μ be the rate of mutation from **A** to **B**,

    $1 - s$ be the fitness of **BB**,

    $1 - hs$ be the fitness of **AB**,

    1 be the fitness of **AA**,

    q_e be the equilibrium frequency of **B**,

and f_e be the equilibrium frequency of affected individuals.

The equilibrium frequencies are as follows:

h	Model	s	q_e	f_e
0	**B** is fully recessive	$0 < s < 1$	$\sqrt{(\mu/s)}$	μ/s
0	**B** is fully recessive	1 (lethal homozygote)	$\sqrt{\mu}$	μ
1	**B** is fully dominant	$0 < s < 1$	μ/s	$2\mu/s$
1	**B** is fully dominant	1 (lethal trait)	μ	2μ

If **B** is partially dominant, q_e is the solution to

$$q\{1 - 2hsq(1 - q) - sq^2\} = q\{1 - sq - (1 - q)sh\} + \mu(1 - q)(1 - qhs)$$

Example 4.2.3 Estimation of the mutation rate using disease frequencies

(a) Recessive disorder albinism has a population frequency of 1/20,000 and fitness 0.9 (Cavalli-Sforza and Bodmer, 1971).
Thus, as shown in Box 4.2.9,

$$s = 0.1,$$
$$h = 0,$$
$$f = 1/20,000 = 5 \times 10^{-5}.$$

Thus we have

$$f_e = \mu/s = \mu/0.1 = 5 \times 10^{-5},$$

and therefore

$$\mu = 5 \times 10^{-6}.$$

(b) Dominant disorder chondrodystrophy has a population frequency 10^{-4} and fitness of 0.2 (Cavalli-Sforza and Bodmer, 1971).
Thus, using the table in Box 4.2.9,

$$s = 0.8, h = 1.0, f_e = 10^{-4}.$$

Thus we have

$$f_e = 2\mu/s = 2\mu/0.8 = 10^{-4},$$

and therefore

$$\mu = \frac{0.8 \times 10^{-4}}{2} = 4 \times 10^{-5}.$$

(c) Recessive disorder galactosaemia (Hansen *et al.*, 1964) has a population frequency of 5.6×10^{-5} and fitness of 0.
Thus, similarly to the above,

$$s = 1, h = 0, f_e = 5.6 \times 10^{-5}.$$

Then

$$f_e = \mu/s = \mu/1 = 5.6 \times 10^{-5}$$

and therefore

$$\mu = 5.6 \times 10^{-5}.$$

estimate the mutation rate of alleles for dominant and recessive traits. Since chromosomal aberrations are essentially dominant 'mutations', one can use the results of Box 4.2.9 to estimate their frequency.

It has been pointed out by Cavalli-Sforza and Bodmer (1971) that in the case of recessive disorder we are probably overestimating the mutation rate since the frequency of affected individuals is inflated by the assumption that all heterozygotes are completely normal. Furthermore, we assume no inbreeding. It can be shown that in situations where we have inbreeding we will overestimate the mutation rates on using the relationships given in Box 4.2.9. Finally, we have the problem that whenever we estimate the mutation rate by the method given above, we are assuming that an equilibrium has been reached between mutation and selection. In the case of a deleterious dominant allele, an alternative estimate of

---

Box 4.2.10 Equilibrium gene frequency for those loci where polymorphism results from balanced mutation pressure (Cavalli-Sforza and Bodmer, 1971)

Let μ_i be the frequency of mutation to allele A_i,
and v_i be the frequency of mutation to alleles other than A_i.
Then the equilibrium frequency of A_i is p_{ei} where

$$p_{ei} = \frac{\mu_i}{\mu_i + v_i} \qquad (4.2.25)$$

Box 4.2.11 Equilibrium genotype frequencies assuming a selective advantage to the heterozygote (Cavalli-Sforza and Bodmer, 1971)

For the model:

Genotype	Fitness of genotype
AA	$1 - t$
AB	1
BB	$1 - s$

(where $0 < t < 1$ and $0 < s < 1$).
The equilibrium gene frequencies are:

Genotype	Frequency without inbreeding	Frequency with inbreeding
AA	$p^2(1 - t)$	$(p^2 + Fpq)(1 - t)$
AB	$2pq$	$2pq(1 - F)$
BB	$q^2(1 - s)$	$(q^2 + Fpq)(1 - s)$
Total	$1 - (tp^2 + sq^2)$	$1 - (tp^2 + sq^2) - (pqs + pqt)F$

Load without inbreeding $(L_0) = tp^2 + sq^2$.
Load with inbreeding $(L_F) = tp^2 + sq^2 + (pqs + pqt)F = L_0 + Fpq(s + t)$.

the mutation rate can be made directly by counting the number of affected offspring born to normal parents.

It should be clear from the preceding discussion that if an allele is deleterious, it will ultimately have a very low relative frequency. Thus alternative models for selection and mutation are used to account for the existence of polymorphic genetic loci; i.e. those loci in which several alleles occur at relatively high frequency. One hypothesis is that there is no selective advantage to any genotype, and the observed relative frequencies of the alleles reflect the relative frequencies of their mutation rates. This is summarized in Box 4.2.10. Another hypothesis for the existence of polymorphism which is more widely accepted is heterozygous advantage. Under this hypothesis, it is assumed that the heterozygote, **AB** say, has fitness one and the two alternative homozygotes, **AA** and **BB**, have intermediate fitnesses $1 - s$ and $1 - t$ respectively. This model is presented in Box 4.2.11 along with the expected genotype frequencies and expressions for genetic load with and without inbreeding. In Box 4.2.12 the equilibrium frequencies of the alleles for the case of heterozygote advantage are given. The classic example of a balanced polymorphism due to selective advantage to the heterozygote is the locus for sickle cell anaemia (Vogel and Motulsky, 1979) which is presented as Example 4.2.4. Cavalli-Sforza and Bodmer cite Allison (1954, 1964) as one who has made a considerable contribution to this subject.

Box 4.2.12 (a) **Equilibrium frequencies of alleles assuming a selective advantage to the heterozygote** (Cavalli-Sforza and Bodmer, 1971)

(b) **Segregational load with and without inbreeding** (Cavalli-Sforza and Bodmer, 1971)

Let the fitness of **AA**, **AB** and **BB** be as given in Box 4.2.11.
Let p_e and q_e be the equilibrium frequencies of alleles **A** and **B** respectively.
Then

$$p_e = \frac{s}{s+t}, \tag{4.2.26}$$

$$q_e = \frac{t}{s+t}, \tag{4.2.27}$$

and the equilibrium load due to selective advantage, the segregational load, is

$$L = \frac{st}{s+t} + F\frac{st}{s+t} \tag{4.2.28}$$

Example 4.2.4 Sickle cell anaemia: a balanced polymorphism due to heterozygote advantage (Cavalli-Sforza and Bodmer, 1971)

Consider a two-allele model, **A** and **S**, as follows:

Genotype	Phenotype	Fitness (African data)
AA	Normal	0.85
AS	Normal; malaria resistant	1
SS	Sickle cell anaemia	0

Comparing with the nomenclature in Box 4.2.11, we have

$s = 1, t = 1 - 0.85 = 0.15.$

By Box 4.2.12, the equilibrium gene frequency of S is given by

$$q_e = \frac{t}{s+t} = \frac{0.15}{1.0 + 0.15} = 0.13.$$

This is consistent with the reported range of estimates for gene frequency of **S**, from affected individuals, of 0.10 to 0.15.

4.3 COMPARISONS OF POPULATIONS: GENETIC DISTANCE, RELATIVE RISK AND LINKAGE DISEQUILIBRIUM

Genotypic distributions in two populations are compared for many reasons. Depending on the populations being compared, different questions can be considered. For example, gene frequencies in populations separated racially, geographically or culturally can be used to obtain information on their similarities, origins and migration pattern (Roychoudhury, 1978; Ryder, Anderson and Svejgaard, 1978). They might also give information on selection and mutation of the genes being studied. On the other hand, gene frequencies can be obtained by comparing information on the relative risk of certain genotypes in two populations, one consisting of individuals having a disorder and the other of individuals who do not have the disorder. These latter comparisons may provide evidence of linkage disequilibrium between an allele for disease susceptibility and the allele at some known marker. Finally, the joint distribution of alleles at linked loci gives information on linkage disequilibrium between alleles (Mattuiz 1970; Cavalli-Sforza and Bodmer, 1971).

Depending on the populations we choose to study, observed genetic differences will have different implications. In this section we consider some mathematical and statistical procedures used to quantify genetic difference in terms of genetic distance, linkage disequilibrium and relative risk. Before doing this, however, we introduce the methods usually employed at the beginning of any study to compare populations in order to determine whether, in fact, there is evidence of genetic difference.

4.3.1 The comparison of genotypic distributions in samples

There are several methods for comparing the genotypic distribution of two populations. Probably the most frequently used is that of comparing the distribution of the associated phenotype frequencies. This is done because the statistical evaluation of phenotype frequencies is more straightforward than evaluation of estimates of gene frequencies. Moreover, under equilibrium conditions, statistical evidence in favour of a difference in phenotype frequency is sufficient and necessary evidence for a difference in gene or genotype frequency. When one considers a genetic locus which has relatively few alleles and hence few phenotypes, such as the A, B, O locus, one can simply consider the appropriate contingency table of the distribution of the phenotypes using a χ^2 statistic (see Section 1.3.10) as illustrated in Example 4.3.1. However, for loci with many alleles, and hence many phenotypes, a more sensitive method for detecting differences in genotype frequencies involves considering each allele separately and looking for differences in the overall frequency of those phenotypes indicating that the allele is present. Thus a 2×2 contingency table [see VI, §

Example 4.3.1 Comparison of ABO phenotype frequencies of Finnish speakers (Kokko, 1940) **and Swedish speakers** (Sievers, 1931) **in Turku-Pori, Finland** (Mourant, Kopic and Domanieluska-Solezak, 1976)

	Frequency in Finnish speakers		Frequency in Swedish speakers		Total	
AB	0.074	(11)	0.033	(4)	0.056	(15)
A	0.493	(73)	0.367	(44)	0.437	(117)
B	0.182	(27)	0.167	(20)	0.175	(47)
O	0.250	(37)	0.433	(52)	0.332	(89)
Total	1.00	(148)	1.00	(120)	1.00	(268)

Analysing these data as a 4×2 contingency table we obtain

$$X^2 = \frac{[11 - (148 \times 15/268)]^2}{148 \times 15/268} + \ldots + \frac{[52 - (120 \times 89/268)]^2}{120 \times 89/268} = 11.22.$$

Referring this value to the chi-square distribution with 3 d.f. we obtain $0.01 < P < 0.025$ and, thus, we conclude that there is a significant difference in **ABO** allele frequencies between these two groups.

§7.5.1] is generated corresponding to the phenotypic data for each allele. There are statistical problems with this approach, notably that, for k alleles, the k comparisons are not independent [see II, §3.5]. An increase in the frequency of one allele could necessarily result in a decrease in the frequency of another. Also, the overall level of significance of k statistical tests, each at the α level of significance, is much more than α [see VI, §5.11]. Investigators frequently adjust for these problems through either computing a 'total χ^2' for the locus (Smouse, 1979) or by computing a 'corrected level of significance' (Walford, Smith and Waters, 1971; Kreisler *et al.*, 1974; Gazit, Orgad and Pras, 1977; Hammond, Appadoo and Brain, 1977; Ivanyi, Ivanyi and Zemak, 1977). In computing a total χ^2 for the locus, one adds all the individual χ^2 values. A conservative estimate of the significance of this statistic could be obtained by comparing it to the chi-square distribution with k degrees of freedom [see VI, Chapter 7], where k is the number of phenotypic distributions compared. Using the second approach, investigators compute a corrected level of significance for each of the observed

---

Example 4.3.2 Comparison of HLA-A phenotype frequencies of people from Brazil with those of people from the United States (Ferreira, Ward and Amos, 1975)

Phenotype indicating presence of	Brazil: observed frequency, %	United States: observed frequency, %	X^2
A1	23.38	25.97	0.14
A2	53.25	48.05	0.42
A3	23.38	19.48	0.35
A9	3.90	1.30	1.03
A10	2.60	5.19	0.73
A11	10.39	12.99	0.25
Aw33	3.90	3.90	0.00
Aw23	2.60	1.30	0.34
Aw24	10.39	6.49	0.76
A25	3.90	9.09	1.71
A26	3.90	7.79	1.06
A28	9.09	3.90	1.71
A29	6.49	3.90	0.53
Aw30	6.49	3.90	0.53
Aw31	12.99	14.29	0.55
Aw32	1.30	5.19	1.89
Total in sample	77	77	11.45

The individual X^2 values are calculated for sixteen contingency tables of the following form (using counts, not percentage frequency, as shown).

	Brazil	United States	
HLA-A1 +	18	20	38
HLA-A1 −	59	57	116
	77	77	154

$$X^2 = \frac{[(18 \times 57) - (20 \times 59)]^2 \times 54}{38 \times 116 \times 77 \times 77} = 0.14.$$

The total X^2 for the sixteen antigens considered = 11.45.

Referring to the chi-square distribution with 16 d.f., $P > 0.70$ indicating that the distribution of HLA-A alleles does not differ significantly between the two populations.

To reject the null hypothesis of equal allele frequencies for a particular allele such as HLA-A1 we would require $P < 0.05/16 = 0.003$, as discussed in the text.

chi-squared values equal to the observed level of significance times the number of phenotypes considered (Svejgarrd and Ryder, 1977). This is also an unduly conservative estimate and if it is less than, say, the 5 per cent level one can feel fairly sure that there is a difference in the corresponding allele frequency. In Example 4.3.2 we indicate how these methods have been used to compare the distribution of alleles at the HLA-A locus of two samples of individuals from Brazil and the United States.

4.3.2 Measures of genetic distance

Having established a difference in the allele frequencies of two or more populations, one measure of difference between populations is genetic distance. This quantity is of interest since with it one can summarize genetic differences at several loci in terms of a single value. The quantity has been shown to be functionally related to the time of divergence between populations, the nature of the relationship being dependent on whether the observed differences in gene frequencies result from *drift* or *selection* (Cavalli-Sforza and Bodmer, 1971). Equations for computing genetic distance, as given by Cavalli-Sforza and Bodmer (1971), are shown in Box 4.3.1. In Example 4.3.3 we consider the computation of genetic distance using allele frequencies estimated for the HLA-A locus and the HLA-B locus in two populations, namely Samoans and Fiji Islanders. The allele frequencies can be estimated either by gene counting, as covered in Box 4.2.5, or by assuming Hardy–Weinberg equilibrium and using the relationships given in Box 4.2.3.

Box 4.3.1 Computation of genetic distance between populations as suggested by Cavalli-Sforza and Bodmer (1971)

Let N be the number of populations being studied,

M be the number of marker loci studied,

K_j be the number of alleles at marker j for $j = 1, 2, \ldots, M$,

and p_{ijs} be the frequency of allele i at marker j in population s ,

(where $s = 1, 2, \ldots, N; j = 1, 2, \ldots, M; i = 1, 2, \ldots, K_j$).

Using information taken from marker j alone, the distance between populations s and t is measured by

$$d_{stj} = \frac{4(1 - \cos \theta_{st\,j})}{K_j - 1}, \tag{4.3.1}$$

where $\cos \theta_{st\,j} = \sum_{i=1}^{K_j} \sqrt{p_{ijs}p_{ijt}}.$ $\qquad$ (4.3.2)

Using M markers, the genetic distance is the weighted average of the distance observed at each marker. Thus the genetic distance is measured by

$$d_{st} = \frac{\sum_{j=1}^{M} (K_j - 1)d_{stj}}{\left(\sum_{j=1}^{M} K_j\right) - M}. \tag{4.3.3}$$

The standard error of d_{st} can be estimated by

$$SE(d_{st}) = \sqrt{\frac{\sum_{j=1}^{M} d_{stj}^2 - \left(\sum_{j=1}^{M} d_{stj}\right)^2 \Big/ M}{(M)(M-1)}}. \tag{4.3.4}$$

Example 4.3.3 Estimating the genetic distance between Oceanic populations
MacQueen *et al.* (1979) cite the following HLA-A, HLB-B allele frequencies for two Oceanic populations of Western Samoa and Fiji:

	Western Samoa[a] ($\hat{p}_{i11}$)	Fiji[b] ($\hat{p}_{i12}$)	$\sqrt{\hat{p}_{i11}\hat{p}_{i12}}$
HLA-A1	0.006	0.00	0.00
HLA-A2	0.212	0.08	0.1302
HLA-A3	0.018	0.00	0.00
HLA-A9	0.216	0.59	0.3570
HLA-A10	0.033	0.04	0.0363

HLA-A11	0.115	0.13	0.1223
HLA-Aw28	0.018	0.00	0.00
HLA-A undefined	0.372	0.16	0.2440

	$(\hat{p}_{i21})$	$(\hat{p}_{i22})$	$\sqrt{\hat{p}_{i21}\hat{p}_{i22}}$
HLA-B5	0.003	0.01	0.00548
HLA-B7	0.012	0.00	0.00
HLA-B8	0.001	0.00	0.00
HLA-B12	0.007	0.00	0.00
HLA-B13	0.038	0.04	0.0390
HLA-Bw35	0.008	0.00	0.00
HLA-B40	0.295	0.21	0.2489
HLA-B14	0.00	0.00	0.00
HLA-B15	0.019	0.19	0.0601
HLA-B17	0.010	0.01	0.01
HLA-Bw22	0.213	0.13	0.1664
HLA-B27	0.013	0.02	0.0161
HLA-Bw16	0.008	0.11	0.0297
HLA-B undefined	0.373	0.22	0.2865

[a] Batchelor *et al.* (1973).
[b] Crosier and Douglas (1976).

Using the notation of Box 4.3.1, from the table above we have:
For HLA-A, $j = 1$, $K_1 = 8$.
Thus, by (4.3.1) and (4.3.2),

$$d_{121} = \frac{4[1 - (0.00 + 0.1302 + \cdots + 0.2440)]}{8 - 1} = \frac{4(1 - 0.8898)}{7} = 0.0630.$$

This is the genetic distance between Fiji and Western Samoa at HLA-A.

For HLA-B, $j = 2$; $K_2 = 14$.
Thus, by (4.3.1) and (4.3.2),

$$d_{122} = \frac{4[1 - (0.00548 + 0.00 + \cdots + 0.2865)]}{14 - 1} = \frac{4(1 - 0.8621)}{13}$$

$$= 0.0424, \text{ the genetic distance at HLA-B.}$$

Using (4.3.3), we estimate genetic distance between Western Samoa and Fiji as

$$d_{12} = \frac{(8 - 1)(0.0630) + (14 - 1)(0.0424)}{8 + 14 - 2} = 0.0496.$$

MacQueen *et al.* (1979) chose to give equal weight to the A and B (i.e. treat them as though $K_1 = K_2 = 2.0$) loci and thus reported the genetic distance as

$$d_{12} = \frac{0.0630 + 0.0424}{2} = 0.0527.$$

In this case, the standard error of d_{12} as given by (4.3.4) is

$$SE(d_{12}) = \sqrt{\frac{0.0424^2 + 0.0630^2 - (0.1054)^2/2}{2}} = 0.01.$$

Box 4.3.2 (a) **Estimating the degree of admixture**
              (b) **The relationship between the degree of admixture and genetic distance**

(a) Let $\hat{p}_A$ denote the estimated frequency of an allele in population A,
    $\hat{p}_B$ denote the estimated frequency of this allele in population B,
    and $\hat{p}_M$ denote the estimated frequency of this allele in population M.
    If population M is a mixture of individuals from population A and population B then the degree of admixture of A in M (m) is estimated by

$$\hat{m} = \frac{\hat{p}_M - \hat{p}_B}{\hat{p}_A - \hat{p}_B}, \tag{4.3.5}$$

and the standard error of M is estimated by

$$\widehat{SE}(\hat{m}) = \sqrt{\frac{1}{(\hat{p}_A - \hat{p}_B)^2}[\widehat{SE}^2(\hat{p}_M) + \hat{m}^2\widehat{SE}^2(\hat{p}_A) + (1 - \hat{m})^2\widehat{SE}^2(\hat{p}_B)]}.$$

$$\tag{4.3.6}$$

(b) Let population M consist only of a mixture of population A and population B.
    Let d_{ij} denote the genetic distance between populations i and j, and m the admixture of A in M.
    Then (Cavalli-Sforza and Bodmer, 1971):

$$d_{AM} = md_{AB}, \tag{4.3.7}$$

$$d_{BM} = (1 - m)d_{AB}, \tag{4.3.8}$$

and $d_{AM} + d_{BM} = d_{AB}.$ $\tag{4.3.9}$

Other slightly different measures of genetic distance are often used (Roychoudhury, 1978; Ryder, Anderson and Svejgaard, 1978). However, the measure we give here has been shown (Cavalli-Sforza and Bodmer, 1971) to be equivalent to the *coefficient of kinship*, f, between two populations. If all genetic divergence is due to drift alone, then f (through its relationship to a third quantity, Wahlund's variance) can in turn be shown to increase linearly with time of divergence, T, if T is large. The transformed variable $-[\log(1-f)]$ increases linearly with T if T is small. If both selection and drift are involved in the genetic distance between populations, then the quantity f should increase linearly with T. Since T is frequently known, the observed values of distance can be examined to see if there is a linear, log-linear or square root relationship with time. The nature of the relationship determines whether selection, drift or selection and drift

---

Example 4.3.4 Computation of the degree of Caucasian admixture (m) in US Negroes using the frequency of the Fy^a allele (Reed, 1969)

Using the notation of Box 4.3.2 the data on the frequency of the Fy^a allele are as follows:

			Population	
			US Negroes	
	African Liberians ($x = $ B)	US Caucasians ($x = $ A)	Non-Southern New York ($x = $ M)	Southern Charleston ($x = $ M)
Allele frequency ($\hat{p}_x$)	0.000	0.429	0.0809	0.0157
SE of allele frequency [$\widehat{SE}(\hat{p}_x)$]	0.000	0.0058	0.0147	0.0039
Sample size (N_x)	661	5046	179	515
Estimate of $m \pm$ SE(m)			$0.189^a \pm 0.034^b$	0.0366 ± 0.0091

[a] By (4.3.5) with $\hat{p}_B = 0$ we have

$$\hat{m} = \frac{\hat{p}_M}{\hat{p}_A} = \frac{0.0809}{0.429} = 0.189.$$

[b] By (4.3.6) we have

$$\widehat{SE}(\hat{m}) = \sqrt{\frac{1}{0.429^2}[0.0147^2 + (0.189^2 \times 0.0058^2) + (0.811^2 \times 0.0^2)]}$$

$$= 0.034.$$

determine the differences. Another useful measure of the genetic distance (Reed, 1969; Cavalli-Sforza and Bodmer, 1971) is that of *admixture* due to Glass and Li (1953), as given in Box 4.3.2. In Example 4.3.4 we indicate how one can measure the degree of Caucasoid admixture in a sample of American negroes.

Frequently a direct statistical method is needed for evaluating whether observed differences in genotype frequencies between two populations are in excess of those differences one would expect due to drift alone. Cavalli-Sforza and Bodmer (1971) indicate that after g generations of separation the chi-square test statistic computed to evaluate the observed difference in gene frequencies at a locus with k alleles would follow the distribution with $(k - 1)g$ degrees of freedom. This result is summarized in Box 4.3.3 and its use in evaluating observed differences at the HLA-A locus in a Surinam isolate (de Vries *et al.*, 1979) is given in Example 4.3.5.

4.3.3 Testing for linkage disequilibrium and the estimation of relevant parameters

We address ourselves here to the situation in which we have data on the joint distribution of phenotypes at two known linked genetic markers. An association between a phenotype at one locus and any phenotype at the second linked locus indicates that there is linkage disequilibrium between the alleles corresponding to these phenotypes. In these situations it is desirable to quantitate the linkage disequilibria between all pairs of alleles at the two loci and to obtain estimates of the haplotype frequencies of these pairs.

Box 4.3.3 Evaluation of an observed genetic difference between two populations with adjustment for genetic drift

Let O_{i1} and O_{i2} denote the frequency of phenotypes corresponding to the presence of allele $\mathbf{A}_i$ in a sample of N_1 from population 1 and N_2 from population 2.

Suppose population 1 and population 2 stemmed from a common population g generations back.

As a result, we would expect a divergence in genotypic distributions due to genetic drift. This divergence is such that a chi-square test statistic used to compare O_{i1} with O_{i2} follows the χ^2 distribution with g degrees of freedom. Similarly, if we compare the frequencies of k genotypes (or k genes) in population 1 with those in population 2 by analysis of the appropriate $k \times 2$ contingency table, the test statistic follows the χ^2 distribution with $(k - 1)g$ degrees of freedom.

Example 4.3.5 Evaluation of the observed differences between descendants of Dutch colonists in Surinam and present-day Dutch people with adjustment for genetic drift (de Vries *et al.*, 1979)
(a) GLO allele frequency by gene counting (sample size × 2):

Genotype	Dutch colonists	Dutch controls	
GLO 1	33	688	721
GLO 2	81	826	907
	114	1,514	1,628

We use a χ^2 test to analyse this contingency table, testing the null hypothesis that there is no difference in the proportions of GLO 1 and GLO 2 allele frequencies in the two groups.
We obtain $\chi^2 = 11.69$ and from tabulation of the χ^2 distribution with 1 d.f. we find that $P < 0.0009$. We thus reject the null hypothesis.
(b) The Surinam isolate diverged from the Dutch population of Holland four generations ago. Using the approach outlined in Box 4.3.4, d.f. = $1 \times 4 = 4$ and $P < 0.03$. Thus we conclude that the GLO difference exceeds that expected due to drift alone.

First consider a situation in which marker A has two alleles, **A** and **a**, and marker B has two alleles, **B** and **b**. Our data consist of phenotype information only; i.e. we know only whether an individual has allele **A** or not and whether or not he also has allele **B**, but we do not know whether **A** and **B** are in coupling or repulsion. The frequency of individuals positive for **A** in the group of those positive for **B** can be compared to that in the group of those negative for **B** using the usual 2×2 contingency table analysis as shown in Box. 4.3.4. If a significant association is observed, it has been shown by Mattiuz *et al.* (1970) that under Hardy–Weinberg equilibrium the *gametic association* between alleles **A** and **B** is estimated by the quantity D or Δ computed using (4.3.11). Its standard error is given by (4.3.12). The χ^2 test of association between phenotypes for allele **A** and those for allele **B** is the test of the hypothesis $D = 0$. The standard error estimates give a good idea of the precision of the estimates of D. Moreover, one is probably justified in using them for comparing estimates of D obtained in different studies from different pairs of markers. However, since D is a measure of the strength of an association between two loci, the appropriate test of no difference between D values should probably involve one of the procedures available for simultaneous analysis of more than two categorical variables (Fleiss, 1981; Fienberg, 1980).

Box 4.3.4 (a) **Testing for linkage disequilibrium**
    (b) **Estimating gametic association D or Δ and its standard error**
        (Mattiuz *et al.*, 1970)
    (c) **Testing the significance of D**
    (d) **Comparing estimates of D**

Let the observed phenotype frequency data be denoted as follows:

Genotype	Observed phenotypes	Observed frequency	Observed relative frequency (O_{ij}/N)
AB/AB, AB/aB, Ab/AB, AB/ab, Ab/aB	$A + B +$	O_{++}	$\hat{f}_{++}$
Ab/Ab, Ab/ab	$A + B -$	O_{+-}	$\hat{f}_{+-}$
AB/aB, aB/ab	$A - B +$	O_{-+}	$\hat{f}_{-+}$
ab/ab	$A - B -$	O_{--}	$\hat{f}_{--}$
	Total	N	

(a) The contingency table chi-square test statistic for linkage disequilibrium between A and B is

$$X^2_{AB} = \frac{(O_{++}O_{--} - O_{-+}O_{+-})^2 N}{(O_{++} + O_{+-})(O_{-+} + O_{--})(O_{++} + O_{-+})(O_{+-} + O_{--})}.$$

(4.3.10)

(b) The estimate of D is

$$\hat{D} = \sqrt{\hat{f}_{--}} - \sqrt{(\hat{f}_{+-} + \hat{f}_{--})(\hat{f}_{-+} + \hat{f}_{--})}.$$

(4.3.11)

We estimate $SE(\hat{D})$ by

$$\widehat{SE}(\hat{D}) = \sqrt{\frac{(\hat{f}_{++} + \hat{f}_{+-})(\hat{f}_{-+} + \hat{f}_{++})}{4N}}.$$

(4.3.12)

(c) We test the null hypothesis $H_0 : D = 0$ at the α level of significance by observing whether X^2_{AB} is greater than the $1 - \alpha$ percentile of the chi-square distribution with 1 d.f.

One can also estimate the frequency of those haplotypes containing **A** and **B** (i.e. in coupling) using phenotype data. Under Hardy–Weinberg equilibrium these estimates would be obtained using the equations given in Box 4.3.5. It is easy to generalize this method to a situation in which there are more than two

---

Box 4.3.5 Estimation of the haplotype frequency and its standard error

Let $\hat{p}_A, \hat{p}_B$ be estimates of the frequencies of alleles **A** and **B**,

$\hat{D}_{AB}$ be the estimate of D obtained using (4.3.11)

and x_{AB} denote the frequency of the haplotype AB.

Then we estimate x_{AB} by

$$\hat{x}_{AB} = \hat{p}_A \hat{p}_B + \hat{D}_{AB} \qquad (4.3.13)$$

and the standard error of $\hat{x}_{AB}$ is estimated by

$$\widehat{SE}(\hat{x}_{AB}) = \sqrt{\widehat{SE}^2(\hat{D}_{AB}) + \widehat{SE}^2(\hat{p}_A)\hat{p}_B^2 + \widehat{SE}^2(\hat{p}_B)\hat{p}_A^2}. \qquad (4.3.14)$$

Thus if p_A and p_B are estimated from the observed phenotype frequencies of allele **A** and allele **B** ($\hat{f}_{+.} = \hat{f}_{++} + \hat{f}_{+-}; \hat{f}_{.+} = \hat{f}_{++} + \hat{f}_{-+}$, respectively) using (4.2.3), and then (4.3.12) and (4.3.15), we have

$$\widehat{SE}(\hat{x}_{AB}) = \sqrt{\frac{1}{4N}(\hat{f}_{+.}\hat{f}_{.+} + \hat{f}_{+.}\hat{p}_B^2 + \hat{f}_{.+}\hat{p}_A^2)}. \qquad (4.3.15)$$

---

alleles at one or both loci. One simply considers in turn all possible pairs of alleles at the two loci.

The above methods have been necessary when only phenotype data were available (Gleichmann, 1974; Hammond, Appadoo and Brain, 1974; Kastelan et al., 1974; Moreno and Kreisler, 1977). In Example 4.3.6 we consider the results of

---

Example 4.3.6 Estimation of HLA-A3, B7 haplotype frequencies, D values and allele frequencies from the distribution of HLA-A and HLA-B antigen in a Basque village

Dausset *et al.* (1972) reported their estimates of haplotype frequencies, D values and allele frequencies of the HLA-A and HLA-B alleles in a Basque village. We give a partial table of their results showing estimated haplotype frequencies, D values $\times 10^3$ (in parentheses), allele and phenotype frequencies.

| | Estimated haplotype frequency $\hat{x}$ and ($\hat{D}$ values $\times 10^3$) | | | B locus | |
| | | | | Allele frequency $\hat{p}_{.j}$ | Phenotype frequency $\hat{f}_{.j}$ |
	HLA-A1	HLA-A2	HLA-A3		
HLA-B5	0.00 (25)	0.068 (37)	0.013 (5)	0.113	0.204
HLA-B7	0.025 (10)	0.035 (3)	0.020 (12)	0.115	0.204
HLA-B8	0.030 (23)	0.004 (19)	0.00 (−9)	0.083	0.147

Allele frequency ($p_i.$)	0.092	0.280	0.077
Phenotype frequency ($\hat{f}_i.$)	0.193	0.496	0.181

The allele frequencies at each locus were obtained by gene counting, but the estimates of D values and haplotype frequencies ($x_{ij}: i = 1, 2, 3; j = 5, 7, 8$) were obtained by (4.3.11) and (4.3.13) respectively. Thus, for the HLA-A3, B7 haplotype, the original data were (using the notation of Box 4.3.4):

Phenotype	Number observed	Notation	Observed relative frequency	Notation
A3 + B7 +	5	O_{++}	0.057	$\hat{f}_{++}$
A3 + B7 −	13	O_{+-}	0.148	$\hat{f}_{+-}$
A3 − B7 +	11	O_{-+}	0.125	$\hat{f}_{-+}$
A3 − B7 −	59	O_{--}	0.670	$\hat{f}_{--}$
Total	88	N	1.0	100

$$\hat{D}_{3,7} = \sqrt{\frac{59}{88}} - \sqrt{\frac{11 + 59}{88} \times \frac{13 + 59}{88}} = 0.012,$$

as given in the table. The significance of $D_{3,7}$ is tested using (4.3.10) and we calculate

$$X^2 = \frac{[(5 \times 59) - (13 \times 11)]^2 \times 88}{18 \times 70 \times 16 \times 72} = 1.401, \qquad P > 0.1.$$

Thus we conclude there is no A3, B7 disequilibrium in the Basque village population. By (4.3.11),

$$\widehat{SE}(\hat{D}_{3,7}) = \sqrt{\frac{(0.057) + 0.148)(0.125 + 0.057)}{4 \times 88}} = 0.010.$$

By (4.3.13) and, substituting the gene counting estimates of p_3 and p_7,

$\hat{x}_{3,7} = D_{3,7} + \hat{p}_3 \hat{p}_7 = 0.012 + (0.077)(0.115) = 0.020$, as given.

Since $\hat{p}_3$ and $\hat{p}_7$ are estimated by gene counting of $2N = 2 \times 88$ gametes, we have

$$\widehat{SE}(\hat{p}_3) = \sqrt{\frac{\hat{p}_3(1 - \hat{p}_3)}{2N}} = \sqrt{\frac{0.077 \times 0.923}{2 \times 88}} = 0.020,$$

$$\widehat{SE}(\hat{p}_7) = \sqrt{\frac{\hat{p}_7(1 - \hat{p}_7)}{2N}} = 0.059,$$

and by (4.3.14),

$$\widehat{SE}(\hat{x}_{3,7}) = \sqrt{0.010^2 + (0.059^2)(0.077^2) + (0.020^2)(0.115^2)}$$
$$= 0.011.$$

a study of the joint distribution of the HLA-A and B phenotypes in a sample from the Basque population (Dausset *et al.*, 1972). We compare the results for HLA-A3, HLA-B7 to those observed in the Amish isolate (Ward *et al.*, 1972).

4.3.4 Studies of the distribution of genetic markers in individuals with diseases

The studies of the distribution of genetic markers in individuals with diseases, such as those done by McMichael and DeWitt (1977) and Aird, Bentall and Roberts (1953) (and many others cited by Vogel and Motulsky, 1979) have led to some provocative hypotheses (McDevitt and Bodmer, 1974; Doherty and Zinkernagel, 1975; Svejgaard and Ryder, 1977). Several diseases which have, for quite some time, been thought to be mainly environmental, or at best of complex genetic aetiology, have been shown to be highly associated with such markers as the ABO system (Cavalli-Sforza and Bodmer, 1971; Vogel and Motulsky, 1979) and the HLA system (McMichael and DeWitt, 1977; Vogel and Motulsky, 1979). The most striking such association to date is the increase in HLA-B27 in patients with ankylosing spondylitis, first observed by Brewerton *et al.* (1973) and later by at least seventeen others (McMichael and De Witt, 1977). These results are of clinical interest in their own right since, wherever a characteristic (be it due to none, one, or many genes) is highly associated specifically with a disease process, one can use this information to identify those individuals who are more likely to have the disease. The ratio of the risk to individuals with the phenotype and the risk to individuals without the phenotype is called the relative risk. In Box. 4.3.6 we present a method for using the sample odds ratio to estimate relative risk from retrospective data. In Example 4.3.7 we indicate how one would first assess data for an association between a disease and a locus and then estimate the relative

---

Box 4.3.6 Use of the sample odds ratio to estimate relative risk of a phenotype associated with a rare disease.
Consider a sample of n_d individuals with a disease, n_c healthy controls and a genetic locus at which there is an allele, **A** say.
Let O_{++} denote the frequency of individuals positive (+) for the disease having allele **A**,

O_{+-} denote the frequency of individuals positive for the disease and negative for the allele **A**,

O_{-+} denote the frequency of individuals in the control population having allele **A**,

and O_{--} denote the frequency of individuals in the control population negative for the allele **A**.

(a) We evaluate the association of allele **A** with the disease by computing the chi-square test statistic associated with the above frequencies, where

$$X^2 = \frac{(O_{++}O_{--} - O_{+-}O_{-+})^2(n_c + n_d)}{n_c n_d (O_{++} + O_{-+})(O_{+-} + O_{--})}. \tag{4.3.16}$$

(b) If the disease is rare then the relative risk (RR) is approximately equal to the odds ratio (ω). Hence we compute an estimate of the relative risk of the disease for individuals positive for allele A using the sample odds ratio ($\hat{\omega}$); i.e.

$$\widehat{RR} = \hat{\omega} = \frac{O_{++}O_{--}}{O_{-+}O_{+-}}.$$

(c) If X^2 of (4.3.16) is significant at the α level (1 d.f.), we conclude that RR is significantly different from unity.

(d) We can estimate the standard error of the relative risk by

$$\widehat{SE}(\widehat{RR}) = \widehat{SE}(\hat{\omega}) = \hat{\omega}\sqrt{\frac{1}{O_{++}} + \frac{1}{O_{+-}} + \frac{1}{O_{--}} + \frac{1}{O_{-+}}}$$

Example 4.3.7 Computation of the sample odds ratio as an estimate of the relative risk and comparison of two relative risk estimates: an evaluation of observed associations between HLA-Dw3 and HLA-Dw4 and juvenile onset diabetes (Nerup *et al.*, 1977)

Results reported were as follows:

	Frequency in patients	Frequency in controls	Relative risk $\pm$ SE
HLA-Dw3	46/100 (46%)	33/176 (18.8%)	3.69 $\pm$ 1.03
HLA-Dw4	64/125 (51–)	31/176 (51–)	4.91 $\pm$ 1.31

(a) Using the nomenclature and results of Box 4.3.6, for Dw3, $O_{++} = 46, O_{+-} = 54, O_{-+} = 33, O_{--} = 143$.

(b) We test the hypothesis that the relative risk for

Dw3 is equal to 1 by the χ^2 test (4.3.17):

$$X^2 = \frac{[(46 \times 143) - (54 \times 33)]^2 276}{100 \times 176 \times 79 \times 197} = 23.177.$$

This value is highly significant and we conclude that the relative risk due to Dw3 is greater than 1; and similarly for Dw4.

(c) Since juvenile diabetes is a relatively rare disease, we assume that the odds ratio (ω) is approximately equal to the relative risk (RR). Hence the relative risk for Dw3 can be estimated by (4.3.17) as

$$\widehat{RR} = \hat{\omega} = \frac{O_{++}O_{--}}{O_{+-}O_{-+}} = \frac{46 \times 143}{54 \times 33} = 3.69$$

Similarly, for Dw4 it is estimated to be 4.9.1.

(d) The standard error of the relative risk for Dw3 is estimated by (4.3.18) as

$$\widehat{SE}(\widehat{RR}) = 3.69 \sqrt{\frac{1}{46} + \frac{1}{54} + \frac{1}{33} + \frac{1}{143}} = 1.03$$

risk corresponding to an observed association. It is important to note that an assumption inherent in using the equations of Box 4.3.6 to estimate relative risk is that the disease is sufficiently rare that the frequency of the marker in the normal population is essentially the same as that in the total population. Certainly, the ideal design for obtaining assumption free estimates of relative risk would be a prospective study in which samples of individuals were selected for the presence of each of the marker genotypes, and the incidence of the disease in those with and without each genotype was observed. However, since there are so many possible genetic phenotypes and the diseases are of such low frequency, an informative prospective study is often not feasible. Of more concern, however, than the assumptions required to estimate relative risk with a retrospective study is the possibility of obtaining spurious results due to inadequate design. Specifically, one could have chosen a set of normal controls which does not represent the population from which the diseased individuals are sampled. If the disease occurs with higher frequency in people from some racial, ethnic or socioeconomic group or geographic location, it is very important that the normal controls be chosen from these groups at the same relative frequency that the groups are present in the diseased sample. It is, of course, very important that every individual in the study should be totally unrelated to all other individuals in the study and that large enough samples be drawn from both the diseased and control populations to ensure adequate power to detect a difference, bearing in mind the need to account for the number of phenotypes considered (see 4.3.1). However, the samples should not be so large that even the smallest disturbance in relative risk is statistically significant. The null hypothesis that the relative risk equals one is tested by the chi-square test. However, it should be noted that due to the inherent nature of the design of most relative risk studies (i.e. the sample of non-affected individuals is usually larger than the sample of diseased individuals) and because the frequency of each marker allele is less than 50 per cent, one is more likely to detect those marker genotypes which are **positively** associated with the disease than those which are negatively associated with the disease (Kidd and Ceppellini, 1977). Thus, if a marker phenotype is associated with disease resistance, we are less likely to detect this fact than to find those marker phenotypes which are associated with disease susceptibility.

A further issue to consider is whether the observation that an allele is positively associated with a disorder in fact indicates that those individuals with the allele are at greater risk. There is the possibility, if the disease can be fatal, that the associated allele is related to disease survival. Thus the diseased sample, consisting solely of survivors, would have an increased frequency of individuals with the disease survival allele. Yet, this observation could be misinterpreted as indicating an allele associated with susceptibility. Two observed estimates of relative risk might be compared using one of the many statistical tests for comparison of two-sample odds ratios (Fleiss, 1981) and/or assessing the relationship between more than two categorical variables (Fienberg, 1980). However, comparison of odds ratios, or in this case, relative risks has been criticized since the number of cases due to the associated factor is not considered. Fleiss (1980) cites some interesting counter-examples and suggests that statistics such as *attributable risk* and *relative difference* may sometimes be more appropriate.

Finally, one should be careful when making elaborate genetic speculations on the basis of observed disease associations, and conversely one should not reject a genetic aetiology if no associations are observed. Associations between a known genetic marker and a disease, when established by an appropriately designed study, probably do indicate that a disease susceptibility gene is either in linkage disequilibrium with the associated genotype or the associated genotype itself is a factor causing the disease. However, it is important to realize that the converse does not hold; i.e. the absence of observed associations between a disease and the alleles at a locus in no way proves that there is no major disease susceptibility gene linked to the locus. One could simply have a disease susceptibility gene linked to the marker with no linkage disequilibrium.

Because an association between a marker and a disease is of genetic significance, methods have been proposed (Thomson and Bodmer, 1977) for using observations on the association between marker phenotypes and the disease to determine whether the hypothetical susceptibility (or resistance) gene is dominant and to estimate its frequency. These methods might be appropriate if in fact the underlying assumptions are correct; namely that there is a major susceptibility gene with full penetrance in linkage disequilibrium with the marker phenotype. However, the validity of these assumptions can only be established through a well-designed family study in which several hypotheses of both genetic and non-genetic modes of transmission are considered and a linkage analysis of the distribution of the disease and marker phenotypes in the family is performed. In the following section we consider these types of studies and the methods used to extract the information from them.

4.4 INTRODUCTION TO GENETIC STUDIES OF HUMAN DISORDERS

In studying any disorder the first question which should be asked is 'To what extent is the disorder genetic?' The question is phrased in this way because there is probably some genetic component to every human disorder or attribute. Consequently, the first step in studying diseases involves taking large random samples of affected individuals from the population at large (Myrianthopoulos and Aronson, 1966; Myrianthopoulos and Leyshon, 1967; Woolf, Koehn and Coleman, 1968; Emanuel *et al.*, 1973). In these studies, where one determines the correlations with, for example, race, region, socioeconomic class, birth order, maternal age, inbreeding and known genetic markers, one looks for evidence of involvement of specific genetic and environmental factors. In another type of population study, investigators often examine twin pairs in which one twin is known *a priori* to be affected (Shields, 1962; Harvald and Hauge, 1965; Pikkarainen, Takkunen and Kulonen, 1966; Hay and Wehrung, 1970; Fischer, 1973). Alternatively, other relatives of affected individuals, such as their mother, father, siblings or first cousins, are examined (Woolf, Woolf and Broadbent, 1963; Woolf, Koehn and Coleman, 1968; Woolf, 1971; Dodge, 1972; Bear, 1976; Lynch, Lynch and Guirgas, 1976).

Population studies of these kinds are often used to determine whether genetic factors are important in the disease and to quantitate their influence. They are also sometimes mistakenly used, in the absence of hypothesis testing (see Section 1.3.2), as evidence in favour of a specific genetic (usually multifactorial) hypothesis. Alternatively, when hypothesis testing has been done, it sometimes turns out that, even with an enormous sample, one cannot discriminate between genetic hypotheses (Chung, Ching and Morton, 1974; Curnow and Smith, 1975). Simulation studies by Smith (1971) and Kruger (1973) indicate that this may often be the case in studying a disease with reduced penetrance. Recently, methods have been developed for testing several more general hypotheses of transmission using either data taken from many nuclear families (parents and all of the offspring) (Morton and MacLean, 1974) and/or data on transmission of the disorder through several generations of a few families (Elston and Stuart, 1971).

Another development in the genetic analysis of disorders has been the realization that, in considering a hypothesis of a single autosomal (or X-linked) gene, one need not categorize individuals as being with or without the disorder (Elston and Stuart, 1971; Morton and MacLean, 1974; MacLean, Morton and

Lew, 1975; Elston and Rao, 1978). In fact, if one has a continuous measure of the disease, one may be better off analysing the distribution of this measure in families rather than categorizing individuals as affected or unaffected. Because of the greater power (MacLean, Morton and Lew, 1975), one can discriminate between a single gene and many genes with fewer individuals using a continuous measure.

In Sections 4.5 and 4.6 we consider some methods which have been proposed for simultaneously testing major gene, multifactorial and environmental transmission of disorders. In doing so, we indicate how these methods have been used in the analysis of both continuous and categorical disease phenotypes. While these new methods have more general application, they require more advanced computational facilities. Thus, we present first some experimental designs and methods of analysis which have been used to estimate the *segregation frequency* under single-gene models and the *heritability* and *variance components* under a simple multifactorial model. Since a very powerful method for proving the existence of a major gene for a disease is a *linkage study*, methods for testing the hypothesis of linkage between a trait (disease) and a genetic marker and methods for estimating the *frequency of recombination* are also presented.

4.5 ESTIMATION OF PARAMETERS AND TESTING OF SOME SIMPLE GENETIC HYPOTHESES

4.5.1 Estimating the probability of ascertainment

In general, rigorous testing of any genetic hypothesis involves first the design of a study from which one can ultimately obtain unbiased estimates of the relevant parameters [see VI, Chapter 5]. One method of doing this is to sample individuals at random in the population at large and consider the distribution of the relevant parameters in some *a priori* defined set of relatives. However, for disorders which occur at low frequency, such a design would not result in any information. In fact, the genetics of most diseases have been determined through the study of families of affected individuals (in the case of a continuous trait, the study of families of individuals having extreme values of the phenotype). This is done either through the study of the offspring of couples, in which one or both is affected, or the study of siblings of affected individuals. In the first situation we have complete *ascertainment* and the *frequency of transmission* is estimated through the observed frequencies in the offspring. These follow the binomial distribution [see II, §5.2.2] and the estimates of transmission frequencies and their standard errors are quite striaghtforward.

Such a design can be used successfully to study the genetics of a trait for which there is no overwhelming effect on reproduction. However, in the case of disorders such as cystic fibrosis, in which affected individuals rarely reproduce, one must study siblings of affected individuals. In addition, sibling data may be more readily available or more reliable than data on the offspring of affected individuals. For example, in the case of birth defects such as cleft lip and cleft palate, pyloric stenosis, and clubfoot, sibling data may be more readily available because one is more likely to encounter affected individuals when they are very young and have not yet had offspring. On the other hand, sibling data are more reliable in delayed onset disorders such as Huntington's chorea, diabetes, familial polyposis or psoriasis since one is more likely to know whether a middle aged sibling is truly unaffected than whether or not a very young offspring is affected.

A problem in any study involving the siblings of affected individuals is that the probability that a family will be sampled may be correlated with the number of affected family members. This probability that an affected individual will be a *proband* is called the *probability of ascertainment* and is usually denoted by π. It must be taken into account and estimated whenever one is estimating the frequency of affected offspring in families with at least one affected offspring.

To some extent the value of π depends on the nature of the disease, the definition of the population to be studied and the sampling design. We may have a situation in which all other affected family members are also probands ($\pi = 1$; truncate selection), or none of the other family members are probands ($\pi = 0$; single selection), or in which in some cases the other family members are probands and in others they are not ($0 < \pi < 1$; multiple selection) (Cavalli-Sforza and Bodmer, 1971). In Box 4.5.1 we give the equations (Morton, 1959) used under multiple selection to express the probability of observing r affected individuals in sibships of size s. The equations under truncate and single selection can be obtained on setting $\pi = 1$ and $\pi = 0$ respectively.

Box. 4.5.1 The probability of observing r affected siblings in a family with s offspring in families ascertained through an affected individual (as derived by Morton, 1959) ·

Let π be the probability an affected individual is ascertained,
  p be the probability an individual in such a family will be affected,
  s be the number of offspring,
and r be the number of affected offspring.
The probability of observing r out of s affected individuals is

$$p(r,s) = \frac{\binom{s}{r} p^r (1-p)^{s-r} [1 - (1-\pi)^r]}{1 - (1 - p\pi)^s} \qquad (4.5.1)$$

where $\binom{s}{r}$ is the binomial coefficient, $\dfrac{s!}{(s-r)!\,r!}$.

Another design for a genetic study involves studying the distribution of disease in more distant relatives as well as in the parents and siblings of affected individuals; i.e. obtaining *pedigree information* as opposed to information from *nuclear families*. The method of sampling the pedigree must be taken into account during data analysis. There is no *ascertainment bias* if we study random families, but, if a family is studied because there is at least one affected individual, ascertainment bias needs to be determined. Probably the best approach, when studying pedigrees ascertained through an affected individual, is to decide *a priori* to study each of these pedigrees regardless of whether it contains other affected individuals.

4.5.2 Testing the hypothesis of a single gene with full penetrance using information about the immediate families of affected individuals

We consider here a trait with two phenotypes, 'affected' and 'unaffected'. We have collected data on the siblings and parents of a population of patients and we wish to test the hypothesis that the disorder results from a recessive gene, A, with full penetrance. If we consider only those sibships in which both parents are unaffected, then, under this hypothesis and using the notation of Box 4.5.1, the expected risk to each offspring in these families is $p = 1/4$. The first step in this analysis is to obtain maximum likelihood estimates of π, the ascertainment probability, and p, the segregation frequency [see VI, §6.2]. The second step is to test the hypothesis that the estimates are not significantly different from 0.25 (see Section 1.3.2). Since the likelihood is calculated using (4.5.1), one could obtain maximum likelihood estimates of π and p by using some computer algorithm to maximize likelihoods (Mi, 1966; Morton, 1969; Kaplan and Elston, 1972) or obtain approximations to maximum likelihood estimates through a scoring method (Morton, 1959; Cavalli-Sforza and Bodmer, 1971). In Box 4.5.2 we show an alternative method for obtaining approximations to the maximum likelihood estimates of π and p and their standard errors which, according to Cavalli-Sforza and Bodmer (1971), was originally proposed by Weinberg (1927) and modified by

---

Box 4.5.2 Approximate maximum likelihood estimates of ascertainment probability and segregation frequency derived by Weinberg (1927) and Fisher (1934) as presented by Cavalli-Sforza and Bodmer (1971)

Consider a situation in which we ascertain sibships containing at least one affected individual.

Let M be the maximum sibship size in our sample,

r_{is} be the number of affected individuals in sibship i of size s ($s = 2, 3, 4, \ldots, M$),

a_{is} be the number of probands in sibship i of size s,

and n_s be the number of sibships of size s ($s = 2, 3, \ldots, M$).

Then let

$$T_s = (s-1) \sum_{i=1}^{n_s} a_{is} \qquad (s = 2, 3, \ldots, M), \qquad (4.5.2)$$

$$R_s = \sum_{i=1}^{n_s} a_{is}(r_{is} - 1) \qquad (s = 2, 3, \ldots, M), \qquad (4.5.3)$$

$$A_s = \sum_{i=1}^{n_s} a_{is}(a_{is} - 1) \qquad (s = 2, 3, \ldots, M). \qquad (4.5.4)$$

We estimate ascertainment probability by

$$\hat{\pi} = \frac{\sum_{s=2}^{M} A_s}{\sum_{s=2}^{M} R_s}. \qquad (4.5.5)$$

We then obtain our first approximation to the maximum likelihood estimate of the segregation frequency as

$$\hat{p}_0 = \frac{\sum_{s=2}^{M} R_s}{\sum_{s=2}^{M} T_s}. \qquad (4.5.6)$$

Our final estimate of the segregation frequency is obtained by setting

$$\frac{1}{C_s} = 1 + \hat{\pi} + \hat{\pi}\hat{p}_0(s-3) \qquad (4.5.7)$$

and computing

$$\hat{p} = \frac{\sum_{s=2}^{M} R_s C_s}{\sum_{s=2}^{M} T_s C_s}. \qquad (4.5.8)$$

Then our estimate of the standard error of $\hat{p}$ is obtained as

$$\widehat{SE}(\hat{p}) = \sqrt{\frac{\hat{p}(1-\hat{p})}{\sum_{s=2}^{M} T_s C_s}}. \qquad (4.5.9)$$

We can test the null hypothesis $H_0 : p = p'$ by computing

$$Z = \frac{\hat{p} - p'}{\widehat{SE}(\hat{p})} \qquad (4.5.10)$$

where Z is distributed as the standard Normal deviate.

Fisher (1934). Cavalli-Sforza and Bodmer describe it as a method which can be used without the aid of computer software. Other methods for estimating p are available for those situations in which the value of π is known to be either zero or one (Li and Mantel, 1968; Sutton, 1975; Vogel and Motulsky, 1979).

In Example 4.5.1 we present an analysis of families of individuals having cystic fibrosis. This analysis is given as an example by Cavalli-Sforza and Bodmer (1971) and is taken from data presented by Crow (1963). In the example we present the detailed data on the sibships having seven or more offspring and a summary of Crow's (1963) analysis of all of the sibships. In these families the evidence is in favour of a simple Mendelian recessive gene with full penetrance. Danke, Allen and Anderson (1965) used $\hat{p}_0$ of (4.5.6) and obtained a 95 per cent confidence interval of 0.211 to 0.275 for the segregation frequency of cystic fibrosis.

Example 4.5.1 Segregation analysis of cystic fibrosis (Crow, 1963) **using the Weinberg (1927) method**

Cavalli-Sforza and Bodmer (1971) cite Crow's (1963) analysis of cystic fibrosis data. We give here a partial table from Crow's paper showing in detail only the results for sibships having seven or more offspring.

Sibship number	Number in sibship (s)	Number affected (r_{is})	Number of probands (a_{is})
1	10	3	1
2	9	3	1
3	8	4	1
4	7	3	2
5	7	3	1
6	7	2	1
7	7	1	1

Using the notation of Box 4.5.2, $M = 10$, $n_7 = 4$, $n_8 = 1$, $n_9 = 1$ and $n_{10} = 1$. For $s = 7$ we can compute the necessary quantities.

By (4.5.2),

$$T_7 = (7 - 1) \sum_{i=1}^{4} a_{i7} = 6(2 + 1 + 1 + 1) = 30.$$

By (4.5.3),

$$R_7 = \sum_{i=1}^{4} a_{i7}(r_{i7} - 1)$$

$$= (2)(2) + (1)(2) + (1)(1) + (1)(0) = 7$$

By (4.5.4),

$$A_7 = \sum_{i=1}^{4} a_{i7}(a_{i7} - 1)$$
$$= 2(2 - 1) + 1(1 - 1) + 1(1 - 1) + 1(1 - 1) = 2$$

Similarly, Crow (1963) computed T_s, R_s and A_s for $s = 2, 3, \ldots, 10$ and obtained the following results:

$$\sum_{s=2}^{10} T_s = 218, \qquad \sum_{s=2}^{10} R_s = 59 \qquad \text{and} \qquad \sum_{s=2}^{10} A_s = 22.$$

Thus, by (4.5.5),

$$\hat{\pi} = \frac{22}{59} = 0.373,$$

and, by (4.5.6),

$$\hat{p}_0 = \frac{59}{218} = 0.271.$$

Using (4.5.7), they then computed

$$1/C_7 = 1 + \hat{\pi} + \hat{\pi}\hat{p}_0(s - 3) = 1 + 0.373 + (0.271)(7 - 3) = 1.78$$

or

$$C_7 = 0.56.$$

Thus

$$C_7 T_7 = (0.56)(30) = 16.85$$

and

$$C_7 R_7 = (0.56)(7) = 3.93.$$

Adding $C_7 T_7$ and $C_7 R_7$ to the terms for $s = 2, 3, \ldots, 10$ they obtained

$$\sum_{s=2}^{M} R_s C_s = 38.61,$$

$$\sum_{s=2}^{M} R_s T_s = 141.85.$$

Thus by (4.5.8) they obtained a final estimate of the segregation ratio,

$$\hat{p} = \frac{38.607}{141.85} = 0.272.$$

Applying (4.5.9),

$$\widehat{SE}(\hat{p}) = \sqrt{\frac{(0.272)(1 - 0.272)}{141.85}} = 0.037.$$

Thus using (4.5.10) we test the hypothesis that $p' = 0.25$ by calculating

$$Z = \frac{0.272 - 0.25}{0.037} = 0.595$$

and from the standard Normal distribution conclude that $P > 0.4$ and therefore that we cannot reject the hypothesis $p' = 0.25$.

The maximum likelihood estimate of p, the risk to siblings of affected individuals, is essentially the estimate of risk of recurrence after adjusting for ascertainment. To test a genetic model, one compares this estimate to the hypothesized value under the model. The hypothesis of recessive inheritance is tested by assessing the significance of the difference between the observed estimate of p and the value 0.25. This might be done using (4.5.10). Alternatively, one could compute the likelihood under the hypothesis that $\pi = \hat{\pi}$ and $p = \hat{p}$ using (4.5.1) and compare it to that observed under the alternative hypothesis that $p = 1/4$ and $\pi = \hat{\pi}$, using the likelihood ratio test [see VI, §5.5]. However, these two approaches should give equivalent results in large samples. One should also reach similar conclusions by comparing the observed distribution of affected and unaffected individuals to the expected distribution (with $p = 1/4$ and $\pi = \hat{\pi}$) using a chi-square test with 1 d.f. One can use the same method to test the hypothesis that the disorder is 'dominant' in a sample of families in which exactly one parent is affected (by testing the hypothesis that $p = 1/2$) or that the disorder is X-linked (by testing $p = 1/2$ and studying only the male offspring). However, inherent in the testing of a hypothesis of autosomal dominance is the assumption that all affected parents are heterozygous (**AB**), i.e. that the homozygous genotype is very rare.

4.5.3 Estimation of parameters assuming polygenic transmission

The polygenic hypothesis involves the assumption that instead of one major gene determining the phenotype there are several genes with essentially small, equal and additive effects. The result of such an aetiology would be a continuum of phenotypes reflecting the number of disease-predisposing alleles each individual has. However, several disorders with no known continuum of severity (or for which severity does not appear to be genetically determined) are considered to be polygenic. For these disorders we assume that there is an underlying continuum of 'liability' to the disorder which is polygenic and individuals with liability above some threshold value are the ones who are affected (Falconer,

1965; Edwards, 1969; Curnow and Smith, 1975). One can further generalize the polygenic model and allow for environmental factors. In this case we consider the phenotypes to be *multifactorial*. In Box 4.5.3 we define some of the parameters which have traditionally been considered in studying traits which are polygenic and present some equations one might use to estimate parameters of interest.

An assumption inherent in these equations is that all correlation (see Section 1.3.15) between family members (of either the phenotype itself or the liability to the phenotype) is due to correlation in genotype; i.e. that any environmental factors involved are not more highly correlated in two related individuals than in two unrelated individuals. It is also assumed that there is random mating (marriage) with respect to the phenotype. However, modifications for situations in which there is assortative marriage and inbreeding are reasonably straightforward (Cavalli-Sforza and Bodmer, 1971; Vogel and Motulsky, 1979). Cavalli-Sforza and Bodmer (1971) indicate that the relationships of Box 4.5.3 were originally proposed by Fisher (1918). They have been used in the analysis of ridge counts by Loesch (1971) and according to Vogel and Motulsky (1979) by many investigators of the inheritance of IQ.

Estimating variance components and heritability for traits with a threshold defining the 'normal' and 'affected' phenotypes has long been a problem.

Box 4.5.3 The model for a polygenic hypothesis and some relationships for the study of correlations observed in pairs of related individuals (Cavalli-Sforza and Bodmer, 1971)

We assume that an individual's phenotype, x, can be expressed as

$$x = \mu + e + g + d, \tag{4.5.11}$$

where μ is the population mean value of x,

e is the observed departure from the mean due to environmental factors,

g is the observed departure from the mean due to effects of many codominant factors,

and d is the observed departure due to dominant effects of genes.

We also assume that e, g and d have mean zero and variances σ_e^2, σ_g^2 and σ_d^2, respectively, and that the covariance among e, g and d is zero. Then the variance of x is

$$\sigma_p^2 = \sigma_e^2 + \sigma_g^2 + \sigma_d^2.$$

Some parameters of interest in studying polygenic disorders are:

(a) Heritability (h^2), where

$$h^2 = \frac{\sigma_g^2}{\sigma_p^2}. \tag{4.5.12}$$

(b) Correlation in phenotypes of pairs of siblings ($r_{s/s}$), which can be shown to be related to σ_e^2 and σ_g^2 in the form

$$r_{s/s} = \frac{\frac{1}{2}\sigma_g^2 + \frac{1}{4}\sigma_d^2}{\sigma_p^2}. \tag{4.5.13}$$

(c) Correlation in phenotypes between parents and offspring ($r_{p/o}$) which has been shown to be:

$$r_{p/o} = \frac{\frac{1}{2}\sigma_g^2}{\sigma_p^2}. \tag{4.5.14}$$

Thus, by equation (4.5.12), (4.5.13) and (4.5.14),

$$h^2 = 2r_{p/o}, \tag{4.5.15}$$

$$\sigma_d^2/\sigma_p^2 = 4(r_{s/s} - r_{p/o}), \tag{4.5.16}$$

$$\sigma_e^2/\sigma_p^2 = 1 - h^2 - \frac{\sigma_d^2}{\sigma_p^2}. \tag{4.5.17}$$

(d) It has also been shown that, in general, the correlation in phenotype of two related individuals (x and y) with coefficient of relationship ($\mathscr{R}$) is related to heritability as

$$r_{x/y} = h^2\mathscr{R}, \tag{4.5.18}$$

whenever $\sigma_d^2 = 0$.
For pairs of cousins, where $\mathscr{R} = 1/8$ (Falconer, 1960), we have

$$r_{c/c} = \frac{h^2}{8}. \tag{4.5.19}$$

Crittendon (1961) suggested a method for estimating heritability using the frequencies of the disorder observed (a) in relatives of affected individuals and (b) in relatives of unaffected individuals or in the general population. This method was later presented in the genetic literature with many detailed examples by Falconer (1965); it is outlined in Box 4.5.4. If one had samples of cousins of probands, siblings of probands, aunts and uncles of probands, one could obtain several independent estimates of the heritability and its standard error. Alternatively, one could obtain estimates of heritability at each age and determine whether or not the early and late onset forms of the disorder have a common genetic aetiology, using equations given by Falconer (1967) to estimate a quantity called *genetic correlation*.

Box 4.5.4 Falconer's method (1965, 1967) for estimating heritability of a disorder under a multifactorial hypothesis

Let q_P denote the prevalence of the disorder in the general population from which we take our probands,

    q_R denote the prevalence of the disorder in the general population from which we take relatives,

    q_{R+} denote the prevelance of the disorder in relatives of affected individuals,

    $\mathcal{R}$ denote the coefficient of relationship between the relatives and affected individuals.

Then heritability under the threshold model is the value of h^2 which satisfies the equation:

$$q_R = \frac{1}{q_P}\left[\int_{XR}^{\infty}\int_{XP}^{\infty}\psi(y_1, y_2, \mathcal{R}h^2)\,dy_1\,dy_2\right.$$

where $\psi(a,b,e) = \dfrac{1}{2\pi\sqrt{1-e}}\exp-\dfrac{1}{2}\left(\dfrac{a^2+b^2-2eab}{1-e}\right),$ (4.5.20)

and where X_i is the Normal deviate corresponding to $1 - q_i (i = R, P, R+)$.

    (4.5.21)

Falconer's approximation to h^2 is obtained as

$$h^2 = \frac{x_R - x_{R+}}{a_P \mathcal{R}}, \tag{4.5.22}$$

where

$$a_i = \frac{1}{\sqrt{2\pi}}\frac{\exp(-x_i^2/2)}{q_i} \qquad (i = P, R, R+). \tag{4.5.23}$$

The standard error of the estimate of h^2 obtained using (4.5.22) and (4.5.23) and estimates of q_P and $q_R (\hat{q}_P$ and $\hat{q}_R)$, based on samples N_P from the general population representing probands, N_R from the general population representing relatives and N_{R+} relatives of probands, is derived by Falconer (1965) to be:

$$\widehat{SE}(h^2) = \frac{1}{\mathcal{R}}\sqrt{h^2\mathcal{R}(a_P - x_P)^2 V_P + \left(\frac{1}{a_P}\right)^2 (V_R + V_{R+})}, \tag{4.5.24}$$

where

$$V_i = \frac{1 - q_i}{a_i N_i q_i} \qquad (i = P, R, P+). \tag{4.5.25}$$

This approach has been used to analyse empirical risk data obtained from studies of relatives of individuals having cleft lip (Woolf, 1971; Bear, 1976; Melnick *et al.*, 1980), pyloric stenosis (Falconer, 1965) and diabetes (Simpson, 1969). There are several problems with this approach (Curnow and Smith, 1975), some of which were noted by Falconer himself (1965). If there are any dominant genes, one obtains an overestimate of heritability from sibling data. A more important problem is that it is often not recognized that h^2, as calculated by (4.5.22), is an approximation to the maximum likelihood estimate (Mendell and Elston, 1974). In the case of a rare disease, it is a biased overestimate. Thus, the observation of an estimated heritability greater than one obtained using (4.5.22) could merely reflect failure of the approximation rather than an inappropriate model. Several approximations to the tetrachoric correlation (which does provide a maximum likelihood estimate) have been proposed (Smith, 1970; Mendell and Elston, 1974). However, computation of the ML estimate itself, the tetrachoric correlation, is now available in some statistical packages and these rather than (4.5.22) should be used for estimating heritability and testing specific hypotheses. An additional problem recognized to some extent by Reich, Games and Morris (1972), Kidd and Spence (1976), Mendell and Spence (1979) and Melnick *et al.* (1980) is that the fact that one obtains estimates of heritability which appear to be in an appropriate range does not constitute a test of goodness of fit to a multifactorial hypothesis. Finally, these analyses, which are based on prevalence in relatives of patients, make no adjustment for the fact that we might have single ascertainment in the case of cousins and complete ascertainment in the case of siblings and, hence, observe unequal or high estimates of heritability. Gladstien, Lange and Spence (1978) have developed methods for simultaneously estimating ascertainment probability and heritability and for testing goodness of fit to a simple multifactorial threshold model using nuclear family data on pyloric stenosis. These methods have been used to establish a good fit for cleft lip and/or cleft palate (Mendell *et al.*, 1980) and a poor fit for multiple sclerosis (Sadovnick, Spence and Tideman, 1980). In Box 4.5.4 we present Falconer's method of

---

Example 4.5.2 Use of Falconer's method to estimate heritability of pyloric stenosis (Falconer, 1965)

The following information is given on pyloric stenosis (see Box 4.5.4 for notation):

Population	i	q_i	Sample size
Males	R	0.005	—
Females	P	0.001	—
Brothers of affected females	R^+	0.1707	82

To obtain the heritability estimate for brothers of affected females we first note that, for siblings, the coefficient of relationship ($\mathscr{R}$) is 0.5. The Normal deviates corresponding to $(1 - q_i)$—i.e. 0.995, 0.999 and 0.8293—are $x_R = 2.576$, $x_P = 3.090$ and $x_{R+} = 0.951$ respectively.

We then substitute x_P and q_P into (4.5.23) and obtain

$$a_P = \frac{1}{\sqrt{2\pi}} \frac{\exp(-3.090^2/2)}{0.001} = 3.370.$$

Similarly, $a_{R+} = 1.487$. Then, by (4.5.22),

$$h^2 = \frac{x_R - x_{R+}}{\mathscr{R} a_P} = \frac{2.576 - 0.951}{(1/2)(3.370)} = 0.97.$$

Since q_P and q_R are given as vital statistics (N_P, $N_R = \infty$), we have, from (4.5.25), $V_R = V_P = 0$ and

$$V_{R+} = \frac{1 - q_{R+}}{a_{R+}^2 q_{R+} N_{R+}} = \frac{1 - 0.1707}{(1.487)^2 (0.1707)(82)} = 0.0268.$$

We estimate $\mathrm{SE}(h^2)$ by (4.5.24) as

$$\widehat{\mathrm{SE}}(h^2) = \frac{1}{\mathscr{R}} \sqrt{\left(\frac{1}{a_P}\right)^2 V_{R+}}$$

$$= 2 \sqrt{\frac{1}{3.370^2} \times 0.0268} = 0.10.$$

estimating heritability and its standard error (on one of four sampling situations he considered in his 1965 paper), along with the expression for the maximum likelihood estimate of heritability. In Example 4.2.2 we show a portion of his analysis of data on pyloric stenosis. However, we feel that these estimates can be biased for the many reasons given above.

4.6 TESTING MORE COMPLEX GENETIC HYPOTHESES

4.6.1 Methods for testing a more general major gene hypothesis for qualitative traits

Having tested and rejected the hypothesis of a Mendelian autosomal gene with full penetrance, there are many possible alternative genetic hypotheses. A trait might be dominant (or recessive) with reduced penetrance or it might be multifactorial. In fact, even if one does not reject the hypothesis of a major gene with full penetrance, one should still consider whether a better fit is possible to these alternative models. It has been pointed out by Curnow and Smith (1975) that one is more likely to accept a major gene hypothesis for a multifactorial trait than to accept a multifactorial hypothesis for a disorder due to a major gene. There is also the issue of genetic heterogeneity; i.e. a disorder might be due to an autosomal gene segregating in some families, a second gene segregating in others and environmental factors in a third set of cases.

One approach to this problem has been to estimate simultaneously the frequency of sporadic cases and the penetrance of the disorder along with the segregation frequency and the ascertainment probability, using sibship data. Expressions for the likelihood of the data under these more complex models were derived by Morton (1959). Maximum likelihood estimates were obtained through taking the first derivative of the log likelihood with respect to each parameter and using iterative procedures to obtain the values at which all desired expressions were equal to zero. One can now write computer programs for obtaining maximum likelihood estimates (Morton, 1962, 1969) of the parameters of interest. One tests a hypothesis of a major gene by first letting the segregation frequency take on an arbitrary value between zero and one and then assuming that it is functionally related to penetrance, frequency of sporadic cases and number of affected parents. The differences in log likelihoods [see VI, §§5.5, 6.2.1] under these hypotheses might be used to test goodness of fit. In this manner, Chung, Ching and Morton (1974) analysed their data on the distribution of cleft lip and cleft palate in Hawaiian families and concluded that, on allowing for sporadic cases, these data fit a simple recessive gene model better than a simple dominant gene model. Chung and Brown (1970) have used these methods to study early childhood deafness and have concluded that there appear to be different modes of inheritance in sibships of those probands having affected second and third degree relatives and in those having no affected aunts, uncles, etc. Boughman, Conneally and Nance (1980) used these methods to estimate the frequency of retinitis pigmentosa due to a dominant gene, a recessive gene and an X-linked gene, and concluded that in the United States none of the cases are sporadic.

This approach to genetic analysis has required huge databases on the distribution of the trait in immediate families of affected individuals. Another approach has been to study a few large pedigrees of affected individuals (Gardner and Plenk, 1951; Cross, Lerberg and McKusick, 1968). The equations for computing the likelihoods of the distributions of phenotypes in a pedigree under various modes of transmission were derived by Elston and Stewart (1971). In doing so, they considered a major gene hypothesis as a null hypothesis to be tested against a more general alternative in which transmission of a character can occur with any probability between zero and one. Similarly, dominance (or recessivity) of the disorder is considered as a null hypothesis that the penetrance of the heterozygote is equal to the penetrance of the homozygote and tested against the alternative hypothesis that the penetrance of the disorder in the heterozygote is any value between zero and one (Elston and Yelverton, 1975; Elston and Namboodiri, 1977). Programs have been created to compute the maximum likelihood estimates of transmission probabilities, gene frequencies and penetrance, under hypotheses that the trait is dominant or recessive (either X-linked or autosomal) and that transmission is either genetic, environmental or random (Kaplan and Elston, 1975). These have been used to analyse large pedigrees of families of individuals with retinitis pigmentosa (Spence, Elston and Cedarbaum, 1974), schizophrenia (Elston and Namboodiri, 1977; Elston *et al.*, 1978), ragweed sensitivity (Mendell *et al.*, 1978) and many other familial diseases. In these studies, investigators computed the maximum likelihood under each hypothesis and compared these likelihoods to those obtained under some less restrictive alternative hypothesis. It has been proposed that twice the difference in the natural logarithm of these likelihoods follows a chi-square distribution with the number of degrees of freedom equal to the difference in the numbers of parameters estimated (Spence, Elston and Cedarbaum, 1974; Elston *et al.*, 1978; Mendell *et al.*, 1978). Thus, since the Elston and Stewart (1971) model for random transmission involves ten functionally independent parameters and the model for Mendelian transmission involves seven parameters, one tests the hypothesis of Mendelian segregation with a likelihood ratio statistic for which minus twice its natural log follows the χ^2 distribution with 3 d.f. Similarly, the hypothesis of a Mendelian dominant (or recessive gene) involves the estimation of three parameters whereas, on dropping this assumption, one has four parameters. Thus the test of dominance (or recessivity) of the disorder involves a likelihood ratio statistic where twice its natural log follows the chi-square distribution with 1 d.f.

4.6.2 Methods for testing a major gene hypothesis for quantitative traits

Both Elston and Stewart (1971) and MacLean, Morton and Lew (1975) have derived expressions for the likelihood of pedigrees for those situations in which the phenotype is continuous. They used conditional probabilities [see II, §§3.9.1 and 6.5.1] while Morton and MacLean (1974) used a combination of path analysis and conditional probabilities (Elston and Rao, 1978). The most general model considered by Elston and Stewart (1971) involves three types of individuals, **AA**, **AB** and **BB** say, each occurring in the general population with frequency f_{AA}, f_{AB} and f_{BB} and for which the phenotypes in each type are normally distributed with means μ_{AA}, μ_{AB} and μ_{BB} and variance σ^2. One can then test dominance of a high phenotype by restricting $\mu_{AA} = \mu_{AB} > \mu_{BB}$ (and the recessivity of the high phenotype by restricting $\mu_{AA} > \mu_{AB} = \mu_{BB}$) and comparing the likelihood to that obtained on allowing μ_{AA}, μ_{AB} and μ_{BB} to take on any value. A major gene hypothesis is tested, as in the case of a categorical phenotype, by testing the hypothesis that individuals of type **AA** have a probability of transmitting **A** of 1, those of type **AB** have a transmission probability of 0.5 and those of type **BB** have a transmission probability of 0 (Morton and MacLean, 1974). MacLean, Morton and Lew (1975) introduced a different set of parameters, some of which can be shown to be functionally related to those of Elston and Stewart (1971) (Elston *et al.*, 1980). Their most general model, a 'mixed model', assumes that the phenotype, x, is due to environment, polygenes and a major gene having frequency, q. The major gene hypothesis is tested by considering the hypothesis $q = 0$, and the multifactorial hypothesis by setting the heritability (H) equal to zero. Analysis under the model of MacLean, Morton and Lew also allows one to estimate the ascertainment probability and the sibling–environment correlation.

The methods of Elston and Stewart (1971) have been used in the genetic analysis of several traits previously believed to be purely polygenic. These include hypercholesteraemia and hypertriglyceridaemia (Elston *et al.*, 1975), blood clotting factor X levels (Siervogel *et al.*, 1979) and dopamine β-hydroxylase activity (Elston, Lamboodiri and Hanes, 1979). the methods of MacLean, Morton and Lew have also been used extensively; one example being the analysis of height and weight by Rao *et al.* (1978) and another that of IgE levels (Gerrard, Rao and Morton, 1978) as outlined in Example 4.6.1. Their model can also be

---

Example 4.6.1 Analysis of IgE levels Gerrard, Rao and Morton (1978) using Morton and MacLean's (1974) mixed model

In their study of 173 nuclear families, Gerrard, Rao and Morton (1978) tested the hypothesis of a major gene mechanism determining levels of serum IgE. After log-transforming the IgE level, their results were as follows:

Genetic model	$-2\log_e$ likelihood	Notation	χ^2	d.f.	P-value
(i) General.	1,116.99	$-L_{GEN}$			
(ii) No major gene: completely polygenic.	1,129.24	$-L_{POL}$	12.25 $(L_{GEN} - L_{POL})$	3	$\langle 0.001$
(iii) Completely recessive: no environmental correlation between siblings ($d = 0$).	1,116.99	$-L_{REC}$	0.00 $(L_{GEN} - L_{REC})$	2	> 0.99
(iv) No polygenes ($H = 0$).	1,124.47	$-L_{MAJ}$	7.48 $(L_{GEN} - L_{MAJ})$	1	< 0.01

The authors results and conclusions were summarised as follows:

(a) The model with 'no major gene' is rejected; there is thus evidence that a major gene is responsible for the IgE levels.

(b) The hypothesis $H = 0$ ('no polygenes' model) is also rejected; there is evidence that the trait is also polygenic.

(c) The hypothesis $d = 0$ is accepted and they include that high IgE is recessive to low IgE.

used in the analysis of categorical traits as in the investigation of tongue pigmentation (Rao and Lew, 1978).

Both methods have advantages and disadvantages (Elston, 1979). To date, the mixed model can be used only to analyse data on parents and offspring or small pedigrees, whereas the Elston model can be used to analyse pedigrees of any size. The limitation in studying only nuclear families is that one is unlikely to be able to establish genetic heterogeneity (different models of inheritance in different families) with such data. The Elston model directly tests the goodness of fit to Mendelian transmission ratios and the conclusions are independent of the scale on which one considers the phenotype in the analysis. There is some concern that the latter may not be true in the case of the method of MacLean, Morton and Lew (Elston, 1979; Rao *et al.*, 1980), i.e. one might reach different conclusions on analysing the log of the phenotype rather than the phenotype itself. On the other hand, the Elston model does not distinguish between polygenic and single gene transmission (Elston, 1979). The analyses of data using the approach of MacLean, Morton and Lew include estimates of the ascertainment parameter, when necessary, whereas those using Elston's methods do not. However, modifications for including ascertainment probability for the case of a continuous variable have been derived (Elston and Sobel, 1979).

In summary, one should realize that there are several maximization procedures available for testing a major gene hypothesis. Using these procedures one can obtain estimates of gene frequency and the distribution of the phenotypes corresponding to each genotype. It should also be realized that, at present, each approach has its advantages and disadvantages. While one simultaneously considers both major gene and polygenic transmission, the other has the advantage that pedigree information can be used and it may be more powerful (Curnow and Smith, 1975). Both have proven useful models in the genetic analysis of diseases. It is very likely that in the near future computer software will be available such that neither approach will be limited.

4.6.3 Linkage studies

If one can show that a major disease (or phenotype) gene is linked to some known marker, then one has definitive evidence for the existence of the gene. Such information has been used to determine the genetics of haemochromatosis (Kravitz *et al.*, 1979) and to provide evidence for the genetic heterogeneity of elliptocytosis (Morton, 1956b). It is essential to know the linkage relationship of a disease with a known marker for antenatal diagnosis or genetic counselling. Thus, established linkages between myotonic dystrophy and ABH secretor (Harper *et al.*, 1971, 1972), between haemophilia and glucose-6-phosphate dehydrogenase C (Edgell *et al.*, 1978) and between HLA and 21-hydroxylase deficiency (Dupont *et al.*, 1977; Levine *et al.*, 1978; Weitkamp, Bryson and Bacon, 1978) can be used for these purposes.

Linkage studies are done by recording the information on the distribution of both the marker and the disease in families of affected individuals. In this situation, one is better off sampling families with several affected individuals (*multiplex families*) in order to obtain as much information about linkage as possible. There is probably no need to worry about a bias unless for some reason all of the isolated cases are due to another unlinked gene. There are several methods for detection of linkage between a marker and a phenotype (Maynard-Smith, Penrose and Smith, 1961, cite Fisher, 1935, Finney, 1940, and Haldane, and Smith, 1947, for some of the earliest investigations). Since that time, many methods have been proposed to detect linkage between a marker and a continuous phenotype (Elston, 1979, cites Haseman and Elston, 1972; Smith, 1975) and between a marker and a discontinuous type (Penrose, 1953; Day and Simons, 1976; and Suarez, Hodge and Reich, 1978). However, for both detecting linkage and estimating the recombination frequency, one usually uses the *lods score*, a sequential likelihood ratio procedure proposed by Morton (1956a). The hypothesis of no linkage is tested by computing the likelihood of each sibship under the hypothesis of no linkage, $L(0.5)$, and comparing it to the likelihood under the hypothesis of linkage with a recombination frequency equal to θ, $L(\theta)$), where θ is some value between 0.0 and 0.5.

Traditionally the logs to base 10 of these likelihood ratios are calculated for each sibship as it enters the sample for $\theta = 0.0, 0.1, 0.2, 0.3, 0.4, 0.5$ and added to any existing sub totals. This quantity is called the *lods score* ('lods' being a contraction of 'log odds') and is denoted $z(\theta)$. The criterion for linkage is an observed total value of the lods score greater than 3.0 for some value of the recombination frequency less than 0.5 (Morton, 1956b). Definitive evidence against linkage is an observed value of the minimum lods score less than -3.0. The value of θ at which the maximum lods score is observed is the ML estimate of the recombination frequency. One can also allow for unequal recombination frequencies in the two sexes (i.e. $\theta_M \neq \theta_F$) and obtain the corresponding lods score in this situation ($z(\theta_M, \theta_F)$). If this is significantly greater than the lods score assuming unequal recombination frequency (i.e. $-2.3\{z(\theta_M, \theta_F) - z(\theta)\} > 3.84$) and also greater than 3.0 then one would conclude that there is linkage and $\theta_M \neq \theta_F$.

In Box 4.6.1 we give the expression for the lod score corresponding to the situation in which we have an autosomal dominant disorder which we wish to test for linkage with a marker having two codominant alleles (**A** and **B**). We use, as our sample sibships, those in which one parent is an affected heterozygote at both loci and the other parent is normal and either homozygous at the marker locus or heterozygous for two other alleles. We also give the expression for the lods score in the case where the disease is recessive, both parents are unaffected and one is heterozygous at both loci. One can show that, in the case in which it is known whether the alleles are in coupling or repulsion, the value of the recombination frequency at which the lods score is maximized, $\hat{\theta}$, is the observed frequency of

Box 4.6.1 Expressions for the lods scores (Morton, 1956a) **which may be used for estimating the recombination frequency between** (a) **a rare autosomal dominant disorder and a known marker and** (b) **a rare autosomal recessive disorder and a known marker.**

(a) **Dominant disorder**

Consider a family in which we have an affected parent and an unaffected parent, where the affected parent is doubly heterozygous (**Gg**) for a dominant disorder and a codominant marker ($\mathbf{M_1 M_2}$). The other parent is a normal homozygote.

Let a be the number of offspring who are normal and inherit allele $\mathbf{M_1}$ from the doubly heterozygous parent,

      b be the number of offspring who are normal and inherit allele $\mathbf{M_2}$ from the doubly heterozygous parent,

      c be the number of offspring who are affected and inherit allele $\mathbf{M_1}$ from the doubly heterozygous parent,

      d be the number of offspring who are affected and inherit allele $\mathbf{M_2}$ from the doubly heterozygous parent,

and $s = a + b + c + d$, the sibship size.

Then, if the phase of the parent is not known, the likelihood of the sibship is

$$L(\theta) = \frac{s!}{a!b!c!d!}\left(\frac{1}{2}\right)^{s}\left[\tfrac{1}{2}\theta^{a+d}(1-\theta)^{b+c} + \tfrac{1}{2}\theta^{b+c}(1-\theta)^{a+d}\right], \qquad (4.6.1)$$

where θ is the recombination frequency. Substituting $\theta = 1/2$ into (4.6.1) we have

$$L(1/2) = \frac{s!}{a!b!c!d!}\left(\frac{1}{2}\right)^{2s-1} \qquad (4.6.2)$$

Thus the lods score in this situation, denoted $z_1(\theta)$ (Maynard-Smith, Penrose and Smith, 1961), is

$$z_1(\theta) = \log_{10}\left[\frac{L(\theta)}{L(1/2)}\right] \qquad (4.6.3)$$

$$= \log_{10}(2^{s-1}) + \log_{10}[\theta^{a+d}(1-\theta)^{b+c} + \theta^{b+c}(1-\theta)^{a+d}].$$

(b) **Recessive disorder**

Consider a family in which we have two unaffected parents and s offspring, of which $c + d$ are affected. Suppose the disorder is due to a recessive allele, **g**, and both parents are **Gg**. Suppose exactly one parent is heterozygous at the marker ($\mathbf{M_1 M_2}$). Let a, b, c, d and s be defined as for the dominant disorder.

Then the likelihood in this case is

$$L(\theta) = \frac{s!}{a!b!c!d!}\left(\frac{1}{4}\right)^s \left[\tfrac{1}{2}(2-\theta)^a(1+\theta)^b(\theta^c)(1-\theta)^d\right.$$

$$\left. + \tfrac{1}{2}(2-\theta)^b(1+\theta)^a(\theta^d)(1-\theta)^c\right]. \tag{4.6.4}$$

Assuming $\theta = 1/2$ we have

$$L(1/2) = \frac{s!}{a!b!c!d!}\left(\frac{3}{8}\right)^{a+b}\left(\frac{1}{8}\right)^{c+d}. \tag{4.6.5}$$

Thus the lods score is

$$z_2(\theta) = \log_{10}\left[\frac{L(\theta)}{L(1/2)}\right] = \log_{10}(2^{s-1}3^{-a-b})$$

$$+ \log_{10}[(2-\theta)^a(1+\theta)^b(\theta^c)(1-\theta)^d$$

$$+ (1+\theta)^a(2-\theta)^b(1-\theta)^c\theta^d] \tag{4.6.6}$$

known recombinants. Expressions for the lods score in several other situations have been derived and the scores have been tabulated for sibships of size 2 through 8 (Morton, 1956a; Maynard-Smith, Penrose and Smith, 1961). The lods score corresponding to data taken from several unrelated sibships is obtained by adding the scores obtained in each sibship. In Example 4.6.2 we present linkage analysis of HLA types and 21-hydroxylase deficiency reported by Weitkamp, Bryson and Bacon (1978) to confirm the observations first reported by Dupont *et al.* (1977).

Example 4.6.2 Linkage analysis of 21-hydroxylase deficiency to HLA-B (Weitkamp, Bryson and Bacon, 1978)

Weitkamp, Bryson and Bacon (1978) consider the families of Dupont *et al.* (1977) as well as three of their own to confirm linkage of HLA-B with 21-hydroxylase deficiency, a recessive autosomal trait. We consider, as an example, the data for Dupont's family 4. In terms of the notation in Box 4.6.1, the father has HLA haplotypes M_1 = Aw24, Bw35, Cw4 and M_2 = A29, B8, (Cw4). The mother's haplotypes are M_3 = A1, B8, (Cw6) and M_4 = A3, B7, Cw6. Two children are affected and are $M_1 M_3$. One is affected and are $M_1 M_4$. Since both parents are heterozygous at the marker locus, they calculate the lods score for $\theta = 0$ directly. The likelihood, assuming no linkage, is

$$L(0.5) = \frac{3!}{2!1!}\left(\frac{3}{16}\right)\left(\frac{1}{16}\right)^2,$$

and the likelihood assuming $\theta = 0$ for both males and females is

$$L(0.0) = \frac{3!}{2!1!}\left(\frac{1}{4}\right)^3\left(\frac{1}{4}\right).$$

Thus the lods score is

$$\log_{10}\frac{L(0.0)}{L(0.5)} = \log_{10}\frac{4^{-4}}{16^{-3}(3)} = \log_{10}\frac{16}{3} = 0.727.$$

On considering Dupont's five other families and their own three families they obtain a total lods score of 6.456 at $\theta = 0$, thus establishing linkage. They then obtain the following lods score for other low values of θ:

Total of lods scores for nine families:

θ	0.0	0.01	0.02	0.03	0.04	0.05
Lods score	6.456	6.272	6.086	5.902	5.718	5.533

They conclude that $\theta = 0.0$ is the maximum likelihood estimate of the recombination frequency.

While the lods score can easily be calculated through sampling unrelated sibships, more information is obtained through considering the distribution of two traits in several generations of a pedigree. Also, the expression for the hand computation of the lods score is quite straightforward in those situations in which only one parent is heterozygous for both traits. However, in the case in which both parents are heterozygous for the disease locus and heterozygous at a marker locus of a codominant trait (such as HLA), the computations must be done directly, as in Example 4.6.2. Renwick and Schultz (1961) devised a program for linkage analysis in these situations and it has been widely used (Harper *et al.*, 1972). There are many situations in which one cannot deduce one or both genotypes in the parents. In these cases the likelihoods of interest are functions of the frequencies of each allele at each locus. One might also want to do a linkage study for some disease which is age-dependent, for a disease which does not have full penetrance or for a disorder which has a continuum of phenotypes for which the mean and variance corresponding to each genotype are known. Finally, one might want to allow for differences in male and female recombination frequency. One of the major contributions to this area of linkage analysis has been the development of a computer program by Ott (1974). With this program one can obtain the values of the lods score for large or small pedigrees of varying complexity. One can consider diseases for which there is not full penetrance and continuous traits or incorporate information on gene frequency in situations where the parental genotypes are unknown. This program is readily available and well documented. It has been extensively used in many of the more recent linkage studies such as the study of the linkage of HLA with spino-cerebellar ataxia, (Jackson *et al.*, 1977), the study of the linkage of HLA with muscular dystrophy, (Tiwari *et al.*, 1980) and other studies in which several markers on different chromosomes are considered for each trait (Hamerton *et al.*, 1978).

Hodge *et al.* (1979) have modified Ott's program to compute lods scores for traits having age-dependent penetrance. One problem of these computer programs is that one needs to know, *a priori*, the mode of inheritance and all of the relevant genetic parameters. Kravitz *et al.* (1979) suggest correctly that the lods score should be obtained by first computing maximum likelihood estimates of all parameters (gene frequency, genotypic means and variances, or penetrance and recombination frequency) and then comparing this likelihood to the maximum likelihood obtained assuming that the recombination frequency is 0.5. Using this approach, they determined, through a linkage study with HLA, that haemochromatosis is recessive whereas the segregation analysis, ignoring HLA, had given ambiguous results as to the mode of inheritance of this disease.

Estimates of recombination frequencies observed in large families might be compared to test whether there are two modes of inheritance. Morton (1956b) suggested a test of heterogeneity of the lods scores and used it to determine genetic heterogeneity of elliptocytosis. This test might be done whenever one has the full lods score table for every family of interest. Another approach might be to determine the standard error of the estimate of recombination frequency using a method such as that suggested by Cavalli-Sforza and Bodmer (1971), which involves estimating the second derivative of the lods score when considered as a function of the recombination frequencies. This latter approach has the advantage that one need not save lods score tables and one can compare estimates by comparing the observed variance between estimates to the overall mean and standard error.

Keats *et al.* (1979) have indicated that cumulative lods scores, taken from many independent studies, provide information for establishing several new linkage relationships, for settling disputed linkages and for providing information on heterogeneity. Rao *et al.* (1979) have indicated how the information on lods scores obtained from several investigators might be combined to obtain a maximum likelihood estimate of recombination frequency. In doing so they apply their methods to obtain a map of chromosome 1.

N.R.M.
F.E.W.

A SHORT GLOSSARY OF TERMS

allele(s): the form(s) of gene that can exist at a locus.
ascertainment: the method by which a family is sought; the sampling scheme.

assortative mating: a mating system in which individuals tend to mate with those who have the same phenotype.

codominant allelles: two alleles which are both expressed in the heterozygous genotype; A_1 and A_2 are codominant if individuals having the genotype A_1A_2 have both the trait possessed by those who have genotype A_1A_1 and also the trait possessed by those who have genotype A_2A_2.

coefficient of kinship (between individuals): the probability that, at a given locus, an allele found in one individual will be identical, by descent, to the allele found in the other individual. Ignoring mutation, the coefficient of kinship between two individuals is equal to the inbreeding coefficient of their offspring.

consanguinity: having ancestors in common.

continuous trait: an attribute which is represented on some quantitative (rational number) scale (e.g. blood pressure, height, weight).

dominant: the extent to which the heterozygote resembles the homozygote; if A_1A_1 and A_1A_2 have identical phenotypes then A_1 is dominant over A_2.

drift: a change in the gene frequency in small populations which occurs due to the offspring generation being a small random sample and hence very likely to have a gene frequency which is quite different from that of the parental generation.

gamete: sperm or egg.

gene counting: a method for estimating the relative frequency of an allele when the genotypes of the individuals in the sample are known.

gene frequency: the relative frequency of an allele in the total population of all alleles.

genetic distance: a measure of genetic difference between populations based on the differences in allele frequencies at several loci.

genetic marker: a gene whose chromosomal location is known.

genotype: the two alleles that an individual has; if there are two alleles **A** and **a**, say, then the three genotypes are **AA**, **Aa** and **aa**.

haplotype: a particular set of alleles at several loci on a single chromosome; if loci for two genes are side by side on the same chromosome and the alleles are A_1 and A_2 for the first locus and B_1 and B_2 for the second, then possible haplotypes are A_1B_1, A_1B_2, A_2B_1 and A_2B_2.

heritability: the proportion of the variability in the phenotype due to variability in genotypes.

heterozygote (at a locus): Individuals carrying two different alleles at a particular locus; if there are three alleles A_1, A_2 and A_3, the heterozygotes are those with genotypes A_1A_2, A_1A_3 or A_2A_3.

HLA-A locus (-B locus; -C locus, etc.): a locus controlling leucocyte antigens of the A series (B series, C series).

homozygote: individuals carrying two alleles of the same type; if a locus has two alleles A_1 and A_2 then individuals homozygous for the gene have genotype A_1A_1 or A_2A_2.

inbreeding coefficient: the probability that, at a given locus, two alleles will be identical and that this identity results from the individual's parents having a common ancestor.

linkage: a measure of the extent to which the alleles at two loci segregate dependently; the occurrence of two loci on the same chromosome.

load: reduction in fitness through the genetic heterogeneity which results from mutation, segregation, recombination and selection where

$$\text{Load} = \frac{\text{maximum possible fitness} - \text{average fitness}}{\text{maximum possible fitness}}.$$

locus: the physical site on the chromosome at which a gene is located.

multifactorial: a phenotype which results from many genes and environmental factors.

mutation: a spontaneous change in an allele.

mutational load: decrease in fitness due to the mutation of alleles to forms where the resultant genotypes are less fit.

nuclear family: family defined by the parents and their offspring; immediate family.

penetrance: the relative frequency with which a person with a genotype manifests a phenotype.

phenotype: how the individual appears. This can be due to genotype and/or environment.

phenotype frequency: the relative frequency of individuals having a particular attribute.

proband: the person through whom a family (or pedigree) is obtained.

recessive: the extent to which the homozygote differs from the heterozygote; if genotypes A_1A_1 and A_1A_2 have identical phenotypes then A_2 is recessive to A_1.

relative risk: the ratio of the incidence of a disorder among individuals having some attribute to the incidence of the disorder among those who do not have the attribute.

segregation: the separation of a pair of alleles when the gametes are formed.

selective advantage (usually of a heterozygote): increase in fitness of individuals with a certain genotype relative to individuals having some other genotype.

trait: an attribute of interest; colour blindness, specificity to the HLA-A antigen and brown eyes are all traits.

transmission: the passing of an allele from one generation to the next.

REFERENCES

Aird, I., Bentall, H. H., and Roberts, J. A. F. (1953). A relationship between cancer of the stomach and the ABO groups, *Brit. Med. J.*, **1**, 799–801.

Allison, A. C. (1954). The distribution of the sickle cell trait in East Africa and elsewhere and its apparent relationship to incidence of subtertian malaria, *Trans. Roy. Soc. Tropi. Med. Hyg.*, **48**, 312–318.

Allison, A. C. (1964). Polymorphism and natural selection in human populations, *Cold Spring Harbor Symp. Quant. Biol.*, **24**, 137–149.

Batchelor, J. R., Morris, P. J., Walford, R. L., Dumble, L., Law, W., Kirk, R., and Case, J. (1973). Studies on HLA-A in a Fijian population, (Eds J. Dáusset and J. Columbani) in *Histocompatibility Testing* 1972, pp. 283–286, Munksgaard, Copenhagen.

Bear, J. C. (1976). A genetic study of facial clefting in Northern England, *Clin. Genet*, **9**, 277–284.

Bernstein, F. (1930). Fortgesetzte Untersuchungen aus der Theorie der Blutgruppen, *Z. Ind. Abst. Vereb. Lehre*, **56**, 233–273.

Boughman, J. A., Conneally, P. M., and Nance, W. (1980). Population genetics of retinitis pigmentosa, *Am. J. Hum. Genet.*, **32**, 223–235.

Brewerton, D. A., Caffrey, M., Hart, F. D., James, D. C. O., Nicholls, A., and Sturrock, R. D. (1973). Ankylosing spondylitis and HLA-B27, *Lancet*, **1**, 904.

Cavalli-Sforza, L. L., and Bodmer, W. F. (1971). *The Genetics of Human Populations*, W. H. Freeman and Company, San Francisco.

Chung, C. S., and Brown, K. S. (1970). Family studies of early childhood deafness ascertained through the Clarke School for the Deaf, *Am. J. Hum. Genet.*, **22**, 630–644.

Chung, C. S., Ching, G. H., and Morton, N. E. (1974). A genetic study of cleft lip and palate in Hawaii. II. Complex segregation analysis and genetic risks, *Am. J. Hum. Genet.*, **26**, 177–184.

Crittendon, L. B. (1961). An interpretation of familial aggregation based on multiple genetic and environmental factors, *Ann. NY Acad. Sci.*, **91**, 769–788.

Crosier, P. S., and Douglas, R. (1976). The distribution of HLA in a Polynesian population of Western Samoans, *Tissue Antigens*, **8**, 173–180.

Cross, H., Lerberg, D., and McKusick, V. (1968). Type II syndactyly, *Am. J. Hum. Genet.*, **20**, 368–380.

Crow, J. (1963). Problems of ascertainment in the analysis of family data, in *Symposium on Contributions of Genetics to Epidemiologic Studies of Chronic Disease* (Eds J. Neel, M. Shaw and W. Schull), pp. 23–44, US Dept. of HEW, Washington.

Cruden, D. (1949). The computation of inbreeding coefficients in closed populations, *J. Hered.*, **40**, 248–251.

Curnow, R. N., and Smith, C. (1975). Multifactorial models for familial disease in man, *J. Roy. Stat. Soc. A*, **138**(2), 131–169.

Danke, D. M., Allen, J., and Andersen, C. M. (1965). A genetic study of fibrocystic disease of the pancreas, *Ann. Hum. Genet.*, **28**, 323–356.

Dausset, J., Legrand, L., Levine, M., Quilici, J. C., Colombani, M., and Ruffie, J. (1972). Genetic distribution of HLA-A antigens in a Basque village, in *Histocompatibility Testing 1972* (Eds J. Dausset and J. Columbani), pp. 99–106, Munksgaard, Copenhagen.

Day, N. E., and Simons, M. J. (1976). Disease suseptibility genes—their identification by multiple case family studies, *Tissue Antigens*, **8**, 109–119.

de Vries, R. R. P., Meera Kahn, P. M., Bernini, L. F., van Loghen, E., and van Rood, J. J. (1979). Genetic control of survival in epidemics, *J. Immunogenetics*, **6**, 271–287.

Dodge, J. A. (1972). Infantile pyloric stenosis: A multifactorial condition, in *Proceedings of the Fourth Conference of the Clinical Delineation of Birth Defects Part XIII* (Ed. D. Bergsma), Williams and Wilkins, Baltimore.

Doherty, P. C., and Zinkernagel, R. M. (1975). A biological role for the major histocompatibility system, *Lancet*, **1**, 1406–1409.

Dupont, B., Oberfield, S. E., Smithwick, E. M., Lee, T. D., and Levine, L. S. (1977). Close genetic linkage between HLA and congenital adrenal hyperplasia (21-hydroxylase deficiency), *Lancet*, **2**, 1309–1317.

Edgell, J. S., Kirkman, J., Clemons, E., Buchanan, P. D., and Miller, C. H. (1978). Prenatal diagnosis by linkage. Hemophilia A and polymorphic glucose-6-phosphate dehydrogenase C, *Am. J. Hum. Genet.*, **30**, 80–84.

Edwards, J. H. (1969). Familial predisposition in man, *Brit. Med. Bull.*, **25**, 58–64.

Elston, R. C. (1979). Major locus analysis for quantitative traits, *Am. J. Hum. Genet.*, **31**, 655–661.

Elston, R. C., and Namboodiri, K. K. (1977). Family studies of schizophrenia, *Bull. Int. Stat. Inst.*, **XLVIII**, 683–697.

Elston, R. C., Namboodiri, K. K., Glueck, C. J., Fallat, R., Tsang, R., and Leuba, V. (1975). Study of the genetic transmission of hypercholesterolemia and hypertriglyceridemia in a 195 member kindred, *Ann. Hum. Genet.*, **39**, 67–87.

Elston, R. C., Namboodiri, K. K., and Hanes, C. G. (1979). Segregation and linkage analyses of dopamine-β-hydroxylase activity, *Hum. Hered.*, **29**, 284–292.

Elston, R. C., Namboodiri, K. K., Spence, M. A., and Rainer, J. D. (1978). A genetic study of schizophrenia pedigrees. II One locus hypotheses, *Neuropsychobiology*, **4**, 193–206.

Elston, R. C., and Rao, D. C. (1978). Statistical modeling and analysis in human genetics, *Ann. Rev. Biophys. Bioeng.*, **7**, 253–286.

Elston, R. C., and Sobel, E. (1979). Sampling considerations in the gathering and analysis of pedigree data, *Am. J. Hum. Genet.*, **31**, 62–69.

Elston, R. C., and Stewart, J. (1971). A general model for the genetic analysis of pedigree data, *Hum. Hered.*, **21**, 523–542.

Elston, R. C., and Yelverton, K. C. (1975). General models for segregation analysis, *Am. J. Hum. Genet.*, **27**, 31–45.

Emanuel, I., Culver, B., Erickson, D., Guthrie, B., and Schuldberg, D. (1973). The further epidemiological differentiation of cleft lip and palate: A population study of clefts in Kings County, Washington, 1956–1965, *Teratology*, **7**, 271–282.

Falconer, D. S. (1960). *Introduction to Quantitative Genetics*, Chap. 5, Oliver and Boyd, London.

Falconer, D. S. (1965). The inheritance of liability of certain diseases estimated from the incidence in relatives, *Ann. Hum. Genet.*, **29**, 51–76.

Falconer, D. S. (1967). The inheritance of liability to diseases with particular reference to diabetes mellitus, *Ann. Hum. Genet.*, **31**, 1–20.

Ferreira, E., Ward, F. E., and Amos, D. B. (1975). HLA in a Brazilian population evidence for new HLA specificities, in *Histocompatibility Testing* 1975 (Ed. F. Kissmeyer-Nielsen), pp. 226–232, Munksgaard, Copenhagen.

Fienberg, S. E. (1980). *The Analysis of Cross-Classified Categorical Data*, The MIT Press, Cambridge, Massachusetts.

Finney, D. J. (1940). The detection of linkage, *Ann. Eugen. Lon.*, **10**, 171.

Fischer, M. (1973). Genetic and environmental factors in schizophrenia: A study of schizophrenic twins and their families. *Acta Psychiatr. Scand. Supplement*, **238**, 1.

Fisher, R. A. (1918). The correlation between relatives on the supposition of Mendelian inheritance, *Trans. Roy. Soc. (Edinburgh)*, **52**, 399–433.

Fisher, R. A. (1934). The effect of methods of ascertainment upon the estimation of frequencies, *Ann. Eugen.*, **6**, 339–351.

Fisher, R. A. (1935). The detection of linkage with 'dominant' abnormalities, *Ann. Eugen. Lond.*, **6**, 187.

Fleiss, J. L. (1981). *Statistical Methods for Rates and Proportions*, Wiley, New York.

Gardner, E. J., and Plenk, H. P. (1951). Hereditary pattern for multiple osteomas in a family group, *Am. J. Hum. Genet.*, 167–176.

Gazit, E., Orgad, S., and Pras, M. (1977). HLA antigen in familial Mediterranean fever, *Tissue Antigens*, **9**, 273–275.

Gerrard, J. W., Rao, D. C., and Morton, N. E. (1978). A genetic study of immunoglobulin E, *Am. J. Hum. Genet.*, **30**, 46–58.

Gladstien, K., Lange, K., and Spence, M.A. (1978). A goodness of fit test for the polygenic threshold model, *Am. J. Med. Genet.*, **2**, 7–13.

Glass, B., and Li, C. C. (1953). The dynamics of racial admixture. An analysis based on the American Negro, *Am. J. Hum. Genet.*, **5**, 1–20.

Gleichmann, H. (1974). HLA phenotype and haplotype frequencies in a German population, *Tissue Antigens*, **4**, 157–165.

Haldane, J. B. S. (1956a). The estimation and the significance of the logarithm of a ratio of frequencies, *Ann. Hum. Genet.*, **20**, 309–311.

Haldane, J. B. S. (1956b). Almost unbiased estimates of function of frequencies, *Sankhya : Indian J. Stat.*, **17**, 201–208.

Haldane, J. B. S., and Smith, C. A. B. (1947). A new estimate for the linkage between the genes for haemophilia and colour blindness in man, *Ann. Eugen. Lond.*, **14**, 10.

Hamerton, J. L., Donald, L. J., et al. (Eds) (1978). *Human Gene Mapping*, Vol. 4, Karger, New York.

Hammond, M. G., Appadoo, B., and Brain, P. (1974). Subdivision of HLA-A5 and comparative studies of the HLA Polymorphism in South African Indians, *Tissue Antigens*, **4**, 42–49.

Hammond, M. G., Appadoo, B., and Brain, P. (1977). HLA and Cancer in South African Negroes, *Tissue Antigens*, **9**, 1–7.

Hansen, R. G., Bretthauer, R. K., Mayes, J., and Nordin, J. H. (1964). Estimation of frequency of occurrence of galactosemia in the population, *Proc. Soc. Exper. Biol. Med.*, **115**, 560–563.

Hardy, G. H. (1908). Mendelian proportions in a mixed population, *Science*, **28**, 49–50.

Harper, P. S., Bias, W. B., Hutchinson, J. R., et al. (1971). ABH secretor status of the fetus; a genetic marker identifiable by amniocentesis, *J. Med. Genet.*, **8**, 438–440.

Harper, P. S., Rivas, M. L., Bias, W. B., Hutchinson, J. R., Dyken, P. R., and McKusick, V. A. (1972). ABH secretor status of the fetus: genetic linkage confirmed between the locus for myotonic dystrophy and the ABH secretion and Lutheran blood group loci, *Am. J. Hum. Genet.*, **24**, 310–316.

Harvald, B., and Hauge, M. (1965). Hereditary factors elucidated by twin studies, in *Genetics and Epidemiology of Chronic Diseases* (Eds J. V. Neel, M. W. Shaw, and W. S. Schull), Public Health Serv. Publication no. 1163, Washington.

Haseman, J. K., and Elston, R. C. (1972). The investigation of linkage between a quantitative trait and a marker locus. *Behav. Genet.*, **2**, 3–19.

Hay, S., and Wehrung, D. (1970). Congenital malformations in twins, *Am. J. Hum. Genet.*, **22**(6), 662–668.

Hodge, S. E., Morton, L. A., Tideman, S., Kidd, K. K., and Spence, M. A. (1979). Age of onset correction available for linkage analysis (letter), *Am. J. Hum. Genet.*, **31**(6), 761.

Huether, Carl A., and Murphy, E. A. (1980). Reduction of bias in estimating the frequency of recessive genes, *Am. J. Hum. Genet.*, **32**, 212–222.

Ivanyi, P., Ivanyi, D., and Zemak, P. (1977). HLA Cw4 in paranoid schizophrenia, *Tissue Antigens*, **9**, 41–44.

Jackson, J. F., Currier, R. D., Terasaki, P. I., and Morton, N. (1977). Spinocerebellar ataxia and HLA linkage, *N. Eng. J. Med.*, **296**, 1138–1141.

Kaplan, E. B., and Elston, R. C. (1972). A subroutine package for maximum likelihood estimation, University of North Carolina Inst. Stat. Mimeo Series no. 823.

Kaplan, E. B., and Elston, R. C. (1975). GENPED: a general pedigree analysis package (unpubl. program writeup).

Kastelan, A., Brkljacic, Kerhin, Hors, J., Brkljačić, L., and Macasovic, P. (1974). The distribution of HLA antigens and genes in the Yugoslav population, *Tissue Antigens*, **4**, 69–75.

Keats, B. J. B., Morton, N. E., Rao, D. C., and Williams, W. R. (1979). *A Source Book for*

Linkage in Man, Johns Hopkins University Press, Baltimore.

Kidd, K. K., and Ceppellini, R. (1977). A Bayesian method for estimation of HLA-associated illness susceptibility (Is) allele frequencies I. Dominant susceptibility, in HLA and Disease (Eds J. Dausset and A. Svejgaard), pp. 81–83, Munksgaard, Denmark.

Kidd, K. K., and Spence, M.A. (1976). Genetic analysis of pyloric stenosis suggesting a specific maternal effect, J. Med. Genet., 13, 290–294.

Kimura, M. (1961). Some calculations on the genetic load, Jap, J. Genet., 36 (Suppl.), 179–190.

Kokko, U. P. (1940). Weitere Beitrage zur finnischen Blutgruppen Forschung unter Berücksichtigung der M, N und MN Blutgruppen, Acta. Soc. Med. Duodecim SA, 22, 56–62.

Kravitz, K., Skolnick, M., Cannings, C., et al. (1979). Genetic linkage between hereditary hemochomatosis and HLA, Am. J. Hum. Genet., 31, 601–619.

Kreisler, M., Arnaiz, A., Perez, B., Fernandez Cruz, E., and Bootello, A. (1974). HLA antigens in leprosy, Tissue Antigens, 4, 197–201.

Kruger, J. (1973). Discrimination between multifactorial inheritance with threshold characters effect and two allele single locus hypothesis, Humangenetik, 17, 181.

Levine, L., Zachmann, M., New, M., Prader, A., Pollock, M., O'Neill, G. J., Yang, S. Y., Oberfield, S. E., and Dupont, B. (1978). Genetic mapping of the 21-hydroxylase deficiency gene within the HL-A linkage group, New England J. Med., 299 (17), 911–914.

Li, C. C. (1976). First Course in Population Genetics, pp. 21–22, Boxwood Press, Pacific Grove, California.

Li, C. C., and Horvitz, D. G. (1953). Some methods of estimating the inbreeding coefficient, Am. J. Hum. Genet., 5, 107–117.

Li, C. C., and Mantel, N. (1968). A simple method of estimating the segregation ratio under complete ascertainment, Am. J. Hum. Genet., 20, 61–81.

Loesch, D. (1971). Genetics of dermatologlyphic patterns on palms, Ann. Hum. Genet. Lond., 34, 277–293.

Lynch, H., Lynch, J., and Guirgas., H. (1976). Heredity and colon cancer, in Cancer Genetics (Ed. H. Lynch), pp. 327–354, Charles Thomas, Springfield, Illinois.

McDevitt, H. O., and Bodmer, W. F. (1974). HLA, immune response and genes and disease, Lancet, 1, 1269–1275.

McKusick, V. A. (Ed.) (1978). Medical Genetic Studies of the Amish, p. 66, Johns Hopkins University Press, Baltimore.

MacLean, C. J., Morton, N. E., and Lew, R. (1975). Analysis of family resemblance. IV. Operational characteristics of segregation analysis, Am. J. Hum. Genet., 27, 365–384.

McMichael, A. J. and DeWitt, H. (1977). The association between the HLA system and disease, Prog. Med. Genet (New Series), 2, 39–100.

MacQueen, J. M., Ottesen, E. A., Weller, P. F., Ottesen, C., Amos, D. B., and Ward, F. E. (1979). HLA histocompatibility antigens in a Polynesian population-Cook Islanders of Mauke, Tissue Antigens, 13, 121–128.

Mange, Arthur P. (1964). Fortran programs for computing Wright's coefficient of inbreeding in human and nonhuman pedigrees, Am. J. Hum. Genet., 4, 484.

Mattiuz, P. L., Ihde, D., Piazza, R., Ceppellini, R., and Bodmer, W. F. (1970). New approaches to the population genetic and segregation analysis of the HLA system, in Histocompatibility Testing, 1970 (Ed. P. Terasaki), pp. 197–203, Williams and Wilkins Company, Baltimore.

Maynard-Smith, S., Penrose, L. S., and Smith, C. A. B. (1961). Mathematical Tables for Research Workers in Human Genetics, Little, Brown and Company, Boston.

Melnick, M., Bixler, D., Fogh-Andersen, P., and Conneally, P. M. (1980). Cleft Lip ± cleft palate: an overview of the literature and an analysis of Danish cases born between 1941 and 1968, Am. J. Med. Genet., 6(1), 83–98.

Mendell, N. R., Blumenthal, M. N., Amos, D. B., Yunis, E. J., and Elston, R. C. (1978). Ragweed sensitivity: segregation analysis and linkage to HLA-B, *Cytogenet. Cell Genet.*, **22**, 330–334.

Mendell, N. R., and Elston, R. C. (1974). Multifactorial qualitative traits: genetic analysis and prediction of recurrence risks, *Biometrics*, **30**, 41–57.

Mendell, N. R., and Spence, M. A. (1979). Empiric recurrence risks and models of inheritance: Part I, *Birth Def. Orig. Art. Series*, **XV:5c**, 39–49.

Mendell, N. R., Spence, M. A., Gladstein, K., Brunette, J., Georgiade, N., Pickrell, K. L., Serafin, D., and Quinn, G. W. (1980). Multifactorial/threshold models and their application to cleft lip and cleft palate, in *The Etiology of Cleft Lip and Cleft Palate: Proceedings of an NIDR Workshop* (Eds M. Melnick *et al.*), Alan R. Liss, New York.

Mi, M. P. (1966). Segregation analysis, *Am. J. Hum. Genet.*, **19**, 313–321.

Moreno, M. E., and Kreisler, J. M. (1977). HLA phenotype and haplotype frequencies in a sample of the Spanish population. *Tissue Antigens*, **9**, 105–110.

Morton, N. E. (1956a). Sequential tests for the detection of linkage, *Am. J. Hum. Genet.*, 277–318.

Morton, N. E. (1956b). The detection and estimation of linkage between genes for elliptocytosis and the Rh blood type, *Am. J. Hum. Genet.*, **8**, 80–96.

Morton, N. E. (1959). Genetic tests under incomplete ascertainment, *Am. J. Hum. Genet.*, **11**(1), 1–16.

Morton, N. E. (1962). Segregation analysis and linkage, in *Methodology in Human Genetics* (Ed. W. J. Burdette), pp. 17–52, Holden Day, San Francisco.

Morton, N. E. (1969). Segregation analysis, in *Computer Applications in Genetics* (Ed. N. E. Morton), pp. 129–140, University of Hawaii Press, Honolulu.

Morton, N. E., and MacLean, C. J. (1974). Analysis of family resemblance. III. Complex segregation of quantitative traits, *Am. J. Hum. Genet.*, **26**, 489–503.

Mourant, A. E., Kopic, A. C., and Domanieluska-Solezak, K. (1976). *The Distribution of the Human Blood Groups and Other Polymorphisms*, Oxford University Press.

Myrianthopoulos, N. C., and Aronson, S. (1966). Population dynamics of Tay Sachs disease I. Reproductive fitness and selection, *Am. J. Hum. Genet.*, **18**, 313–328.

Myrianthopoulos, N. C., and Leyshon, W. (1967). The relationship of blood groups and the secretor factor to amyotrophic lateral sclerosis, *Am. J. Hum. Genet.*, **19**(5), 607–616.

Nerup, J., Cathelinean, C., Seignalet, J., and Thomsen, M. (1977). HLA and endocrine diseases, in *HLA and Disease* (Eds. J. Dausset and A. Svejgaard), pp. 149–167, Munksgaard, Copenhagen.

Ott, J. (1974). Estimation of the recombination fraction in human pedigrees; efficient computation of the likelihood for human linkage studies, *Am. J. Hum. Genet.*, **26**, 588–597.

Penrose, L. S. (1953). The general purpose sib pair linkage test, *Ann. Eugen (Lond.)*, **18**, 120–124.

Pikkarainen, T., Takkunen, J., and Kulonen, E. (1966). Serum cholesterol in Finnish twins, *Am. J. Hum. Genet.*, **18**(2), 115–126.

Rao, D. C., Keats, B. J., Lalouel, J. M., Morton, N. E., and Yee, S. (1979). A maximum likelihood map of chromosome 1, *Am. J. Hum. Genet.*, **31**, 680–696.

Rao, D. C., and Lew, R. (1978). Complex segregation analysis of tongue pigmentation. A search for residual family resemblance, *Hum. Hered.*, **28**, 317–320.

Rao, D. C., Lalovel, J. M., Morton, N. E., and Gerrard, J. W. (1980). Immunoglobulin E revisited, *Am. J. Hum. Genet*, **32**, 620–625.

Rao, D. C., MacLean, C. J., Morton, N. E., and Yee, S. (1975). Analysis of family resemblance V. Height and weight in Northeastern Brazil, *Am. J. Hum. Genet.*, **27**, 509–520.

Reed, T. E. (1969). Caucasian genes in American Negroes, *Science*, **165**, 762–768.

Reich, T., James, J. W., and Morris, C. A. (1972). The use of multiple thresholds in determining the mode of transmission of semicontinuous traits, *Ann. Hum. Genet.*, **36**, 163–184.

Renwick, J. H., and Schultz, J. (1961). A computer programme for the processing of linkage data from large pedigrees (abst), Excerpta Med. Internat. Congr. Series no. 30 E145.

Roychoudhury, A. K. (1978). Genetic distance between the American Indians and three major races in Man, *Hum. Hered.*, **28**, 380–385.

Ruderman, R. J., and Ward, F. E. (1977). HLA-B27 in Black patients with ankylosing spondylitis, *Lancet*, **1**(8011), 610.

Ryder, L. P., Anderson, E., and Svejgaard, A. (1978). An HLA map of Europe, *Hum. Hered.*, **28**, 171–200.

Sadovnick, A. D., Spence, M.A., and Tideman, S. (1980). A goodness of fit test for the polygenic threshold model: application to multiple sclerosis, Unpublished manuscript.

Schull, W. J. and Neel, J. V. (1970). The effect of parental consanguinity and inbreeding in Hirado, Japan. V. Summary and interpretation, *Am. J. Hum. Genet.*, **22**, 239–262.

Shields, J. (1962). *Monozygotic Twins Brought up Apart and Brought up Together*, Oxford University Press, London.

Siervogel, R. M.; Elston, R. C.; Lester, R. H. and Graham, J. B.: Major gene analysis of quantitatic variation in blood clotting Factor X levels, *Am. J. Hum. Genet.* **31**, 199–213.

Sievers, O. (1931). Die Verteilung der Blutgruppen in der Schwedisch spechen den Bevolkerung Finnlands (in Finnish), *Finska LakSallsk Handl.*, **73**, 960–969.

Simpson, N. E. (1969). Heritabilities of liability to diabetes when sex and age of onset are considered, *Ann. Hum. Genet.*, **32**, 283–303.

Smith, C. (1970). Heritability of liability and concordance in monozygotic twins, *Ann. Hum. Genet.*, **34**, 85–91.

Smith, C. (1971). Discrimination between different modes of inheritance in genetic disease, *Clin. Genet.*, **2**, 303–314.

Smith, C. A. B. (1975). A non-parametric test for linkage with a quantitative marker, *Ann. Hum. Genet.*, **38**, 451–460.

Smouse, P. E. (1979). Statistical analysis of HLA disease associations, *Prog. Clin. Biol. Res.*, **32**, 545–551.

Spence, M.A., Elston, R. C., and Cedarbaum, S. D. (1974). Pedigree analysis to determine the mode of inheritance in a family with retinitis pigmentosa, *Clin. Genet.*, **5**, 338–343.

Suarez, B., Hodge, S., and Reich, T. (1978). A robust method for the detection of linkage in familial diseases, *Am. J. Hum. Genet.*, **30**, 308–321.

Sutton, H. E. (1975). *An Introduction to Human Genetics*, Chap. 17, Holt, Rinehart, and Winston, New York.

Svejgaard, A., and Ryder, L. (1977). HLA and disease, in *HLA System : New Aspects* (Ed. G. B. Ferrara), pp. 143–152, Elsevier, North-Holland Biomedical Press.

Svejgaard, A., and Ryder, L. (1977). Notes on methodology and a report from the HLA and disease registry, in *HLA and Disease* (Eds. J. Dausset and A. Svejgaard), pp. 46–53, Munksgaard, Copenhagen.

Thomson, G., and Bodmer, W. (1977). The genetic analysis of HLA and disease associations, in *HLA and Disease* (Eds J. Dausset and A. Svejgaard), pp. 84–93, Williams and Wilkins, Baltimore.

Tiwari, T., Hodge, S., Terasaki, P., and Spence, M. A. (1980). HLA and the inheritance of multiple sclerosis; linkage analysis of 72 pedigrees, *Am. J. Hum. Genet.*, **32**, 103–111.

van Rood, J. J., and van Leeuwen, A. (1965). Defined leukocyte antigenic groups in man, in *Histocompatibility Testing* (Eds. P. C. Russell, H. J. Winn and D. B. Amos), p. 21, Publication 1229, National Academy of Sciences, National Research Council, Washington, DC.

Vogel, F., and Motulsky, A. G. (1979). *Human Genetics Problems and Approaches*, Springer-Verlag, New York.

Walford, R. L., Smith, G. S., and Waters, H. (1971). Histocompatibility systems and disease states with particular reference to cancer, *Transplant. Rev.*, **7**, 78–109.

Ward, F. E. (1975). Histocompatibility antigens in a North American Black population, in *Histocompatibility Testing 1975* (Ed. F. Kissmeyer-Nielsen), pp. 195–204, Munksgaard, Copenhagen.

Ward, F. E., Bias, W. B., Reisner, E. G., and Amos, D. B. (1972). HLA specificities among Old Order Amish—a genetic isolate, in *Histocompatibility Testing 1972* (Eds J. Dausset and J. Colombani), pp. 93–98, Munksgaard, Copenhagen.

Ward, F. E., and Biegel, A. (1976). HLA antigens in North American Black families, *Am. J. Hum. Genet.*, **28**, 1–8.

Weinberg, W. (1908); Uber den Nachweis der Vererbung bein Menschen, *Jahreshefte des Vereins für vaterlandische Naturkunde in Wurttemburg*, **64**, 368–382.

Weinberg, W. (1927). Mathematische Grundlagen der Probanden-Methode, *Z. Ind. Abst. Vereb. Lehre*, **48**, 179–228.

Weitkamp, L. R., Bryson, M., and Bacon, G. E. (1978). HLA and congenital adrenal hyperplasia linkage confirmed, *Lancet*, **1** (8070), 931–932.

Woolf, C. M., Woolf, R. M., and Broadbent, T. R. (1963). A genetic study of cleft lip and cleft palate in Utah, *Am. J. Hum. Genet.*, **15**, 209–215.

Woolf, C. M., Koehn, J., and Coleman, S. (1968). Congenital hip disease in Utah: the influence of genetic and nongenetic factors. *Am. J. Hum. Genet.*, **20**, 430–439.

Woolf, C. M. (1971). Congenital cleft lip: a genetic study of 496 propositii, *J. Med. Genet.*, **8**, 65–83.

5

Biological Signal Processing

5.1 INTRODUCTION

The techniques of biological signal processing have as their main objective the separation of information which is of use from that which is not. Signal processing techniques make use of the redundancy in the raw data to reduce the effects of noise and confounding mechanisms which are of no interest to the observer. The term redundancy is used here to indicate an excess of informatiin over and above that needed to convey the features of interest.

The information extracted from raw data by signal processing techniques may be useful in making scientific inferences about the nature of the observed biological systems. It may also be clinically useful in reaching diagnostic and therapeutic decisions (Figure 5.1.1).

Signals are often measured in association with an external perturbation or driving force, usually under the control of the observer, where they may be considered as responses to known inputs to the system. Two common properties of signals which are frequently exploited in signal processing techniques are correlation with some other measured phenomenon and the presence in the signal of repetitive or periodic features.

At the same time, the data of interest may be obscured because of variability in the signal, which may stem from various sources. These may be classified in terms of *inter-subject* variability due to genetic make-up, accumulated environmental

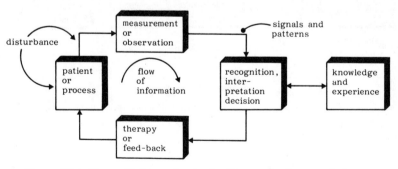

Figure 5.1.1 Flow of information in the diagnostic–therapeutic loop.

influences, age and disease and *intra-subject* variability in time. Reasons for intra-subject variability include *noise*, such as thermal, background, biological and measurement noise; *concurrent processes*, such as the electrical activity of the heart when measuring the electroencephalogram (EEG) or the effect of respiration when measuring the electrocardiogram (ECG); *non-stationary processes*, such as alterations in homeostatic mechanisms under changing environmental influences.

Signal processing may be described in terms of three stages:

(a) *Measurement*, where signals are recorded and observations made;
(b) *Signal transformation*, where known properties of the signals are used to reduce the variability and facilitate analysis;
(c) *Feature extraction and classification* (or interpretation), where key features of the transformed signal are extracted and used to make a decision, such as the recognition of a pattern or diagnostic classification.

As indicated in Figure 5.1.2, there is a strong resemblance between these stages of signal processing and the processes used in pattern recognition techniques. With the advent of cheap microprocessor systems it is becoming increasingly possible to use on-line data acquisition and to integrate the three stages, such as in systems for automated ECG interpretation.

There is no standard method or approach to problems in biological signal processing. It is, rather, a craft which makes use of methods having a rigorous mathematical basis but whose application rests largely on heuristic justification. The signals that we deal with in this chapter are variables in one or more dimensions (scalars or vectors) as functions of time, space, frequency or independent parameters. Such signals can all be considered as time series [see VI, Chapter 18]. We will discuss the different types we may encounter, the superimposed noise and more or less standard processing techniques.

Signals, biological or not, can be divided into *deterministic* and *stochastic*

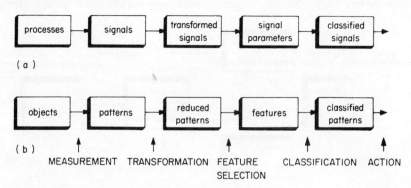

Figure 5.1.2 Stages in (a) signal processing and (b) pattern recognition.

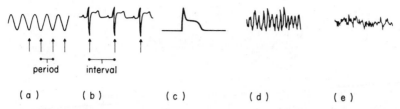

Figure 5.1.3 Types of biological signals: (a) to (c) are deterministic and (d) and (e) are stochastic signals. (a) Sine wave, periodic; (b) ECG, quasi-periodic; (c) cell response, transient; (d) alpha-waves in EEG, stationary; (e) EMG, non-stationary.

signals. With respect to amplitude, we can categorize them as, on the one hand, *analogue* and, on the other hand, discrete or *digital* signals. Another aspect to be taken into account is whether or not the signals are sampled (not necessarily periodically). One category of signals consists of *point processes*, for which it is not the signal shape but the occurrence of a certain event in time that is relevant [see II, Chapter 20]. Deterministic signals may be subdivided into *periodic* signals and *transients*. In Figure 5.1.3 we illustrate these groups of signals with some examples. For instance, the occurrence of the R-wave peak in an ECG can be indicated by a specific point in time, indicating a special event in the biological process. A series of such points in time can be described by a point process, represented by a two-valued series of impulses (known as *Dirac impulses*; see below) where the amplitude is always zero except for the short intervals ε where the events occur.

For a Dirac impulse, we normally define the product of impulse amplitude A and its duration ε in such a way that $A\varepsilon = 1$. In the case of digital processing, we frequently take $A = 1$. We may then represent the point process by a true binary signal, which can be completely represented by the inter-pulse distances.

Many quasi-periodic analogue signals can be reduced to a single *waveshape*, from a very large and repetitive series of events in the recorded waveform, and a point process which 'generates' the signal from this waveshape. We give the mathematical formulation of this concept in the Appendix, when dealing with convolution. Figure 5.1.4 gives an example of a point process derived from an ECG.

We should bear in mind that the biological signals or patterns are the carriers

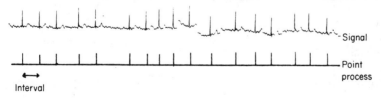

Figure 5.1.4 Point process derived from a continuous (analogue) ECG.

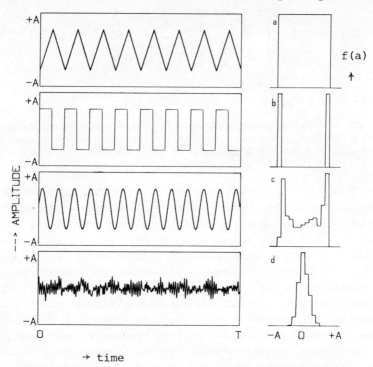

Figure 5.1.5 Signals and amplitude density distribution functions, $f(a)$: (a) triangular signal (uniform distribution); (b) square wave (binary distribution); (c) sine wave (sinusoidal distribution); (d) electroencephalogram (normal distribution). The effect of quantization (see the Appendix) and finite duration is seen in (c) and (d).

Table 5.1.1 Examples of well-known probability density functions, $f(a)$, as illustrated in Figure 5.1.5.

Uniform distribution	$\dfrac{1}{2A}$ if $|a| < A$; 0 elsewhere
Binary distribution	$\tfrac{1}{2}\delta(A - |a|)$ with $\delta(x) = \begin{cases} 1, & x = 0, \\ 0, & x \neq 0 \end{cases}$
Sinusoidal distribution	$\dfrac{1}{\pi\sqrt{A^2 - a^2}}$ if $|a| < A$; 0 elsewhere
Normal distribution	$\dfrac{1}{\sigma\sqrt{2\pi}}$ $\exp\!\left(\dfrac{-a^2}{2\sigma^2}\right)$ where σ is the standard deviation

of the information and that the relevant (semantic) parameters still have to be extracted from them. This means that all operations oriented towards the reduction of data must at the same time also enhance the information content. Such signals can only be obtained by using the correct transducers or sensors, such as electrodes (ECG, EEG, electromyogram — EMG), microphones (phono-cardiogram), crystals (ultrasonic waves), pressure transducers (blood pressure), strain gauges (respiration), electromagnetic coils (blood flow), etc.. This stage is of the utmost importance; everything possible must be done to minimize all disturbing factors during the recording stage, since the information can only tend to be degraded during the further processing.

If we have a deterministic signal with a known waveshape, we have no need to analyse its amplitude properties other than as a function of its independent variable such as time. In these cases the 'behaviour' of the signal as a function of time tells us enough about the state of the process. The response of a cell to a stimulus is an example of such a waveshape. On the other hand, if we have no deterministic waveshape, e.g. if we are dealing with a stochastic signal, we can only describe the amplitude properties in statistical terms. Well-known ampli-tude probability density functions (p.d.f.) are, for instance, those for triangular, rectangular, sinusoidal and Gaussian waveforms [see II, §§10.2 and 11.4.3] (Figure 5.1.5 and Table 5.1.1).

The main mathematical results used in signal processing are summarized in the Appendix to this chapter. More detailed treatments can be found in the appropriate Core Volumes, or in the general reference books such as those by Gold and Rader (1969), Bendat and Piersol (1971), Rabiner and Rader (1972), Beauchamp (1973), Rabiner and Gold (1975) or Schwartz and Shaw (1975).

5.2 EVENT AND BOUNDARY DETECTION

In many instances biological processes deliver (quasi-) periodic signals with more or less repetitive waveforms. In the case of an ECG, a blood pressure or a respiration signal, for example, the events that cause the generation of the signal can be represented by an impulse series, whereas the repetitive signal can be described by a wave contour. Knowledge about this waveshape eases the detection of the events, and knowledge about the time instants facilitates the computation of the waveshape. In real life, we do not know either the time instants or the waveshapes beforehand. Van Trees (1971) and Schwartz and Shaw (1975) give detailed discussions of the detection of events. The detection is usually an iterative process; first, a rough location of the time instants of the events using a general detection scheme; then a rough estimation of the waveshape; thereafter, a refined location of the event, followed by a better shape determination. Figure 5.2.1 shows a processing scheme where we have a so-called strong coupling between event and wave information, the ideal situation for detection. In practice, we try to reach this situation gradually by first gathering

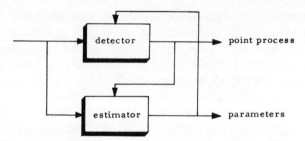

Figure 5.2.1 Strong coupling between signal detection
and estimation.

general information about the process and the signals it generates and later individual knowledge about a specific signal.

The signal detection problem is very similar to that of classification (the discrimination between the presence or absence of diseases or patterns). Here, too, we make use of feedback and training for tuning classifiers to a specific problem.

We first consider the detection problem from the point of view of statistical detection theory (see Section 1.2.8) and therefore briefly discuss Bayes' theorem [see II, §16.4, and VI, §15.2] for a two-class detector. As is well known, Bayes' theorem also plays an important role in medical decision-making (see Chapter 3 of this Guidebook).

5.2.1 Bayes' theorem for a two-class detector

Assume we have a signal $x(t)$ consisting of a waveform of known waveshape $s_1(t)$ and duration T, buried in noise. By means of one of the filtering schemes mentioned in the Appendix to this chapter, we enhance the signal to noise ratio (SNR) as much as we can. We do not know the instants of occurrence of the waveshape. During some observation interval T we have to decide whether $s_1(t)$ was present (decision D_1) or not (D_0).

First, we define probabilities $p(s_1)$, the *prior probability* that s_1 is present, and $p(s_0)$, the prior probability that s_1 is *not* present (or s_0 is present), where

$$p(s_1) + p(s_0) = 1. \tag{5.2.1}$$

Now we have four possible situations which form the *decision matrix*:

CP (correct positive)—decision D_1 is correctly made because s_1 was present,

CN (correct negative)—correct decision D_0 that s_1 was absent (or s_0 present),

FN (false negative)—incorrect decision D_0 that s_1 was absent,

FP (false positive)—incorrect decision D_1 that s_1 was present, also called a 'false alarm' in RADAR terminology.

The *joint probability* of s_1 and a certain signal x may be written as

$$p(s_1, x) = p(s_1)p(x|s_1) = p(x)p(s_1|x) \qquad (5.2.2)$$

[see II, Definition 6.5.1]. In words, the probability that the observed signal x was generated by the waveshape s_1 is equal to the prior probability of s_1 multiplied by the conditional probability of x, given the presence of s_1, or to the prior probability of x multiplied by the conditional probability of s_1, given x. Similarly,

$$p(s_0, x) = p(s_0)p(x|s_0) = p(x)p(s_0|x). \qquad (5.2.3)$$

In most instances, however, we observe x and then have to decide whether s_1 is present. The corresponding *a posteriori probabilities* are $p(s_1|x)$ and $p(s_0|x)$.

From (5.2.2) and (5.2.3) we can write

$$p(s_1|x) = \frac{1}{p(x)}p(s_1)p(x|s_1), \qquad (5.2.4)$$

$$p(s_0|x) = 1 - p(s_1|x) = \frac{1}{p(x)}p(s_0)p(x|s_0). \qquad (5.2.5)$$

From these equations it can easily be derived that

$$p(s_1|x) = \left[1 + \frac{p(s_0)}{p(s_1)}\frac{1}{l(x)}\right]^{-1}, \qquad (5.2.6)$$

where $l(x)$ is the likelihood ratio of $x(t)$ given by

$$l(x) = \frac{p(x|s_1)}{p(x|s_0)}. \qquad (5.2.7)$$

(see Section 1.2.8). Since $l(x)$ is the ratio of two probabilities, we know that $0 \le l(x) < \infty$. In practice we often compute only $l(x)$ or its logarithm [see I, §3.6] instead of the entire expression (5.2.6) and compare $l(x)$ with a threshold value λ. If then, for instance, $l(x) \ge \lambda$, we take the decision D_1, otherwise D_0.

In processing biological signals, one does not very often need to apply Bayes' theorem in this way since frequently one can make use of prior knowledge other than of the signal waveshape, such as the periodicity of the waveform. Nevertheless, the derived formulae do indicate that, in order to decide on the presence or absence of a signal, we have to decide about prior probabilities as such. In practice, we frequently use them in an 'on/off' mode, e.g. in applying a *dead time zone* after having detected a QRS complex in an ECG or applying a *detection window* in searching for the dichrotic notch in an aortic pressure wave. Very often, however, and here again is a parallel with pattern recognition, we devise heuristic and specific alogrithms for the problem at hand. Such specific approaches will be exemplified in the next sections. We will illustrate the detection of P-waves in an ECG, onsets and end-points of waves, and dichrotic notches in arterial pressure waves.

5.2.2 Detection of small P-waves

Our first example is the detection of a *P*-wave in a routine ECG (Hengeveld and van Bemmel, 1976). P-waves are small compared with the QRS complex and of the order of 100 μV or less, whereas the noise in the bandwidth of the ECG (0.10 to 150 Hz) may vary from below 10 to 100 μV or more. However, the frequency of the P-wave itself lies far below this upper limit, between 0.10 and about 8 Hz P-waves may be coupled to QRS-complexes; they commonly occur with a repetition rate lower than 200 per minute. The P-wave duration is about 60 to 100 msec, whereas the range of PR-intervals, in the case of coupling between SA and AV nodes, is less than 30 msec.

The processing of biological signals may require a great deal of computer time—sometimes too much if it is to be done in real-time—unless we make use of data reduction methods and compact algorithms to speed up the analysis. It may be necessary to make a compromise between what is theoretically desirable and what is practically achievable. The detection of P-waves is a representative illustration of such techniques.

First of all, we must discriminate between coupled and non-coupled P-waves. This is important, since regular sinus rhythms are seen in more than 90 per cent of all patients. The detection of non-coupled P-waves requires much more prior knowledge and considerably more computational effort.

The following processing stages are involved in the detection.

(a) Location of signal parts, windows

To enhance the conditional probabilities of finding P-waves, we only search in the regions between the beginning of a QRS-complex and the end of the T-wave of a preceding ECG complex. First of all, the QRS-complexes are detected (for details see van Bemmel, 1982) and a rough indication of the point of QRS onset is computed. The end of the T-wave is either found by a regression formula, based upon the RR-interval, or determined by an algorithm similar to the one discussed in Section 5.2.3 for QRS onset and end-point.

(b) Filtering

After determination of the search interval for detection of the P-waves, the QRS signal following this window is replaced by the value of the last sample point of the P-wave part of the signal (see Figure 5.2.2a and b). The entire signal is then

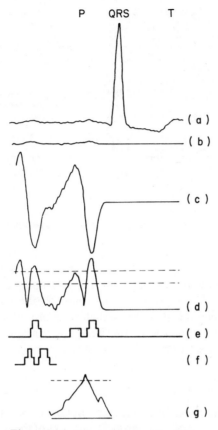

Figure 5.2.2 Processing steps for *P*-wave detection: (a) is the original *PQRST*-complex; in (b) the QRS is cut away; (c) is the amplified and band-pass filtered signal; (d) after rectification with thresholds at 50 and 75 per cent; (e) the ternary signal resulting from (d); (f) the *P*-template; (g) the matching function with a detection level.

low-pass filtered by means of a simple recursive moving average filter after which the derivative is taken by first-order differences (Figure 5.2.2c). The overall result is comparable to band-pass filtering.

(c) Extrema

The next stage is the computation of the maxima and minima [see IV, §3.5] of the filtered signal. At this point we first check the consistency of the PR-intervals by

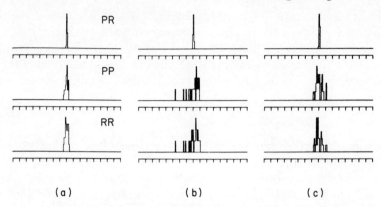

Figure 5.2.3 Examples of *PR*, *PP* and *RR* interval histograms in cases with (a) regular and (b and c) irregular sinus rhythm. The PR intervals remain stable.

computing the range of all intervals between extrema and points of QRS onset. In practice, six such ranges are computed from three simultaneous ECGs (each with a maximum and a minimum per interval). If one of these ranges fulfills the criteria for the PR-interval mentioned above, the detection procedure is terminated since we have found coupled P-waves. Figure 5.2.3 gives examples of such histograms.

Otherwise we proceed to the following stages.

(*d*) *Threshold detection* I

If the criteria of the preceding stage are not met, two threshold levels are applied—one at 50 per cent and one at 75 per cent of the largest extremum in a certain part of the signal (Figure 5.2.2d). The filtered signal is first rectified and a ternary signal is then computed using the two thresholds at 50 and 75 per cent. This gives a waveshape which bears some resemblance to the band-pass filtered and rectified P-wave (Figure 5.2.2e). Only the instants of level crossing are actually stored. In this way we have achieved a considerable data reduction but are left with a rather crude rectified and quantized filtered P-wave, for which the time of occurrence is still unknown.

(*e*) *Cross-correlation*

In the next stage we compute the convolution (see Appendix 5.A.2f) or matching of the above ternary signal with another ternary signal (Figure 5.2.2f) which is a template from a set of P-waves used for setting up the method (a *learning population*). Of course, it would be better if the specific P-wave shape of the individual ECG were known. It would then be possible to design an optimal (in linear terms, matched) filter for the detection of the signal. In this example, a reference P-wave shape is computed (using the band-pass filtering, rectification and ternary level detection) and used as the basis of a general detector. The cross-correlation used, which can be viewed as a convolution with the template signal (see Figure 5.2.2g), only computes the inner products at the instants of change in amplitude, i.e. only at the instants of level crossing. This again saves processing time since the entire convolution can be carried out by additions and subtractions alone.

(*f*) *Threshold detection* II

We now apply a further threshold in order to decide whether a P-wave is present. This threshold (80 per cent of the maximum cross-correlation) was also determined from the learning population of P-waves used for detailed develop-ment and timing of the technique. Further improvements in the method have been made by Talmon (1983).

(*g*) *Evaluation*

The method described has been extensively evaluated by Plokker (1978). We show his decision matrix in Table 5.2.1. False detections or missed P-waves do not necessarily give rise to errors in the arrhythmia diagnosis since multiple criteria are involved and majority rules of decision have been built into the algorithm.

5.2.3 Onsets and end-points of waves

There is a similarity between detection and classification in that both processes concern decisions about the presence of a defined phenomenon, be it a wave, a pattern or a disease. There is also a close connection between detection and parameter estimation. A problem, intermediate between detection and recog-nition, is the estimation of the onset or the end-point of a wave such as a QRS-complex or P-wave in an ECG, an intra-uterine pressure wave or an arterial pulse pressure signal. Having detected the presence of a wave, we are left with two major problems: the estimation of wave duration and the classification of the waveshape.

Table 5.2.1 Decision matrix for the detection of P-waves in a large population of vectorcar-diograms (2,769 cases).

R e f e r e n c e		Computer	
		+	−
+		41.168 (96.6%)	1.072 (3.0%)
−		162 (0.4%)	n.a.

Although no computer pattern-recognition method will perform as intelligently as the most accurate human observer, computer algorithms do at least offer stable results in estimating such points of onset and end-points. We illustrate such a technique using the example of the estimation of the key marker points in P, QRS- and T-waves in a vectorcardiogram van Bemmel, 1973a).

(a) The detection function

From the original vectorcardiogram presented by the vector **h**, where

$$\mathbf{h} = (x_1, x_2, x_3) \tag{5.2.8}$$

[see I, §5.2], we compute a digitally filtered scalar version defined by

$$|\Delta\mathbf{h}| = |\Delta x_1| + |\Delta x_2| + |\Delta x_3|, \tag{5.2.9}$$

where Δ is a differential operator [see IV, §8.1]. The detection function $s = |\Delta\mathbf{h}|/|\Delta\mathbf{h}|_{max}$ is next computed and serves as a basis for the estimation of the points of interest.

(b) Training and templates

For the detection of markers such as wave onset and end-points we make use of a set of training functions, $\{s^k\}$, for which human observers have first recognized the desired points in the original signals $\{\mathbf{h}^k\}$. Around such recognized points, e.g. the QRS-wave onset, we apply windows of a certain size (see Figure 5.2.4) in order to analyse the statistical behaviour of the set $\{s^k\}$ within the window.

Across the region enclosed by the window we determine a multilevel threshold function

$$T_i^k(\lambda) = \text{sign}\,[s_i^k - \lambda], \tag{5.2.10}$$

where λ is an applied threshold. In this function, i is the sample number across the window, k indicates the kth out of K detection functions of the set $\{s^k\}$ and

$$\text{sign}\,[\xi] = \begin{cases} 1, & \xi > 0, \\ -1, & \xi \le 0. \end{cases} \tag{5.2.11}$$

We now define a template g in which the statistical properties of interest of all the T^k are incorporated, where

$$g_i(\alpha) = \frac{1}{K} \sum_{k=1}^{K} T_i^k(\alpha). \tag{5.2.12}$$

It can be shown that $g_i(\alpha)$ is a linear combination of the cumulative density distribution functions [see II, §§10.1.1 and 10.3.1] of the functions s_i^k. Once the template g is obtained, it is cross-correlated with each original individual

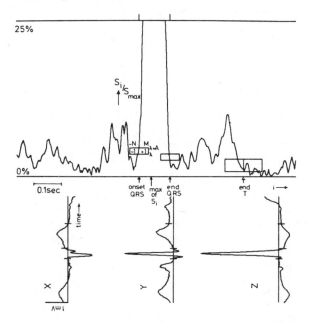

Figure 5.2.4 Detection function s_i for the recognition of the QRS onset and end-point, and the $ST–T$ end-point. Within the three windows, matching is done with a template, with results as shown in X, Y and Z.

template T_i^k of the learning population. The peak of the cross-correlation function enables a revised estimate of the individual marker points in the learning set $\{s^k\}$. These in turn could form the basis for a new template g.

This iterative adaptation may be repeated several times until a stable template results, no longer influenced by the intra-observer variation in the training set. Figure 5.2.5 shows a final P-wave template after the process. This is applied to newly recorded vectorcardiograms by cross-correlation with the derived detection function within the appropriate windows set up around the marker points determined from the learning population. The peak of this cross-correlation function enables the appropriate marker point to be set for each individual waveform.

(c) *Further simplification*

We have already stressed the importance of fast algorithms for biological signal processing. In practice, in the interests of speed, we do not make use of the template g, which can have real values between -1 and $+1$, but a much simpler

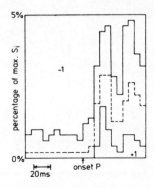

Figure 5.2.5 Template $g_i(\alpha)$ for the recognition of the *P*-wave onset, *i* being the sample index (time scale) and α the amplitude value in the detection functions. The area in between the two solid lines indicates the field where the detection function T_i is most probably located. The dotted line is the most probable function T_i, computed from a learning population. If the detection function does not lie in between the two solid lines the resulting correlation is lower than when there is a good fit.

one, W, where

$$W_i(\alpha) = \begin{cases} \text{sign}\,[g_i(\alpha)], & |g_i(\alpha)| \geq \varepsilon, \\ 0, & |g_i(\alpha)| < \varepsilon. \end{cases} \tag{5.2.13}$$

The value of ε is chosen somewhere between 0.2 and 0.4. The described method is in routine use for the estimation of the key markers in P-, QRS- and T-waves, as part of a system for ECG/VCG processing, discussed briefly in Section 5.5.1 See also Talmon, 1983.

5.2.4 Dichrotic notches in arterial pressure waves

The location of the dichrotic notch in an arterial pressure waveform is of interest for the determination of the mechanical systole and diastole. Some processing algorithms make use of this point for the computation of cardiac output or systolic time intervals. Its determination is the more difficult if we cannot use intra-arterial, let alone intra-cardiac, catheters, but have to rely on non-invasive techniques, such as an external transducer, to pick up the carotid pressure wave.

In estimating the location of the notch we may also make use of the phonocardiogram and the electrocardiogram to find a time window within which the notch is located. The notch itself is caused by the closure of the main cardiac valves to the aorta and the pulmonary circulation.

The change in the slope of the decreasing part of the pressure wave, as shown in Figure 5.2.6, is clearly seen after band-pass filtering of the signal, e.g. by using the filter (operating on sequential sampled values x_i)

$$Y_i = x_{i+2} + x_{i+1} - x_{i-1} - x_{i-2}, \tag{5.2.14}$$

which has the transfer function (see Appendix 5.A.2f)

$$G(f) = 2j[\sin(2\pi f/f_s) + \sin(4\pi f/f_s)]. \tag{5.2.15}$$

Here f_s is the sampling frequency and the filter has a bandwidth between 7 and 23 Hz if the sampling is at 100 Hz.

A simple method for finding the notch within the time window is to look for the instant where the derivative reaches half the minimum (negative) value in the search area, as can be seen in Figure 5.2.6 (Veth and van Bemmel, 1978).

From the foregoing three examples, it should be clear that there can be no standard method for processing biological signals aimed at the detection of events. Numerous other illustrations could be given, but we mention here just one more important aspect of the development of methods for detection, i.e. their evaluation using independent populations of test signals. This is of the utmost importance since many techniques operate satisfactorily in a laboratory environment or on a certain training population but may give considerably different results in clinical practice. This may be because: (a) the practical circumstances with respect to noise and disturbance are quite different from those in the training set, (b) the training set is not representative or is too small or (c) the **a priori** probabilities for certain waveshapes differ from one application area to another, e.g. due to biological variability.

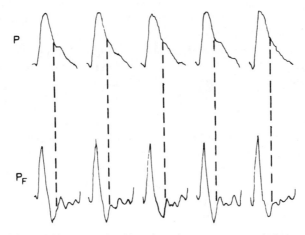

Figure 5.2.6 Example of foetal aortic pressure waves before (P) and after (P_F) digital band-pass filtering between 7 and 23 Hz.

5.3 PATTERNS FROM SIGNALS

We have seen that proper selection of features is the basis for all signal classification and pattern recognition. In the detection stage we determine the signal parts which have to be classified or in which parameters have to be estimated as a function of time. The question then arises: which parameters or features? We have already stressed the need to use as much prior information as possible in deciding which are likely to prove useful parameters. If one were inexperienced, one might easily think that all parameters with discriminating power would automatically be revealed by whatever statistical technique is used for classification. This is not quite true, however. Many parameters, if not all of them, have to be determined by non-linear combinations, or by highly complex algorithms operating on the input samples. Indeed, squares, products, ratios, angles, integrals, differences, time intervals, for example, [see I, §3.1; IV, §4.1], representing important biological parameters, will never 'automatically' arise from even sophisticated non-linear mapping techniques. Sound theoretical reasoning based on fundamental knowledge of the biological process is the only proper way to arrive at the correct features. In this respect, also, many parallels exist between signal processing and pattern recognition (see, for example, Duda and Hart, 1973; Kanal, 1974; Gelsema and Kanal, 1980).

To illustrate certain types of features used in signal classification, we give, as an example, the determination of parameters for QRS typification (van Bemmel, 1973b). For the processing of ECGs it is necessary to know the different types of QRS-complex in the signal. This is needed for rhythm diagnosis as well as for contour classification. For the latter, it is necessary to find the dominant waveshape in the recording. In processing ECG recordings taken during rest, we only have a signal or relatively short length, e.g. 5, 10 or 20 seconds. For such signals a method has been developed which typifies all QRS-complexes present in the recording. Here, again, it is necessary to make a compromise between theory and practice and to have a fast processing algorithm which is able to operate on only a few relevant parameters. The procedure has been devised in such a way that only a single landmark or point of reference in each waveshape is needed.

5.3.1 Frequency spectrum

Since the typification technique has no goal other than the preparation of signals for further diagnostic classification, we assume that the method will work equally well or even better with signals restricted to that part of the frequency spectrum where most of their signal power is usually located—the part between about 10 and 40 Hz. After sampling the ECG and detection of R-waves, the QRS segment is filtered within this bandwidth.

The parameters chosen after filtering are ten instantaneous amplitudes in the filtered signal **h**, defined in the preceding section, which are synchronized with the above-mentioned fiducial points. These instantaneous vectors $\mathbf{v}^k$ are computed at

10 msec intervals. The next step is to reduce the data even further using a cross-correlation or covariance method.

5.3.2 Covariance matrix

If we have a set of L filtered waveforms, then the filtered instantaneous vectors $\mathbf{v}^k$ can be written as

$$\mathbf{v}^k = (v_1^k, v_2^k, \ldots, v_L^k), \tag{5.3.1}$$

where $L = 10$ in our example of Section 5.3.1. From these vectors $\mathbf{v}^k$ we determine the *variance–covariance* matrix [see II, §13.3.1] by

$$\text{cov}(j,k) = (\mathbf{v}^j, \mathbf{v}^k), \tag{5.3.2}$$

where $(\mathbf{a}, \mathbf{b})$ denotes the inner product of the vectors $\mathbf{a}$ and $\mathbf{b}$, and the *cross-correlation* matrix by

$$\rho(j,k) = \text{cov}(j,k)[\text{cov}(j,j)\text{cov}(k,k)]^{-1/2} \tag{5.3.3}$$

[see II, §13.3.3]. These values of ρ are used for typification of the QRS-complexes.

5.3.3 Typification

Two complexes with indices j and k are said to be *identical* (of the same type) if

$$\text{cov}(k,k)/W < \text{cov}(j,j) < W\,\text{cov}(k,k) \tag{5.3.4}$$

and

$$\rho(j,k) > \lambda_\rho. \tag{5.3.5}$$

W is a weighting coefficient and λ_ρ a discrimination level. The proper values of W and λ_ρ can be found using a learning population. The influence of λ_ρ on the typification is shown in Figure 5.3.1. In practice we have chosen $W = 2$ and $\lambda_\rho = 0.8$. Table 5.3.1 gives the results for a large population of ECGs (see Plokker, 1978).

5.3.4 Practical implementation

To speed up computing, we do not determine the upper half of a full covariance matrix of perhaps 20×20 terms, but instead use a sequential method which only needs a small part of that matrix. First, we compute the covariance between the first complex encountered and all others. If, according to the above rules for typification, some complexes appear to differ from the first, we use the same technique for this group alone. This method is repeated until all complexes have been labelled. In routine use, this technique is applied to three simultaneous leads of the ECG signal, using a similar strategy and applying majority rules of decision

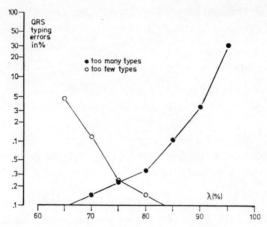

Figure 5.3.1 Determination of a discrimination threshold for *QRS*-typification. If the threshold λ is too low, too many waves are generated, and vice versa.

Table 5.3.1 Classification of QRS-waves according to different types in three different populations. In the learning population, up to four different types were found; ten artifacts were wrongly classified as QRS-waves (not detected by an earlier module as such); the testing population (b) gives an error for only nine out of more than 25,000 complexes; and (c) gives results from a normal population.

Reference	Type	Computer 1	2	3	4		Type	Computer 1	2	3	4	5
	1	7,201	6	—	—		1	24,910	4	—	—	—
	2	13	89	3	—		2	1	177	4	—	—
	3	1	—	7	—		3	—	—	19	—	—
	4	—	—	—	—		4	—	—	—	2	—
	Artifact	—	6	3	1		5	—	—	—	—	1
							Artifact	—	13	3	4	

(a) Learning population (hospital). 455 cases

(b) Testing population (hospital), 1,496 cases

Reference	Type	Computer 1	2
	1	13,320	—
	2	5	26
	Artifact	—	1

(c) Testing population (population survey), 743 cases

if the answers differ. This sequential procedure of typification is based on the assumption that if, for complexes with order i, j and k, it is found that $\rho(i,j) > \lambda_\rho$ and $\rho(i,k) > \lambda_\rho$, then this implies that $\rho(j,k) > \lambda_\rho$.

5.4 DATA REDUCTION AND SEGMENTATION

Data reduction techniques are needed both to facilitate fast processing and also for economical permanent computer storage of biological signals in databases. The central question in this respect is always whether we want to store the original data, the reduced signal aimed at a reliable reconstruction of the original data or only parameters relevant for the classification of the signals.

In the preceding paragraphs we have encountered several forms of data reduction; e.g. the computation of instantaneous vectors of the pre-processed ECG for QRS typification and the computation of a ternary signal for P-wave detection. The purpose of segmentation is to divide a biological signal into logical parts or segments in which we can assume that the signal structure does not change; in other words, the underlying biological process remains stationary. In the following sections we give, as examples, a data reduction algorithm for storage or transmission of ECGs, a segmentation algorithm for the reduction of a foetal heart rate (FHR) pattern and segmentation methods for the processing of electroencephalograms.

5.4.1 Segmentation of the electrocardiogram

We will not here consider the ECG as a continuous signal (repetitive or otherwise) which can be represented by some series of orthogonal functions (see Appendix) but as a chain of events separated by certain epochs where there is no electrical activity. These are the P-wave, the 'silent' PR-interval, the QRS-complex, the ST-T-wave and the baseline between end-of-T and P-onset—five periods altogether.

It makes a considerable difference for data reduction if we make use of the onsets and end-points of the periods, computed as described in section 5.2.3, instead of the original signal. However, in most instances we only have the original signal without such points of reference. The basis of the segmentation method here is the assumption that we can approximate the continuous signal by linear or non-linear segments of varying lengths. One method is the AZTEC algorithm (Cox *et al.*, 1968), which makes use of amplitude changes from point to point within a signal. As soon as the amplitude change in a certain part of a signal is larger than a threshold value, ΔA, the time at which this occurs is stored. Instead of amplitude values, we now only need to store these time instants. An almost complete reconstruction is then possible provided ΔA is within reasonable limits, e.g. of the order of magnitude of natural noise or diagnostically relevant Q-wave amplitudes. For ambulatory monitoring purposes, this data reduction is widely used but, if one wishes to be able to reconstruct the waveform itself, such a reduction still causes difficulties.

5.4.2 Segmentation for reduction of foetal heart rate patterns

A slightly different method is to reduce the information content of the signal with the aid of slope variations (e.g. with second-order differences [see III, §1.4]) instead of amplitude changes. It should be understood that a proper low-pass filter has to precede all segmentation algorithms, especially if we take higher order differences for the determination of the segments. Differentiation of the signal means a multiplication of the frequency spectrum by $2\pi \mathrm{j} f$ [see IV, §§3.1 and 3.2], so that high-frequency noise is amplified with respect to the low-frequency components.

In this second approach we represent a part of the signal by the time series T_k [see VI, Chapter 18] and compute the regression line between $k = k_1$ and $k = k_2$ by the method of least squares. That is, a straight line of the form

$$T_k^e = \alpha(k - k_1) + \beta \tag{5.4.1}$$

for which we minimize the sum of the squared differences between T_k and T_k^e,

$$\mathrm{SQD} = \sum_{k=k_1}^{k_2} (T_k - T_k^e)^2. \tag{5.4.2}$$

By differentiation with respect to the parameters α and β, we easily find the values for the best linear fit [see VI, §6.5]. From the given formula we predict the amplitude $T_{k_2+1}^e$ and compute $\Delta = T_{k_2+1}^e - T_{k_2+1}$ based on these values for α and β. If Δ is small enough (it can have either a fixed or an adaptive threshold), $T_{k_2+1}^e$ is attached to the already existing signal part from k_1 to k_2. New parameters α and β are now computed. The computation is started anew when the threshold level Δ is crossed. Other versions of this algorithm are 'look backward' or 'look forward and backward' methods. The method described looks forward.

A combination of a forward and a backward-looking method is as follows. Starting from a point k_1, over fixed intervals before and after, compute the least squares fitted lines and then compute the angle between these lines or the surface enclosed by them, applying a segmentation threshold as before. Figure 5.4.1 gives an example of this last segmentation algorithm applied to a part of a foetal heart rate pattern.

5.4.3 Segmentation of electroencephalograms

It has been stressed that prior knowledge of the origin of biological signals and patterns as well as a clear view of the purpose of the processing is essential. Many signal processing methods have been developed for EEG analysis (Barlow, 1979). However, if we want to develop segmentation algorithms for the processing of EEGs, we have no clear understanding of the origin of the signal and only few

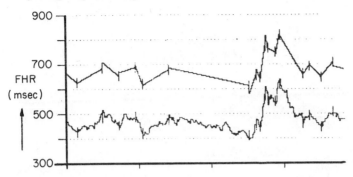

Figure 5.4.1 Segmentation of an FHR pattern by a least squares method.

ideas about the purpose of the processing. Several research groups have developed techniques for EEG segmentation (Bodenstein and Praetorious, 1977; Jansen, Hasman and Lenten, 1981). Our method, summarized here, is based on *state vectors* obtained by *Kalman filtering* [see VI, Chapter 20]. A certain segment of the EEG is used for training, i.e. estimation of the parameters of an autoregressive filter. New parts of the EEG are then 'predicted' by this filter with respect to the state vector. As soon as there is too large a deviation from the preceding state vector, we assume that a new segment is present.

In the formulae

$$\hat{y}_k = \alpha_1 y_{k-1} + \alpha_2 y_{k-2} + \cdots + \alpha_n y_{k-n} = \alpha' \mathbf{y}_{k-1} \qquad (5.4.3)$$

and

$$\varepsilon_k = y_k - \hat{y}_k, \qquad (5.4.4)$$

$\hat{y}_k$ is the predicted sample value and ε_k the deviation from the real sample value. In the Kalman filter, it is assumed that ε_k has a Gaussian distribution with zero mean [see II, §11.4]. We require that the variance of ε_k is equal to or less than the variance of the samples y_k. Using the Kalman filtering approach we are now able to devise a strategy to optimize the vector α for a certain signal part. Many other techniques can be developed, e.g. half-wave analysis, zero-crossing analysis and texture analysis. In Figure 5.4.2 we show a scheme for the estimation of the Kalman parameters computed for segmentation purposes (Jansen, Hasman and Lenten, 1981). With the help of such parameters, we build a cluster of identical EEG patterns in a six-dimensional parameter space. New clusters (EEG patterns) are automatically formed if they fall outside an already existing cluster, with defined boundaries as illustrated in Figure 5.4.3.

5.5 SYSTEMS FOR SIGNAL PROCESSING

In this section we give a compact review of some working computer-assisted systems for the processing of biological signals. Many of the methods used in such systems are based on or are related to the theories and methods discussed in the

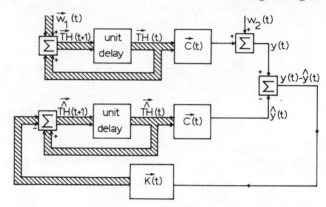

Figure 5.4.2 Model for the segmentation of non-stationary EEGs by autoregressive (Kalman) filtering. The EEG $y(t)$ is thought to be the sum of a predicted value $[C(t) \cdot TH(t)]$, with $C(t) = [y(t-1), \; y(t-2), \ldots, y(t-N)]$ and $TH(t)$ the state vector, and a correction or noise term $w_2(t)$, so that $y(t) = C(t) \cdot TH(t) + w_2(t)$. The state vector $TH(t+1) = TH(t) + w_1(t)$, with w_1 being white noise. The estimated EEG $\hat{y}(t)$ is computed by the model, in which the Kalman coefficients to predict $\hat{w}_2$ are estimated by the error $y(t) - \hat{y}(t)$. In the figure the shaded lines indicate vectors; single lines indicate scalar signals.

preceding sections. We will deal with aspects of systems for function laboratories such as ECG/VCG, exercise ECG (XECG), EEG and catheterization laboratory data; then systems for computer-assisted intensive care in the coronary care unit and for peri- or post-operative care and peri-natal care.

5.5.1 Function laboratories

In contrast to the situation in intensive care, it is not necessary to have a real-time analysis of signals during function testing (Cox, Nolle and Arthur, 1972; van Bemmel, 1977). Most of the processing can be done off-line, although in many instances it is required that the result be available before the patient leaves the examination room or is disconnected from the transducers.

In examining the condition and function of certain organs, the purpose is diagnosis, the basis for further therapy. The departments where such functions are examined may be oriented towards prevention, (early) diagnosis or eva-luation of possible therapy, e.g. after surgery. Further, we can differentiate between so-called passive examinations (i.e. the recording of information which is generated spontaneously by the organism) and active or even provocative examinations. The latter category includes atrial pacing, light flash stimuli for electroencephalography and the use of a tracer such as radioactive xenon for

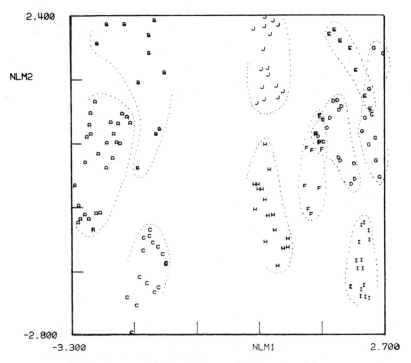

Figure 5.4.3 Non-linear mapping from a six-dimensional feature space to two dimensions in which ten clusters A...J have been built from EEG features (five parameters from a Kalman filter and one signal power parameter). The EEGs were derived from patients during renal dialysis. The two features NLM1 (abscissa) and NLM2 (ordinate) are computed by non-linear mapping from the six original features in such a way that the set of distances computed between points in the two-dimensional plane is as similar as possible to the set of point-to-point distances in six dimensions.

evaluation of the condition of the heart during physical exercise. Although not always allowed for medical reasons, the provocative examination has, nevertheless, many advantages.

In a department where we perform a function test and use a computer for the assistance of the examination, we commonly follow a scheme such as that shown in Figure 5.5.1. The signals are fed to a computer by a telephone line and modems, via a direct connection or via an intermediate storage device such as a tape recorder (AM, FM, PDM or other manner of coding), a floppy disk or a cassette recorder. We often encounter the first of these in departments where EEGs are computer processed or as an input medium for computer-assisted ECG interpretation (van Bemmel and Willems, 1977). The last is used, for instance, in ambulatory ECG monitoring for the detection of arhythmias. The cassette can then be played back at ten to more than one hundred times the original speed and

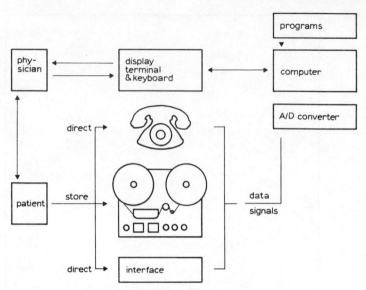

Figure 5.5.1 General scheme for signal processing in a function
laboratory

processed by a dedicated computer. In many instances the output is sent back in an alpha-numeric form. If direct communication is desired, we usually have a visual display unit (VDU).

(*a*) *Heart function*

In cardiology, many applications of information processing are encountered. For example, much research is in progress aimed at early detection of ischaemic heart disease. Many articles and books have been written on ECG/VCG processing (e.g. van Bemmel and Willems (1977), Wolf and Macfarlane (1979), Talmon (1983); see also the chapter devoted to cardiology in Part II of this Guidebook).

Exercise ECG analysis offers an interesting example of signal processing and signal transformation (Simoons, 1975). In one of our earlier studies in this area, we investigated the sensitivity and specificity of an orthogonal system, such as the Frank VCG system, compared to the use of scalar leads such as CC5, CB5, CM5. The problem in processing the Frank VCG, however, is the amount of noise due to exercise and also the fact that the Frank leads are not optimally located with respect to this EMG noise. For this reason, the following technique is applied (Ascoop, 1974):

(i) During rest, the VCG is recorded with four other scalar leads which we know, from anatomical reasoning and from experience, do not generate much 'muscle noise', even during maximal exercise.

We define the vectorcardiogram, as in section 5.2.3, by

$$\mathbf{h} = (x_1, x_2, x_3) \tag{5.5.1}$$

and the four leads by

$$\mathbf{s} = (x_4, x_5, x_6, x_7). \tag{5.5.2}$$

All signals x_k are time series $x_k = x_k(t)$.

(ii) For each individual patient during rest, we define the individual approximated vector $\mathbf{h}$ as

$$\mathbf{h}^* = (x_1^*, x_2^*, x_3^*), \tag{5.5.3}$$

for which we require that

$$\varepsilon^2 = |\mathbf{h} - \mathbf{h}^*|^2 \tag{5.5.4}$$

[see IV, (21.2.6)] be minimal. The transformation from $\mathbf{s}$ to $\mathbf{h}^*$ is defined

$$\mathbf{h}^* = \mathbf{Ls} \tag{5.5.5}$$

[see I, §5.13], so that

$$\varepsilon^2 = |\mathbf{h} - \mathbf{Ls}|^2. \tag{5.5.6}$$

This expression can be differentiated [see IV, §5.5] to give the coefficients for the matrix $\mathbf{L}$, l_{ik}, with $i = 1, 2$ or 3 and $k = 1, 2, 3$ or 4. Thus, the problem resolves into a simple matrix inversion [see III, §4.5].

(iii) In the third step we use the matrix $\mathbf{L}$ to generate the 'simulated' vector cardiogram during exercise, $\mathbf{h}^*$, with the aid of the scalar lead set $\mathbf{s}$. In this way we can avoid the Frank leads during exercise. Figure 5.5.2 shows the comparison of the ST-T loops of the VCG during exercise (a) without and (b) with the use of the transformation matrix $\mathbf{L}$.

(iv) The evaluation of this method for the exercise ECG is different from that for the resting ECG. Our reference here consists of findings from coronary arteriography for detecting obstructions in the coronary vessels. These are classified into categories of severe, moderate or no obstruction and are compared to the findings from exercise ECG analysis.

(b) Catheterization laboratory

Signal analysis in a catheterization laboratory differs from the analysis of ECGs in that the signals have to be analysed on-line, not necessarily in real-time. It is of great importance that the cardiologist should obtain quantitative results for variables such as flows, shunts, pressures and volumes during the catheterization. For that reason, dedicated minicomputer systems have been devised to display the computed results, e.g. on a visual display unit in the laboratory. By

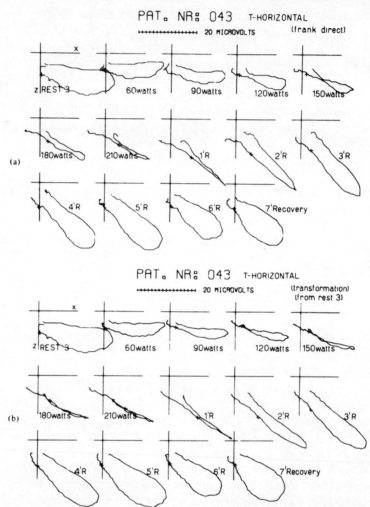

Figure 5.5.2 ST–T loops measured during exercise by direct leads (a) and computed from an individual transformation matrix (b).

this direct feedback to the cardiologist, it is possible to obtain a quick impression of whether the signals are disturbed and whether the catheter is in its proper place or not. The signal processing techniques do not differ appreciably from those described in the preceding sections.

(c) EEG analysis

Analysis of the electroencephalogram is still an area of great difficulty, not so much because the signal offers special processing problems but because the meaning of the EEG for clinical purposes cannot be stated explicitly and so translation into an algorithm is not always possible. We will not, for this reason, mention the numerous approaches that have been undertaken to analyse the EEG with respect to its different components (see, for example, Rémond, 1977; Barlow, 1979). We will, however, treat a very special application of EEG analysis in the next section where we discuss the use of computers in intensive care.

5.5.2 Computer-assisted intensive care

The use of computers for intensive care of patients is one of the most complex areas because of the need for accurate responses in a dynamic and noisy environment. In this area, computers are used for data presentation, documentation, quality control, signal processing and therapeutic measures (Sheppard, 1979). The amount of data to be processed can be enormous. Because of the changing situation, a fast computation of results is required with on-line and real-time feedback to nurse and physician or even patient. We will mention here only a number of signal processing aspects.

(a) *Peri-natal intensive care*

During birth, one may record a huge amount of data from the mother and the foetus, such as the foetal heart rate (from the foetal ECG, an ultrasonic transducer or a phonocardiogram), the intra-uterine pressure and the foetal pH and pO_2 (van Bemmel, de Haan and Veth, 1974). The relationship between heart rate and intra-uterine pressure (a plot is shown in Figure 5.5.3) is of great value for the diagnosis of the condition of the unborn child. Such signals are sampled and digitized, filtered and further analysed. In Section 5.4.2 we have given an example of a data reduction method for such signals.

(b) *Peri-operative intensive care*

An example of the use of signal analysis here is during open-heart surgery. Because respiration and circulation are artificially regulated, we only monitor the brain function of the patient. To that end the EEG is recorded. This stochastic signal reveals some aspects of the brain function influenced, for example, by anaesthetic agents, temperature and hypoxia. This is quantified in terms of the number of waves per time unit as well as by the mean amplitude of the EEG.

In practice, the EEG is filtered and the zero-crossings of the signals are determined, using special hardware, and fed as interrupts to a minicomputer. The task of the computer is then to produce histograms of zero crossings over 30 to 60 second intervals and to plot these histograms on a frequency scale as a function of real-time. By observing such condensed plots, one can quickly see non-stationarities caused by measures taken during the surgery. Such patterns may

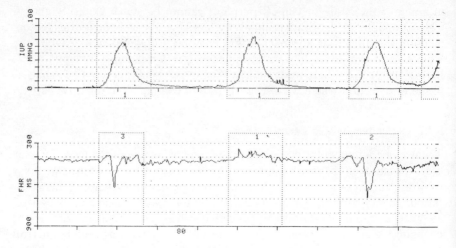

Figure 5.5.3 Computer plot of the intra-uterine pressure with an FHR pattern. The endpoints in the IUP wave form are automatically generated; those in the FHR are indicated by the user.

last for many hours. Figure 5.5.4 shows two series of such histograms for two patients simultaneously (from two operating rooms), each with two EEG leads (Pronk, 1981).

(c) *Coronary care*

One aspect of CCU monitoring is the supervised classification of ventricular waveforms. Of importance are the monitoring of the heart rate or RR-interval and the early detection of ectopic beats or ventricular fibrillation. In a man–machine interaction, the computer is 'taught' the individual waveshapes of a certain patient during the first minutes that the patient is connected to the monitoring equipment. This is done by computing a feature vector of ten instantaneous amplitudes, 10 msec apart, using a method similar to that described in section 5.3. Here, however, no automatic typification takes place, but the waveform, if it cannot be identified by the computer, is offered to a human observer as an unfiltered signal on a CRT. The computer processing operates on a digitally filtered version.

The waveform is labelled by the observer as, say, 'type k', which could be the nodal beat or an extra-systole. If a second beat of this type occurs, the computer compares the latter with the earlier beat(s), but again shows it to the observer if it still cannot classify the waveform. The observer again labels it as 'type k'. During processing of perhaps two to five such waveforms in the training phase, the computer continuously updates several parameters. These are, for cluster k, the

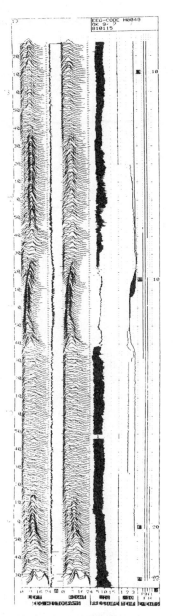

EEG-CODE H0040
OK 9 ?
810115

EEG/ANAESTHESIE DOKUMENTATIE
ST.ANTONIUS ZIEKENHUIS
KLINISCHE NEUROFYSIOLOGIE
MEDISCH FYSISCH INSTITUUT-TNO
UTRECHT
PROGRAM-VERSION: HSD812

NAME   :
BIRTH [YYMMDD]:
SEX   [M/F]: M
STAZU CODE   : G210219M
EEG CODE   : H0040
DATE   [YYMMDD]: 810115
PREM   : 10VIAN 4 HALDOL
SURGERY   : RE-OP. AO-KLEP
OPERATING ROOM: OK 9
SURGEON   : OR
ANAESTH.   : OR
NEUROPHYS.   : OR
TECHNICIAN   :

8:24   START PROGRAM

8:28   N2O ON
8:28   VALIUM 20
8:29   FENTANYL 10
8:29   HALOTHANE 05
8:55   FENTANYL OFF
8:55   INFUSION
8:57   FENTANYL 20
9:21   HALOTHANE OFF
10:32   PERFUSION ON
10:35   COOLING
11:5   REWARMING
11:15   VALIUM 10
11:17   N2O OFF
11:37   WARNING LOW ASYM EEG
11:39   N2O ON
11:42   PERFUSION OFF
11:44   PERFUSION ON
11:45   ARTEFACT OFF
11:45   PERFUSION OFF
11:47   WARNING HIGH ASYM EEG
11:48   END WARNING HIGH ASYM EEG
11:53   WARNING LOW ASYM EEG
12:0   ATT KEY LOW ASYM EEG
12:31   WARNING LOW ASYM EEG

12:42   WARNING HIGH ASYM EEG
12:47   ALARM HIGH ASYM EEG
12:47   ATT KEY LOW ASYM EEG
12:47   END ALARM HIGH ASYM EEG
12:49   WARNING HIGH ASYM EEG
12:51   ALARM HIGH ASYM EEG
12:52   ATT KEY HIGH ASYM EEG
12:54   END ALARM HIGH ASYM EEG
12:59   WARNING HIGH ASYM EEG
12:59   WARNING LOW ASYM EEG
13:1   END WARNING HIGH ASYM EEG
13:10   VALIUM 10
13:11   END WARNING LOW ASYM EEG
13:16   WARNING LOW ASYM EEG
13:21   ATT KEY LOW ASYM EEG
13:27   WARNING SLOW EEG
13:27   END WARNING SLOW EEG
13:28   STOP PROGRAM

Figure 5.5.4 Plot of zero-crossing histograms of EEG's from the two hemispheres of a patient during open heart surgery (see Pronk, 1981). The histograms are computed every 10 sec.; the effects of anaesthesia, perfusion and cooling can be seen in the mean amplitude and the wave frequency of the EEG.
The signals, from the left, are the consecutive histograms (abscissa in cycles/sec.); the arterial bloodpressure (which becomes flat in the middle of the recording because of perfusion); the nasopharyngeal temperature together with the type of cooling and an indication of events occurring. The different codes (P, F, N, H, L) refer to anaesthetic agents such as fentanyl or halothane.

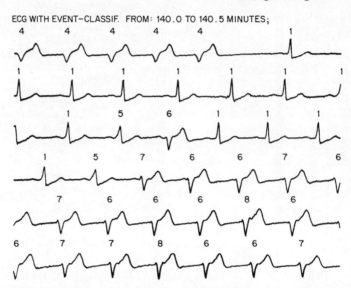

ECG WITH EVENT-CLASSIF. FROM: 140.0 TO 140.5 MINUTES;

Figure 5.5.5 Classification of QRS-complexes and extra-systoles of different (multifocal and supraventricular) origin. The system was trained by the human operator by means of a few (e.g. two to five) waveforms of a certain type. The numbers above the complexes indicate the waveform type number with 1 being the normal complex (Swenne *et al.*, 1977).

centre of gravity

$$\mathbf{m}^k = \sum_{i=1}^{n} \frac{\mathbf{v}_i^k}{n} \tag{5.5.7}$$

and the *dispersion of the cluster*

$$(s^k)^2 = \sum_{i=1}^{n} \frac{(\mathbf{v}_i^k - \mathbf{m}^k)^2}{n-1}. \tag{5.5.8}$$

Cluster k is built by the waveforms of type k and $\mathbf{v}_i^k$ is the ith measured feature vector. A new vector $\mathbf{v}_j$ is allocated to cluster k if it falls within a sphere of radius 5 times the dispersion s^k. However, if this applies for more than one cluster, the cluster with the minimal distance is chosen. A whole series of measures is taken by the program to ascertain that no incorrect human decision can 'pollute' the operation. Figure 5.5.5 shows the effect of human intervention for a patient showing seven types of ventricular complex (Swenne *et al.*, 1977).

5.6 CONCLUDING REMARKS

In this chapter we have stressed the need for a careful and detailed analysis and investigation of the signal and its source. We have seen that processing techniques for biological signals must be tuned to a specific problem through use of prior knowledge gathered about the biological process and its output. We have also observed that many 'standard' mathematical tools are of great use for biological signal processing but that, in many instances, we have to devise special methods for signal analysis which are often of a heuristic character. At the same time, we have to make compromises between what is desirable, from a theoretical point of view, and what is feasible with respect to processing power and time allowed. Nonetheless, it is possible to follow a rather well-founded strategy in the processing, as we have tried to show. Very many examples could have been given; we have given only a few, though representative, examples of the signal processing strategies, the special processing solutions and the compromises involved. We have restricted ourselves to the major issues in this respect: signal detection, wave recognition, feature selection and data reduction or segmentation. In developing the proper techniques there is a great need for well-defined populations of signals for training and testing of algorithms.

APPENDIX 5.A A SUMMARY OF MATHEMATICAL DEFINITIONS AND TECHNIQUES ENCOUNTERED IN SIGNAL PROCESSING

5.A.1 Statistical moments

The nth-order *statistical moment* $(n = 1, 2, \ldots)$ of the probability distribution $f(x)$ of a random variable (or stochastic variable) X, where $f(x)$ denotes the probability density at x, is given by

$$E\{X^n\} = \int_{-\infty}^{\infty} x^n f(x) \, dx, \tag{5.A.1}$$

where $E\{\cdots\}$ denotes the expectation of the variable [see II, §10.4.1].

Intuitively, this is the average of all possible realizations of the random variable at an arbitrary instant of time. The time average, on the other hand, denoted here by $\overline{x^n(t)}$, is the average value of a particular time-dependent trajectory of the signal $x^n(t)$. This is defined by

$$\overline{x^n(t)} = \lim_{T \to \infty} \frac{1}{2T} \int_{-T}^{+T} \{x(t)\}^n \, dt. \tag{5.A.2}$$

For *ergodic signals* the two averages are equal; i.e.

$$\overline{x^n(t)} = E\{X^n\}. \tag{5.A.3}$$

The first-order moment $E\{X\}$ is the mean value of the signal.

The *dispersion* is defined by the standard deviation $\sigma = \sigma(X)$ or equivalently by the variance $\sigma^2 = \sigma^2(X)$, where

$$\sigma^2(X) = E\{(X - E\{X\})^2\} \tag{5.A.4}$$

[see II, Chapters 8, 9 and §10.4].

Again, for ergodic signals,

$$\sigma^2(X) = \sigma^2(x(t)) = \lim_{T \to \infty} \frac{1}{2T} \int_{-T}^{T} [x(t) - \overline{x(t)}]^2 \, dt \tag{5.A.5}$$

where $x(t)$ denotes any particular (time-dependent) trajectory. Wide-sense stationary or *weakly stationary* signals are only ergodic with respect to their first- and second- order moments, i.e. (5.A.3) holds for $n = 1, 2$ only. For fully ergodic or *strongly stationary* signals, (5.A.3) holds for $n = 1, 2, \ldots$.

The same types of definitions can be given for two-dimensional (or multi-dimensional) distribution functions [see II, §13.1].

5.A.2 Signals and noise

The introductory section has mentioned the influence of noise and other disturbances on signal processing methods. Here, we give some relevant mathematical descriptions. First of all, we treat, briefly, the sampling process, which is of great importance if we use digital computers for signal processing. We deal with the degree of quantization and the sampling frequency. Our main goal will be to develop a sampling procedure in such a way that, in principle, a reconstruction of the main features of the original signal is possible. The sampling process with equidistant samples is shown in Figure 5.A.1, which shows a segment of the trajectory of a signal $x(t)$, a continuous function of the time t [see IV, §2.1], observed or sampled at time instants separated by an interval ΔT.

At each of these instants the observer is able to read the magnitude of the signal correct to the nearest sub-unit which the equipment is capable of discerning (just as a person's height may be measured correct to the nearest centimetre). The size of these sub-units is indicated as Δq in Figure 5.A.1. The process of converting a real number, i.e. the actual magnitude of the signal, into the nearest integer multiple of Δq is referred to as *quantization*.

(a) Quantization

For the sampling of a signal, we make use of an *analogue-to-digital converter* (ADC). The most common scheme for this ADC is seen in Figure 5.A.2. The *quantization degree* of an ADC (i.e. the size Δq of the sub-units mentioned above)

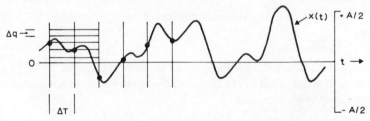

Figure 5.A.1 Sampling and quantization of the signal $x(t)$.

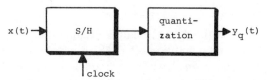

Figure 5.A.2 Sample/hold and quantizer.

with an n-bits output over a range A is

$$\Delta q(n) = \frac{A}{2^n}. \tag{5.A.6}$$

A one-bit ADC, which only takes into account the sign of the signal, has a quantization degree of

$$\Delta q(1) = \frac{A}{2}. \tag{5.A.7}$$

Its output can also be represented by

$$y_q(t) = \text{sign}\,\{x(t) - \lambda\} = \begin{cases} 1, & x(t) \geq \lambda, \\ 0, & x(t) < \lambda. \end{cases} \tag{5.A.8}$$

where λ is an arbitrarily chosen threshold. Usually, for biological signals, we take samples with a six- to twelve-bit ADC. With the last one we reach an accuracy (quantization degree divided by range) of 0.025 per cent. The quantization process causes an extra disturbance on the signals which should preferably be smaller than the 'natural' noise. The quantization noise can then be expressed as

$$n_q(t) = y_q(t) - x(t). \tag{5.A.9}$$

We may remark that for signals with a noise standard deviation in the region of 1 per cent of the signal range, a twelve-bit ADC is an unnecessary luxury. In considering data reduction, while still keeping a high enough accuracy, it is seldom necessary to have a very low quantization noise. For instance, in computing an estimate of variance or mean value (with a thirteen- to fifteen-bit accuracy) we usually do not need an ADC more accurate than eight bits. In many cases, where the signals themselves are of a stochastic nature, as in an EEG, even a four-bit ADC is often sufficient. Sometimes even a one-bit ADC can be of great use, as in the computation of zero-crossing histograms (see Figure 5.5.4).

Without giving proofs, we note that, in computing statistical values from quantized signals,

$$E\{y_q\} = E\{x\}$$
$$E\{y_q^2\} = E\{x^2\} + \tfrac{1}{12}(\Delta q)^2 \tag{5.A.10}$$
$$E\{y_q^4\} = E\{x^4\} + \tfrac{1}{2}(\Delta q)^2 E\{y_q^2\} + O((\Delta q)^4).$$

Such relations are known as *Sheppard's corrections* for grouped data.

(b) *Sampling rate*

The *sampling theorem*, with which the names of Shannon, Weaver and Nyquist are associated (see Shannon and Weaver, 1949), is based on the assumption that we have a signal $x(t)$, confined within a frequency bandwidth W. First, we introduce the *Fourier transform* [see IV, §13.2] (see, for example, Cooley and Tukey, 1966, or Schwartz and Shaw, 1975). For a non-periodic signal $x(t)$, the (complex valued) Fourier transform (FT) is given, as a continuous function of the frequency f, by

$$X(f) = \int_{-\infty}^{\infty} x(t) \exp(-2\pi jft)\,dt, \qquad (5.A.11)$$

where j is the imaginary number $\sqrt{-1}$. The inverse transformation by which the signal may be reconstructed from $X(f)$ is given by

$$x(t) = \frac{1}{2\pi} \int_{-\infty}^{\infty} X(f) \exp(2\pi jft)\,df = \frac{1}{2\pi} \int_{-W}^{+W} X(f) \exp(2\pi jft)\,df, \qquad (5.A.12)$$

the last expression being valid because of the restricted bandwidth W. If the signal is periodic, integrals are replaced by sums and the continuous spectrum (5.A.11) becomes a series of lines. An artificial operation that we apply in order to derive the sampling theorem is to make the spectrum periodic (by repetition), as seen in Figure 5.A.3.

The appropriate replacement for (5.A.11) is then

$$X_p(f) = \sum_{n=-\infty}^{\infty} C_n \exp\left(-2\pi j \frac{n}{2W} f\right), \qquad (5.A.13)$$

with

$$C_n = \frac{1}{2W} \int_{-W}^{W} X(f) \exp\left(2\pi j \frac{n}{2W} f\right) df. \qquad (5.A.14)$$

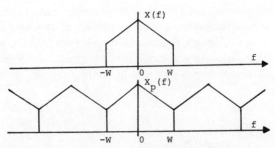

Figure 5.A.3 Frequency spectrum $X(f)$ and its periodic counterpart $X_p(f)$.

Now, if (5.A.12) is valid for all t between $-\infty$ and $+\infty$, it is also valid for $t = n/2W$, whence

$$x\left(\frac{n}{2W}\right) = \int_{-W}^{W} X(f) \exp\left(2\pi j \frac{n}{2W} f\right) df, \tag{5.A.15}$$

so that

$$C_n = \frac{1}{2W} x\left(\frac{n}{2W}\right) \tag{5.A.16}$$

or

$$X_p(f) = \frac{1}{2W} \sum_{n=-\infty}^{\infty} x\left(\frac{n}{2W}\right) \exp\left(-2\pi j \frac{n}{2W} f\right). \tag{5.A.17}$$

$X(f)$ is the part of $X_p(f)$ lying between $-W$ and $+W$, so that

$$x(t) = \int_{-W}^{W} \frac{1}{2W} \sum_{n=-\infty}^{\infty} x\left(\frac{n}{2W}\right) \exp\left(-2\pi j \frac{n}{2W} f\right) \exp(2\pi j f t) df \tag{5.A.18}$$

$$= \sum_{n=-\infty}^{\infty} x\left(\frac{n}{2W}\right) \int_{-W}^{W} \frac{1}{2W} \exp\left(-2\pi j \frac{n}{2W} f\right) \exp(2\pi j f t) df. \tag{5.A.19}$$

The integral in (5.A.19) is the function

$$\frac{\sin(2\pi Wt - n\pi)}{2\pi Wt - n\pi}, \tag{5.A.20}$$

known as a *sinc function* $(\text{sinc}(x) = \sin(x)/x)$, whence

$$x(t) = \sum_{n=-\infty}^{\infty} x\left(\frac{n}{2W}\right) \text{sinc}(2\pi Wt - n\pi). \tag{5.A.21}$$

With respect to (5.A.20), we note that the signal represented by a rectangular frequency spectrum can be written as $x(t) = \text{sinc}(2\pi Wt)$.

The original continuous signal $x(t)$ can be restored from the sampled signal $x(n/2W)$ (i.e. sampled at twice the maximum frequency of interest in the signal, the *Nyquist frequency*) by a convolution with a signal which is rectangular between $-W$ and $+W$.

(c) Covariance and correlation of signals [see II, §§13.1.3 and 22.2]

Random factors play a central role in the behaviour of stochastic signals; their behaviour is not exactly, only statistically, predictable. Nevertheless, there are many properties that can be derived from such signals. Stochastic signals are treated in the same way as other signals as far as their sampling rate is concerned: here, also, we can define a bandwidth upon which the Nyquist frequency is based.

The *covariance* of two variables x and y, with a joint density distribution function $f(x, y)$, is defined as

$$\rho_{xy} = E\{xy\} = \int \int_{-\infty}^{\infty} xy f(x, y) \, dx \, dy. \tag{5.A.22}$$

With respect to the time trajectories $x(t)$, $y(t)$ we define, similarly,

$$R_{xy} = \lim_{T \to \infty} \frac{1}{2T} \int_{-T}^{T} x(t) y(t) \, dt \tag{5.A.23}$$

and if the variables x and y are ergodic, $R_{xy} = \rho_{xy}$ More generally,

$$R_{xy}(\tau) = \lim_{T \to \infty} \frac{1}{2T} \int_{-T}^{T} x(t) y(t + \tau) \, dt. \tag{5.A.24}$$

Obviously, if $x = y$ and $\overline{x(t)} = 0$, then

$$R_{xx}(0) = \sigma_x^2. \tag{5.A.25}$$

We call R_{xx} the *auto-covariance* and R_{xy} the *cross-covariance* function. The covariance function, after normalization with $R(0)$ (i.e. $R(\tau)/R(0)$), is called the *correlation function*.

(d) Periodic components in signals; signal to noise ratio (SNR)

Assume that $x(t)$ consists of a periodic component $s(t)$ (e.g. a sine wave [see IV, §2.12]) and noise $n(t)$ (e.g. wide-band noise with a Gaussian frequency distribution [see II, §11.4]). Then

$$x(t) = a \sin(2\pi f t + \psi) + n(t) = s(t) + n(t). \tag{5.A.26}$$

We define the *signal to noise ratio* (SNR) as the ratio between the variances of signal and noise:

$$\text{SNR} = \frac{E\{(s - E\{s\})^2\}}{E\{(n - E(n))^2\}} = \frac{\overline{(s - \bar{s})^2}}{\overline{(n - \bar{n})^2}} \tag{5.A.27}$$

If the signal has a low amplitude compared with the noise dispersion, it is difficult or even impossible to detect the presence of the signal. The auto-covariance function of $x(t)$, however, can help us to visualize the presence of $s(t)$ in $x(t)$. Assuming $\bar{s} = \bar{n} = 0$, then

$$
\begin{aligned}
R_{xx}(\tau) &= \overline{x(t)x(t + \tau)} \\
&= \overline{s(t)s(t + \tau)} + \overline{s(t)n(t + \tau)} + \overline{s(t + \tau)n(t)} + \overline{n(t)n(t + \tau)} \\
&= \overline{s(t)s(t + \tau)} + \overline{n(t)n(t + \tau)}.
\end{aligned} \tag{5.A.28}
$$

The last expression is valid because of the independence of $s(t)$ and $n(t)$ [see II, §9.6.7], and thus

$$R_{xx}(\tau) = R_{ss}(\tau) + R_{nn}(\tau). \tag{5.A.29}$$

If we compute $R_{ss}(\tau)$ for the sine wave $s(t) = a \sin(2\pi ft + \psi)$, it can be shown that

$$R_{ss}(\tau) = \frac{a^2}{2} \cos 2\pi f\tau. \tag{5.A.30}$$

The *phase angle* ψ has disappeared from the expression. The covariance function R_{nn} for wide-band noise with a rectangular frequency spectrum has the form of a sinc function, which tends towards zero for large τ such that

$$R_{xx}(\tau) \approx \frac{a^2}{2} \cos 2\pi f\tau. \tag{5.A.31}$$

(e) Power spectrum, Wiener–Khintschin relation

The *power spectrum* of a signal, $H(f)$, is defined as the square of the frequency spectrum given by (5.A.11) and so

$$H(f) = |X(f)|^2. \tag{5.A.32}$$

We now derive the *Wiener–Khintschin relation*, which is of great importance for rapid computation. For two signals $x(t)$ and $y(t)$, using (5.A.11) we can write

$$x(t) = \frac{1}{2\pi} \int_{-\infty}^{\infty} X(f) \exp(2\pi j f t) \, df,$$

$$y(t+\tau) = \frac{1}{2\pi} \int_{-\infty}^{\infty} Y(f) \exp[2\pi j f(t+\tau)] \, df. \tag{5.A.33}$$

By analogy with (5.A.32), we define the *cross-spectrum* as

$$H(f) = X(f)Y(f), \tag{5.A.34}$$

with H, X and Y complex variables of f. Then, for the inverse Fourier transform of $H(f)$ [see IV, §13.2.2], we can write

$$h(\tau) = \frac{1}{2\pi} \int_{-\infty}^{\infty} H(f) \exp(2\pi j f\tau) \, df, \tag{5.A.35}$$

which can be expressed as

$$h(\tau) = \int_{-\infty}^{\infty} y(t) \int_{-\infty}^{\infty} X(f) \exp[2\pi j f(t-\tau)] \, df \, dt$$

$$= \int_{-\infty}^{\infty} y(t)x(t-\tau) \, dt. \tag{5.A.36}$$

If in (5.A.34) we replace $Y(f)$ by the complex conjugate spectrum $Y^*(f)$, it follows that

$$\int_{-\infty}^{\infty} X(f)Y^*(f) \exp(2\pi j f\tau) \, df = \int_{-\infty}^{\infty} x(t)y(t+\tau) \, dt = R_{xy}(\tau).$$ (5.A.37)

For $x = y$ and $\tau = 0$, we can write

$$\int_{-\infty}^{\infty} |X(f)|^2 \, df = \int_{-\infty}^{\infty} x^2(t) \, dt = R_{xx}(0).$$ (5.A.38)

This is known as *Parseval's theorem* [see IV, §20.6.3]. It says that the power of a signal measured in the time domain has the same value as when it is measured in the frequency domain. From (5.A.37) we may also write, with $x = y$ and taking the inverse Fourier transform,

$$|X(f)|^2 = \int_{-\infty}^{\infty} R_{xx}(\tau) \exp(-2\pi j f\tau) \, d\tau.$$ (5.A.39)

Since the auto-covariance function is symmetric, $R_{xx}(\tau) = R_{xx}(-\tau)$ [see II, §22.2.2], we can select the symmetric component of (5.A.39) and show that

$$|X(f)|^2 = 2 \int_0^{\infty} R_{xx}(\tau) \cos 2\pi f\tau \, d\tau.$$ (5.A.40)

This is the Wiener–Khintschin relation.

The inter-relationships among the preceding formulae are shown schematically in Table 5.A.1. The Fourier transform is shown as the symbol $\leftrightarrow$ in the table.

Another important property of the covariance function is that the covariance function of sampled continuous signals is equal to the sampled covariance function of continuous signals. For the auto-covariance function of quantized signals, we may write, for example (see also paragraph (a) above),

$$R_{xx}(\tau) = R_{y_q y_q}(\tau) \qquad \text{for } \tau \neq 0.$$ (5.A.41)

(f) Convolution

The *convolution* of $x(t)$ and $g(t)$ is given by the Duhamel (or folding) integral

$$y(t) = \int_{-\infty}^{\infty} x(t-\tau)g(\tau) \, d\tau,$$ (5.A.42)

Table 5.A.1 Relationships between functions in the time and frequency domains.

$x(t)$	$\leftrightarrow$	$X(f)$	$\leftrightarrow$	R_{xx}	$\leftrightarrow$	$|X(f)|^2$
$y(t)$	$\leftrightarrow$	$Y(f)$	$\leftrightarrow$	R_{yy}	$\leftrightarrow$	$|Y(f)|^2$
$\downarrow$		$\downarrow$				
$R_{xy}(\tau)$		$H(f) = X(f) * Y(f)$				

$\leftrightarrow$ stands for Fourier transform. $\rightarrow$ denotes a variance/covariance function.

also written symbolically as

$$y(t) = x(t) * g(t). \tag{5.A.43}$$

Using the formulae of the last paragraph we may derive

$$Y(f) = X(f)G(f), \tag{5.A.44}$$

and

$$G = Y/X. \tag{5.A.45}$$

For linear systems we call $g(t)$ the *impulse response* to a Dirac impulse $\delta(t)$ at the input of the system (Figure 5.A.4). $G(f)$ is called the *transfer function*; it is a complex function of frequency. We next give some examples of the use of G for the design of digital filters for signals.

(g) Digital filtering

Moving average filters A *moving average filter* is defined by the impulse response $g(\tau)$ where

$$g(\tau) = \begin{cases} \dfrac{1}{T}, & \text{for } |\tau| \le T/2, \\ 0, & \text{for } |\tau| > T/2, \end{cases} \tag{5.A.46}$$

so that, with (5.A.42),

$$y(t) = \frac{1}{T} \int_{-T/2}^{T/2} x(t - \tau) \, d\tau. \tag{5.A.47}$$

We have already seen that the frequency spectrum of a rectangular time signal is a sinc function:

$$G(f) = \frac{1}{T} \int_{-T/2}^{T/2} \exp(-2\pi \mathrm{j} f\tau) \, d\tau = \frac{\sin(\pi f T)}{\pi f T}. \tag{5.A.48}$$

This filter has low-pass properties; i.e. it attenuates higher frequency components of the signal.

Auto-regressive filters The output of *auto-regressive* or *recursive* digital filters is determined by a combination of input and previous output, i.e. by feedback. The auto-regressive filter can be written in general terms, with x_i and y_i representing

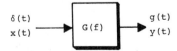

Figure 5.A.4 Impulse response
$g(t)$ of a system G.

the sampled data, as

$$a_0 y_n + a_1 y_{n-1} + a_2 y_{n-2} + \cdots + a_N y_{n-N} = b_0 x_m + b_1 x_{m-1} + \cdots + b_M x_{m-M},$$

(5.A.49)

the a_k and b_k being scalar weights.

A common filter which uses many previous outputs but only one recent input at a time is exemplified by

$$y_n = g x_n + a_1 y_{n-1} + a_2 y_{n-2} + \cdots + a_N y_{n-N}.$$

(5.A.50)

Here g and the a's are scalars.

The FT of (5.A.50) can be written as

$$Y(F) = g X(f) + Y(f) \sum_{k=1}^{N} a_k \exp(-2\pi j f k \Delta t),$$

(5.A.51)

Δt being the sampling interval. In computing transfer functions for sampled digital systems and signals, we commonly use the z transform [see IV, §13.4], related to the FT, but giving a quick insight into zeros and poles of the transfer function [see IV, §9.8].

The z transform for digital filters Digital filters have impulse responses $g(\tau)$ which can be described by a series of weighting coefficients

$$(a_0, a_1, a_2, \ldots, a_N) = a_0 \delta(t) + a_1 \delta(t - \Delta t) + a_2 \delta(t - 2\Delta t) + \cdots + a_N \delta(t - N\Delta t).$$

(5.A.52)

We have seen in the preceding section that the response of this filter to a Dirac impulse can be represented by the Fourier transform. This, of course, could also be done for digital filters, but because of the discrete character we prefer the use of the *Laplace transform* or, based on it, the z transform. In parallel to (5.A.11), the Laplace transform of a function $g(t)$ is defined by

$$L(s) = \int_0^\infty g(t) \exp(-st) \, dt$$

(5.A.53)

[see IV, §13.3]. For the filter of (5.A.52), this is equal to

$$L(s) = \int_0^\infty (a_0, a_1, \ldots, a_N) \exp(-st) \, dt = \sum_{k=0}^{N} a_k \exp(-k\Delta t s).$$

(5.A.54)

The *z transform* $G(z)$ is now defined by letting $z = \exp(\Delta t s)$, so that

$$G(z) = \sum_{k=0}^{N} a_k z^{-k};$$

(5.A.55)

i.e. $G(z)$ is a polynomial in z^{-1} with coefficients given by the coefficients of our original filter impulse response $(a_0, a_1, a_2, \ldots, a_N)$ [see IV, §13.4] and z is a complex parameter. We obtain the frequency behaviour by letting $s = j\omega$ or $z = \exp(j\omega\Delta t)$, with Δt as the sampling interval. As in the case of the Fourier expansion, here convolution in the time domain implies multiplication of functions in the z domain [see IV; §13.5.2].

We now give some examples. For a moving average filter, as defined in (5.A.46), with sampled data, we may write

$$y_k = \frac{1}{2N+1} \sum_{i=-N}^{N} x_{k-i}, \quad \text{with} \quad x_{k-i} = x[(t_0 + k\Delta t) - i\Delta t], \quad (5.A.56)$$

whence the z transform can be written as

$$G(z) = \frac{Y(z)}{X(z)} = \frac{1}{2N+1} \sum_{k=-N}^{N} z^{-k}$$

$$= \frac{1}{2N+1} (z^{-N} + z^{-N+1} + \cdots + z^{-1} + 1 + z + \cdots + z^N) \quad (5.A.57)$$

or

$$G(z) = \frac{1}{2N+1} \frac{1 - z^{2N+1}}{(1-z)z^N}. \quad (5.A.58)$$

This formula can be expressed in the complex z plane by *poles* (where $G(z)$ is infinite) and *zeros* [see IV, §9.8]. There are N poles at $(0,0)$ and one pole at $(1,0)$, and there are $2N + 1$ zeros at the unit circle [see I, §2.7]. Formula (5.A.58) can quickly give the auto-regressive version of this moving average filter by dividing by z^{N+1}; hence

$$G(z) = \frac{1}{2N+1} \frac{z^{-(N+1)} - z^N}{z^{-1} - 1}. \quad (5.A.59)$$

The inverse transformation to the sampled time domain yields

$$y_k = y_{k-1} + \frac{x_{k+N} - x_{k-N-1}}{2N+1} \quad (5.A.60)$$

because

$$y_{k-n} = z^{-n} y_k.$$

In principle, any digital filter can be defined by the z transform. Extensive information about filter design can be found in the standard texts on signal analysis referenced at the beginning of this chapter.

(h) Optimal or 'matched' filters

If we want to filter a signal with a known waveshape of duration T from a noisy mixture—e.g. to find its location in time—we can optimize the filter response to this particular signal. Assume that the original signal can be written as

$$x_0(t) = s_0(t) + n_0(t),$$ (5.A.61)

n_0 being the noise.

Let the filter again have an impulse response $g(\tau)$; then after filtering we obtain

$$x_1(t) = s_1(t) + n_1(t) = \int_{-T/2}^{T/2} x_0(\tau)g(t - \tau)\,d\tau = x_0(t)*g(t).$$ (5.A.62)

Different strategies are now possible in order to optimize $g(\tau)$. We could optimize the similarity between x_1 and s_0, i.e. try to ensure that the output signal shape is identical to the known waveshape $s_0(t)$. To this end we might minimize the cost function C where

$$C = \int_{-T/2}^{T/2} \{x_1(t) - s_0(t)\}^2\,dt.$$ (5.A.63)

Another criterion could be that the output noise be minimal or the signal to noise ratio (SNR_1) maximal. We will not derive all intermediate steps but just state that for signals buried in (white) Gaussian noise this *optimal filter* response $g(\tau)$ is equal to

$$g(\tau) = s_0(t_0 - \tau).$$ (5.A.64)

This means that the matched filter response is the shape of the signal s_0 in reverse order in time. If the noise is not white (coloured), the same derivation applies, if we first of all use a 'pre-whitening' filter to obtain a flat frequency spectrum.

(i) Coherent averaging

In the last paragraph we assumed that we knew the signal shape and wanted to locate it in time. In this paragraph we assume that the reverse holds: we know the locations (points of reference within the signal) in time, i.e. the point process, and we want to find the signal shape. This problem is very common in signal analysis and can be solved by *coherent averaging*. A simple example is the computation of a signal waveform which is buried in Gaussian noise, coloured or not. If the original SNR for a signal as described by (5.A.61) can be written as

$$SNR_0 = \frac{\overline{s_0^2(t)}}{\overline{n_0^2(t)}},$$ (5.A.65)

and if the signal shape $s(t)$ is defined from $-T/2$ to $+T/2$ and occurs N times in the signal $x_0(t)$, then we may write

$$s_0(t) = \psi(t)*s(t),$$ (5.A.66)

which is the convolution of $s(t)$ with the impulse series $\psi(t)$, i.e. the occurrence of the signal $s(t)$ in $x_0(t)$ (see, for example, Figure 5.1.4). If we apply $\psi(t)$ to the noisy signal $x_0(t)$, we can write

$$
\begin{aligned}
x_1(t) &= \psi(t) * x_0(t) \\
&= \psi(t) * s_0(t) + \psi(t) * n_0(t) \\
&= s_1(t) + n_1(t).
\end{aligned}
\tag{5.A.67}
$$

For the new SNR_1 we may write

$$
\mathrm{SNR}_1 = \frac{\overline{s_1^2(t)}}{\overline{n_1^2(t)}} = \frac{N^2 \overline{s_0^2(t)}}{N \, \overline{n_0^2(t)}} = N \times \mathrm{SNR}_0,
\tag{5.A.68}
$$

which means that the SNR (expressed in power terms) increases proportionally with the number of summed complexes, $s(t)$, in the noisy signal. The noise samples may be considered as independent elements in a stochastic Gaussian process.

5.A.3 Transformations

In this section we generalize the (linear) transformations of (biological) signals. We have already introduced the Fourier transform. Other examples of transforms used in biological signal analysis are the Karhunen–Loève expansion, the Chebyshev transformation and the Walsh–Hadamard transformation.

(a) Karhunen–Loève expansion

We now discuss the most general expansion in terms of orthonormal components through which any given signal can be represented [see IV, §20.4]. Let us assume that we have a signal $x(t)$ which is defined for $-T/2 < t \le T/2$. Let there be a set of elementary functions $l_k(t)$ with coefficients c_k such that

$$
x(t) = \sum_{k=-\infty}^{\infty} c_k l_k(t) \qquad \text{for} \quad -T/2 < t \le T/2.
\tag{5.A.69}
$$

(For comparison also see Formula 5.A.13.) Furthermore, let the functions $l_k(t)$ be an orthonormal set with respect to the *inner product*

$$
(l_i(t), l_j(t)) = \frac{1}{T} \int_{-T/2}^{T/2} l_i(t) l_j(t) \, dt = \delta_{ij}.
\tag{5.A.70}
$$

[see IV, §§11.7 and 11.8]. Applying equation (IV. 20.4.10) to (5.A.70) in this guidebook, we are able to find the coefficients c_n in (5.A.69):

$$
\frac{1}{T} \int_{-T/2}^{T/2} x(t) l_n(t) \, dt = \frac{1}{T} \int_{-T/2}^{T/2} \sum_k c_k l_k(t) l_n(t) \, dt = c_n.
\tag{5.A.71}
$$

The elementary functions $l_k(t)$ define a multi-dimensional signal space in which the set of signals $\{x(t)\}$ can be reconstructed.

Many orthonormal sets of basic components $l_k(t)$ obey the equations (5.A.69) to (5.A.71). We introduce the further constraint that the coefficients c_k be independent or, statistically for $\{x(t)\}$,

$$\overline{c_k c_n} = 0. \tag{5.A.72}$$

From (5.A.67), it can be shown that

$$\frac{1}{T} \int_{-T/2}^{T/2} l_k(t) \left[\frac{1}{T} \int_{-T/2}^{T/2} R_{xx}(t-\tau) l_n(\tau) \, d\tau \right] = 0. \tag{5.A.73}$$

This is only true for

$$\frac{1}{T} \int_{-T/2}^{T/2} R_{xx}(t-\tau) l_n(\tau) \, d\tau = \lambda_n l_n(t), \qquad n \neq k. \tag{5.A.74}$$

[see IV, (20.4.7)].

If, on the contrary, $k = n$, we see that

$$\overline{c_k^2} = \lambda_k. \tag{5.A.75}$$

This series expansion is called the Karhunen–Loève expansion. The process is equivalent to a rotation of axes within the multi-dimensional signal space, where the λ's are eigenvalues of the system based on the set $\{l_k(t)\}$ and the new axes are determined by the shape of the cluster $\{x(t)\}$ in the signal space.

If the original signal consists of independent samples of equal variance (e.g. white noise), yielding a diagonal covariance matrix [see II, §13.3.1], the direction of the axes is immaterial.

It must be stressed that the Karhunen–Loève expansion is the only transformation which yields independent coefficients. Other expansions may be orthonormal but do not necessarily give independent c's. Also, the signal components from the Shannon theorem give basic components, although they are not necessarily orthonormal. Every linear transform of a signal can again be transformed to the K–L expansion or some other linear transformation. Each transformation can be seen as a matrix operation on the original set [see I, §5.13]. We must stress here again that a linear transformation does not necessarily offer the right solution to a signal processing problem.

(b) Chebyshev transformation

The *Chebyshev transformation* is another well-known type of transformation where we start from a set of basic components, the Chebyshev polynomials, which have a predefined relationship [see IV, §10.5.3]. Chebyshev polynomials are shown in Figure 5.A.5.

The following relations hold:

$$T_0(\tau) = 1 \qquad \text{(a DC component)},$$
$$T_1(\tau) = \tau. \tag{5.A.76}$$

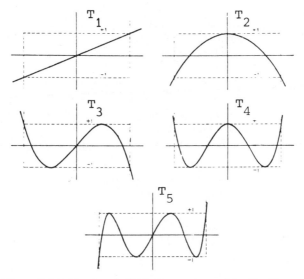

Figure 5.A.5 The first 5 Chebyshev polynomials, T_1–T_5.

The recursion formula for all the T_k is

$$T_{k+1}(\tau) = 2\tau T_k(\tau) - T_{k-1}(\tau) \tag{5.A.77}$$

or, in other terms,

$$T_k(\tau) = \cos[k \arccos(\tau)]. \tag{5.A.78}$$

As seen in Volume IV, Sections 10.5.0 and 10.5.3, the Chebyshev polynomials are orthonormal and so may be used to build an orthogonal basis for $x(t)$. For example, on the interval $t_0 - T/2 < t \le t_0 + T/2$,

$$x(\tau) = \sum_{k=0}^{N} c_k T_k(\tau), \tag{5.A.79}$$

where $\tau = t - t_0$.

(c) Walsh–Hadamard transformation

Another transformation of interest, of much later date than the Fourier transformation, is one based on Walsh functions. These functions can only take the values $+1$ and -1, in contrast to continuous sine and cosine functions. This offers certain advantages for digital processing of biological signals (or images).

It can be shown that Walsh functions form an orthonormal set with respect to the inner product:

$$\left(\text{wal}_k\left(\frac{t}{T}\right), \text{wal}_l\left(\frac{t}{T}\right) \right) = \frac{1}{T} \int_0^T \text{wal}_k\left(\frac{t}{T}\right) \text{wal}_l\left(\frac{t}{T}\right) dt$$

$$= \delta_{k,l} \tag{5.A.80}$$

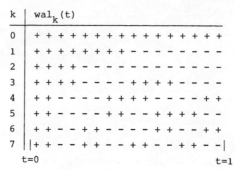

Figure 5.A.6 The first 8 Walsh functions,
$\text{wal}_k(t)$, for the interval $0 \leq t < 1$.

and so [see IV, §20.4] we may write

$$x(t) = \sum_{k=0}^{\infty} c_k \text{wal}_k\left(\frac{t}{T}\right), \tag{5.A.81}$$

and [see IV, (20.4.10)]

$$c_k = \frac{1}{T} \int_0^T x(t) \text{wal}_k\left(\frac{t}{T}\right) dt. \tag{5.A.82}$$

The number of sign changes in wal_k per time unit, $s = k/T$, is called the *sequency* of the function and is illustrated by Figure 5.A.6. Several attempts have been made to store signals with the help of such functions.

Although they seem to be very simple, it turns out that the number of terms c_k necessary to store a signal with bandwidth W far exceeds the number of coefficients when using Fourier components. It has been shown (Blackman, 1974) that for a signal with a spectrum of up to, for example, 2 kHz and requiring an error of less than 1 per cent r.m.s., the number of Walsh terms is over 360 as compared to about 6 for a Fourier expansion when storing a 1-second signal. For this reason a Walsh expansion (obtained, for example, via the fast Walsh transform), although it can operate extremely quickly on a computer, requires much storage.

J.H.vB.

REFERENCES

Ascoop, C. A. (1974). *ST-forces during Exercise*, Thesis, University of Groningen.
Barlow, J. S. (1979). Computerized clinical electroencephalography in perspective, *IEEE Trans. BME*, **26**, 377–391.
Beauchamp, K. G. (1973). *Signal Processing*, George Allen and Unwin, London.

Bendat, J. S., and Piersol, A. G. (1971). *Random Data: Analysis and Measurement Procedures*, Wiley, New York.

Blackman, N. M. (1974). Sinusoids versus Walsh functions, *Proc. IEEE*, **62**, 346–354.

Bodenstein, G., and Praetorius, H. M. (1977). Feature extraction from the EEG by adaptive segmentation, *Proc. IEEE*, **65**, 642–657.

Cooley, J. W., and Tukey, J. W. (1966). An algorithm for machine calculation of complex Fourier series, *Math. Comp.*, **19**, 297–301.

Cox, J. R., Nolle, F. M., and Arthur, R. M. (1972). Digital analysis of the EEG, the blood pressure and the ECG, *Proc. IEEE*, **60**, 1137–1164.

Cox, J. R., Nolle, F. M., Fozzard, H. A., and Oliver, G. C. (1968). AZTEC, a preprocessing program for real time ECG rhythm analysis, *IEEE Trans. BME*, **15**, 128–129.

Duda, R. U., and Hart, P. E. (1973). *Pattern Classification and Scene Analysis*, Wiley, New York.

Gelsema, E. S., and Kanal, L. N. (Eds) (1980). *Pattern Recognition in Practice*, North-Holland Publishing Company, Amsterdam.

Gold, B., and Rader, C. M. (1969). *Digital Processing of Signals*, McGraw-Hill, New York.

Hengeveld, S. J., and van Bemmel, J. H. (1976). Computer detection of *P*-waves, *Comp. Biomed. Res.*, **9**, 125–132.

Jansen, B. H., Hasman, A., and Lenten, R. (1981). Piecewise analysis of EEG's using AR-modeling and clustering, *Comput. Biomed. Res.*, **14**, 168–178.

Kanal, L. N. (1974). *Patterns in Pattern Recognition. IEEE Trans. IT*, **20**, 697–722.

Plokker, H. W. M. (1978). *Cardiac Rhythm Diagnosis by Digital Computer*, Thesis, Free University, Amsterdam.

Pronk, R. A. F., Simons, A. J. R. (1981). Rechnerunterstützte EEG Überwachung Während Operationen an eröffneten Herzen, in *Rechnounterstützte Intensiv Pfluge* (Ed. E. Epple), pp. 27–32, Thieme Verlag, Stuttgart.

Rabiner, L. E., and Gold, B. (1975). *Theory and Application of Digital Signal Processing*, Prentice-Hall, Englewood Cliffs, New Jersey.

Rabiner, L. E., and Rader, C. M. (1972). Digital Signal Processing, IEEE Press Selected Reprint Series no. 25.

Rémond, A. (Ed.) (1977). *EEG Informatics, a Didactic Review and Applications*, North-Holland Publishing Company, Amsterdam.

Schwartz, M., and Shaw, L. (1975). *Signal Processing, Discrete Spectral Analysis, Detection and Estimation*, McGraw-Hill, Tokyo.

Shannon, C. E., and Weaver, W. (1949). *The Mathematical Theory of Communication*, University of Illinois Press, Chicago.

Sheppard, L. C. (1979). The computer in the care of critically ill patients, *Proc. IEEE*, **67**, 1300–1306.

Simoons, M. L. (1975). On-line processing of orthogonal exercise electro-cardiograms, *Comp. Biomed. Res.*, **8**, 105–117.

Swenne, C. A., van Bemmel, J. H., Relik, T. F. M., and Versteeg, B. (1977). A computerized interactive coronary care monitoring system, *IEEE Trans. BMF*, **24**, 63–67.

Talmon, J. L. (1983). *Pattern recognition of the ECG*, Thesis, Free University, Amsterdam.

van Bemmel, J. H. (1973a). Template wave form recognition applied to ECG/VCG analysis, *Comp. Biomed. Res.*, **6**, 430–441.

van Bemmel, J. H. (1973b). Clustering algorithm for QRS and STT waveform typing, *Comp. Biomed. Res.*, **6**, 442–456.

van Bemmel, J. H. (1977). *The Role of Computers in Cardiology and Clinical Physiology*, MEDINFO-77, pp. 819–827, North-Holland Publishing Company, Amsterdam.

van Bemmel, J. H. (1982). Recognition of electrocardiograpic patterns, in *Handbook of*

Statistics (Eds P. R. Krishnaiah and L. N. Kanal), Vol II, pp. 501–526, North-Holland Publishing Company, Amsterdam.

van Bemmel, J. H., Haan, J. de, and Veth, A. F. L. (1974). Instrumentation for obstetrics and gynaecology, in *Medical Engineering* (Ed. C. D. Ray), pp. 548–588, Year Book Medical Publishers, Chicago.

van Bemmel, J. H. and Willems, J. L. (Eds) (1977). *Trends in Computer-processed Electrocardiograms*, North-Holland Publishing Company, Amsterdam.

van Trees, H. L. (1971). *Detection, Estimation and Modulation Theory, I, II and III*, Wiley, New York.

Veth, A. F. L. and van Bemmel, J. H. (1978). The role of the placental vascular bed in the foetal response to cord occlusion, in *Fetal and Newborn Cardiovascular Physiology* (Eds L. D. Longo and D. D. Reneau), pp. 579–614, Garland Press, New York.

Wolf, H. K., and Macfarlane, P. W. (Eds) (1979). *Optimization of Computer ECG Processing*, North-Holland Publishing Company, Amsterdam.

Mathematical Methods in Medicine
Edited by D. Ingram & R. F. Bloch
© 1984 John Wiley & Sons Ltd.

6

Mathematical Aspects of Laboratory Medicine

6.1 INTRODUCTION

6.1.1 The role of the clinical laboratory

Laboratory medicine is concerned with the following sequence of events:

(a) Obtaining a sample from a patient,
(b) Analysing the sample,
(c) Obtaining a result from the analysis,
(d) Interpreting the result in the context of the patient.

The first three items are the responsibility of the clinical laboratory; the last item is the responsibility of the clinician who can be advised by the laboratory.

Mathematics is applied to the sequence of events in three distinct ways:

(a) The application of simple arithmetic; e.g. to transform the raw data of an assay to a result.
(b) The application of statistical techniques to groups of results. This is commonly done by the non-specialist, who takes methods or equations from a book or uses a pre-programmed calculator.
(c) The application of more complex mathematical methods. This is usually done by a specialist with the aid of a computer. A typical example is standard curve analysis.

Mathematical techniques are seldom used by the laboratory analyst or by the clinician who interprets the result. One reason for this is that intrinsic variability in the sample and in the interpretation is often greater than variability in analysis and in derivation of results. A result calculated using sophisticated mathematical techniques is therefore often almost as difficult to interpret as a result obtained by simple arithmetic. A second reason is that clinical laboratories are subjected to

273

pressures of time and cost as well as of accuracy of analysis. It is easy to establish, for example, that technique A for measuring an analyte gives a result in six hours at a cost of £1 with a coefficient of variation [see II, §9.2.6] of 10 per cent and that technique B for the same analyte gives a result in three hours at a cost of £1.50 with a coefficient of variation of 15 per cent. It is not easy to decide whether technique A or technique B should be routinely used.

6.1.2 The place of mathematics in the clinical laboratory

A clinical laboratory is concerned with three factors: accuracy, time and cost of analysis. The main use of mathematical methods is to improve one or more of these without worsening the others. For example, sophisticated standard curve analysis can improve accuracy without impairing time or cost, and critical path analysis can reduce time without impairing accuracy or cost. For a clinical laboratory, questions of time and cost are to some extent dictated by established practice in a hospital or clinic, and the pressure to reduce these comes from outside the laboratory. The question of accuracy is primarily under the control of the laboratory.

It is surprisingly difficult to establish how accurate a result should be. Published guidelines tend to be based on the normal range or on the magnitude of the measured quantity. For example, 'The maximum allowable error should be plus or minus a quarter of the normal range or ten per cent of the actual quantity, whichever is less' (Tonks, 1963). Such guidelines are always inadequate because the purpose of a result is to enable a clinician to make correct clinical decisions. The clinical value of a result depends both on its accuracy and on the skill of the clinician and the adequacy of the supporting information. The less skilled the clinician, the more accurate the result should be.

The assumption underlying this chapter is that any improvement in accuracy leads to a result which is easier for a clinician to interpret, and therefore makes the result more valuable. The chapter reviews some of the mathematical techniques which can be applied to the sequence of work in the clinical laboratory with the aim of improving laboratory efficiency or increasing the accuracy of results. It does not aim to cover all the mathematical techniques which have been applied to laboratory medicine, neither does it cover simple arithmetic operations or standard statistical formulae for assessing results since these are all described in handbooks of laboratory practice (e.g. Dacie and Lewis, 1975; Duguid, Marmion and Swain, 1975; Tietz, 1976).

6.2 DEFINITIONS

Many of the terms used in this chapter have no single commonly accepted definition. The usage adopted here is set out below, together with explanations where appropriate. These are based in the main on *Webster's Third New International Dictionary* (Gove, 1966).

6.2.1 Precision, bias and accuracy

Precision is the degree of agreement of repeated measurements of a quantity. This is usually measured in terms of *imprecision*—the scatter (measured as the standard deviation [see II, §9.1] or coefficient of variation [see II, §9.2.6]) of repeated measurements of the same quantity.

Individual measurements of a quantity are subject to variation from one observation to another. When there is no *bias* the observations are sometimes larger and sometimes smaller than the true value, but on average they are just right.

Accuracy is the degree of conformity to some recognized standard value. It is usually measured in terms of *inaccuracy*, as the combination of bias and imprecision.

6.2.2 Error

Error is the variation in measurements, calculations or observations of a quantity due to mistakes or to (usually) uncontrollable factors. In a clinical laboratory, there are three special uses of the term:

(a) *Intrinsic error* (or *inherent error*) is the variability in results caused by the innate imprecision of each analytical step.
(b) *Systematic error* is the difference in results caused by the bias of an assay.
(c) Finally, there is error arising from the occasional *gross mistake* which occurs in every analytical process; e.g. failure to add a reagent or incorrect reading of a scale.

6.2.3 Assay and assay run

An *assay* is a test to determine the presence or absence or, more often, the quantity of one or more components of a material. 'Assay' can be used as a descriptive term for a type of test, or can be used to indicate a single test on one sample. An *assay run* is a set of consecutive measurements, readings or observations all based on the same batch of reagents.

Intra-assay is within an assay run; *inter-assay* is between successive runs.

6.2.4 Quality control

Quality control is an aggregate of functions designed to ensure adequate quality of analytical results by a critical study of instruments, materials, processes, equipment and human performance followed by periodic inspection and analysis of the results of inspection to determine causes for deficiencies, and by removal of such causes (Fleck *et al.*, 1974).

6.2.5 Normal and reference ranges

Traditionally, the *normal range* of an analyte is the range within which 95 per cent of values occur, obtained on samples from a group of selected individuals. Such a range has certain problems. First, there is a tacit assumption that every value outside it is abnormal, even though by definition 5 per cent of the selected individuals tested fall outside the range. Second, the calculation of the range has frequently been based upon the mean value plus or minus two standard deviations [see II, §9.4 and VI, §4.1.2], and the problems of non-Gaussian distribution [see II, §11.4] and, more important, sampling error have often been ignored. Third, the selection of individuals has frequently been based upon what is readily obtainable rather than what is desirable. Thus, many published normal ranges have been based on samples obtained from laboratory staff, medical students or the general hospital inpatient population (Pryce, Haslam and Wootton, 1969).

There is a tendency to avoid the use of the term and the concept of normal range, and to replace it by the term *reference range*, a range of values characteristic of a defined population. The population definition may be in terms of disease, age, sex, ethnic group or any other combination of characteristics (Dybkaer, 1972; Grasbech, 1972). The derivation of reference ranges and their applications in laboratory testing have been discussed by Galen and Gambino (1975).

In calculating a normal range or a reference range, it seems best to transform the values so that they approximate to a Gaussian distribution, for example, by working with the logarithm of the values rather than the values themselves (Bliss, 1967) [see VI, §2.7]. This is likely to be statistically more efficient than using non-parametric (i.e. distribution-free) methods (Healy, 1969) [see VI, Chapter 14], but in some circumstances the latter may be more accurate (Reed, Henry and Mason 1971). Both normal and reference ranges are, of course, affected by laboratory bias and imprecision as well as by the distribution of values in the sampled population (Gowenlock, 1969; Krause *et al.* 1975). This is not of major consequence except, for example, when laboratories use linear discriminant functions [see VI, §16.6] derived in other centres to aid in differential diagnosis (Holland and Jacobs, 1982).

6.3 LABORATORY LOGISTICS

Laboratory logistics are concerned with the workload to be analysed and the organization of analysis. It is necessary for a laboratory director both to predict the workload and to organize it in the most effective manner.

The major influence on the total workload is the test with the largest single workload. In the case of clinical chemistry, the predominant influence on workload has been the group of tests on urea, sodium, potassium and bicarbonate which tend to be measured together. The total workload of a clinical chemistry department increased exponentially when this group of tests was in a period of rapid growth, and the increases slowed when these tests reached a plateau (Sanders, 1980).

Since the advent of automation, the demand on a laboratory is governed more by the range of tests which are requested and the frequency of each assay run than by the number of samples analysed. To decide what resources are necessary to run a laboratory, the growth curve of each test or group of tests must be examined separately.

Every director of a clinical laboratory has at some point faced the problem of coping with increased demand on services while operating with limited resources in time, staff and space. In this situation either efficiency or resources must be increased, or staff morale and analytical accuracy will decrease. *Operational research* techniques have been applied to assist with planning and reorganization of work in clinical laboratories (Carruthers, 1970; Rath *et al.*, 1970; Cundy, 1972; Barber, 1978).

There are two main types of operational research: direct measurement and a theoretical approach, usually based on simulation. Both depend on the ability to define a quantitative measure of efficiency, with the aim of maximizing this. In practice there are no agreed values which can be placed on changes in laboratory accuracy, on the time needed to generate a result or on benefits to patient care.

In some circumstances the method of *simulation* provides a useful technique (Tocher, 1963). In simulation, the effect of possible changes in organization, staffing or equipment is predicted. Applications range from simple (e.g. the amount of work that could be undertaken) to complex (e.g. the numerical simulation of a whole department).

Full theoretical specification of a complex system often leads to sets of equations that are intractable. In simulation, criterion variables are calculated repeatedly, choosing random values from the frequency distributions known or assumed for the input and resource variables. This enables a frequency distribution of the criterion variables to be built up, even when it is not possible to solve the equations directly.

For simulation techniques to be useful, the assumptions underlying the representation must of course be realistic. The largest uncertainty in any description of a laboratory is how best to measure performance. Without an appropriate definition of this, there is little to be gained from a complex analysis (Peto, Whitby and Finney, 1972).

6.4 VARIATION IN BIOLOGICAL SAMPLES

6.4.1 Sampling and the combination of errors

In a clinical laboratory, most problems with biological samples are due to error. Is the sample from the right patient? Was it taken at the correct time of day? Is the preservative appropriate? If an error occurs, generally speaking it is better to

Table 6.4.1 The combination of errors

Assume a result, z, is calculated from two independent variables, x and y, each of which has an error, characterized by the standard derivations σ_x and σ_y.
For $z = x + y$ and for $z = x - y$,

$$\sigma_z^2 = \sigma_x^2 + \sigma_y^2.$$

For $z = xy$ and for $z = x/y$,

$$\left(\frac{\sigma_z}{z}\right)^2 = \left(\frac{\sigma_x}{x}\right)^2 + \left(\frac{\sigma_y}{y}\right)^2.$$

repeat the sampling correctly rather than to carry out corrections of doubtful validity, e.g. based on the degree of haemolysis of the sample.

Convenience and established practice have been the predominant influences in establishing both the nature and the timing of samples. Many studies have compared measurements of the same analyte in different biological fluids, but these have all demonstrated feasibility rather than established the best. To define which is best is difficult, since this involves accuracy, time, cost and convenience. But the mathematics of *combination of errors* [see VI, §2.7.1(b)] can be used to answer some of the questions of accuracy (see Table 6.4.1). For example, it is widely believed that the excretion of many metabolities is approximately constant from day to day (except as discussed in Section 6.4.2 below), and therefore a 24-hour urine collection is a desirable sample for minimizing sampling imprecision. However, the collection of a 24-hour urine sample is tedious and can be difficult to arrange. An alternative is to collect a single random urine sample and to measure both the analyte concentration and the creatinine concentration within it (Dickey *et al.*, 1966). Since normal adults excrete approximately one gram of creatinine daily, the daily analyte excretion can be established by calculating the excretion per gram of creatinine.

For both of these procedures, the daily analyte excretion is determined by multiplying together the 24-hour urine volume and the analyte concentration. The coefficient of variation (CV)—i.e. the ratio of standard deviation to mean value [see II, §9.2.6]—of analyte excretion is therefore approximately equal to the square root of the sum of the squares of the CVs of the two components (see Table 6.4.1). For the former procedure, the error in 24-hour urine volume is due to the imprecission of collection (and the imprecision of volume measurement, which is likely to be small). For the latter procedure, the 24-hour volume is calculated in appropriate units as

$$\text{24-hour volume} = \frac{\text{creatinine excretion per day}}{\text{creatinine concentration in sample}}.$$

The CV of the 24-hour volume is approximately equal to the square root of the sum of the squares of the CVs of creatinine excretion and creatinine concentration. It may therefore be possible to calculate which procedure gives the more precise determination. However, there is a further error in the latter procedure, since it assumes that the pattern of excretion of the analyte throughout the day exactly mimics the pattern of creatinine excretion. This is unlikely to be true, particularly for analytes which show a significant diurnal variation in serum concentration. In practice, there seem to be large discrepancies between the actual analyte excretion and the excretion calculated from a creatinine ratio (Shelley *et al.*, 1970).

6.4.2 Biological rhythms

Many analytes show a rhythmical variation in their blood or urine con-centrations (Simpson, 1976). In humans, the most obvious of these are hormones, many of which show well-defined circadian or longer-term variations (Figure 6.4.1). In the presence of disease, the variations may change or disappear.

When the amplitude of a circadian rhythm is large, it can readily be demonstrated by analysing samples taken every few hours. A statistically significant difference between peak and trough values is evidence of an underlying

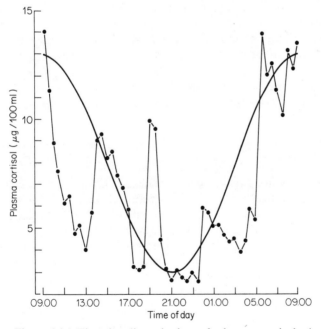

Figure 6.4.1 The circadian rhythm of plasma cortisol. A cosine wave has been superimposed upon sequential cortisol estimations. The episodic nature of the rhythm is clearly shown.

rhythm. In this way, plasma cortisol was shown to have a circadian rhythm (Tyler *et al.*, 1954) which was changed or abolished in Cushing's syndrome (Tournaire *et al.*, 1971; Sederberg-Olsen *et al.*, 1973).

To give an accurate quantitation of rhythm parameters, *time series analysis* can be used [see VI, Chapter 18]. A useful technique for biological time series is least squares spectral analysis (Simpson, 1976) [see VI, §18.10]. A spectrum of time periods are selected around the presumed time period of the rhythm, and cosine waves [see VI, §2.12] of these time periods are fitted to the raw data by least squares regression techniques.

Many circadian rhythms have been shown to be episodic with a series of pulses superimposed on a smooth rhythm (Weitzman, Fukushima and Nogeire, 1971; see Figure 6.4.1). This type of pattern has been analysed using a model based upon pharmacodynamic concepts (Jusko, Slaunwhite and Aceto, 1975). Least squares spectral analysis [see VI, §18.10] can reveal several coexisting rhythms of different amplitudes (Halberg *et al.*, 1965) and there is not usually a need to use the more complex Fourier analysis [see IV, Chapter 20] in these systems. However, between individuals, circadian rhythms may vary in the clock times of peaks and troughs. An extension of least squares spectral analysis, cosine vector analysis (Halberg, Tong and Johnson, 1976), can accommodate this, but it is often simpler to relate circadian rhythms to mid-sleep time rather than to clock time (Simpson, 1976).

The use of biological rhythms as a medical tool is unlikely to become widespread owing to the need for frequent sampling. However, these studies are valuable and may give guidance on the best time for taking a single or limited series of samples for clinical purposes. The best time is usually the time associated with minimum inter- and intra-individual variability, and maximum change in disease.

6.4.3 Dynamic tests

Many tests in laboratory medicine involve measuring the response of an analyte to a stimulus; e.g. the rise of blood glucose following an oral glucose load (Figure 6.4.2). Little work has been done on the factors governing optimum timing and number of samples, or on the best way of expressing results. Consequently, different laboratories frequently perform the same test in different ways. For example, the TRH (thyroliberin) test involves measuring serum thyrotropin (TSH) after the injection of TRH (Hall, 1971; Pickardt *et al.*, 1972). Some laboratories perform this test with three samples, others with six; some laboratories take the peak sample at twenty minutes after injection, others at thirty minutes; some laboratories define the response in terms of the peak TSH concentration, others in terms of the difference between basal and peak concentrations.

It is possible that dynamic function tests could give more information if the

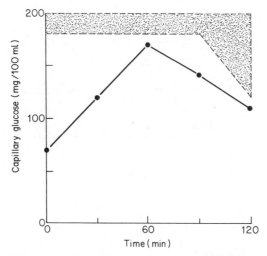

Figure 6.4.2 The glucose tolerance test. This test consists of the measurement of blood (usually capillary) glucose in five samples taken before and at half-hourly intervals after the administration of 50 g of glucose orally. A typical response is shown. A diabetic response can be defined as any result falling into the shaded area.

response could be better quantified. For many tests, the total response, defined as the area under the response curve, is considered a good clinical index. Finding the area under a curve is a problem which occurs in many sections of laboratory medicine and is of particular importance in chromatography. Rule-of-thumb methods include drawing the area on good quality graph paper and counting the squares. Simpson's rule [see III, §7.1.5] or the trapezium rule [see III, §7.1.3] are also often used (Kynch, 1955). In chromatography, micro-computer-based algorithms are used to filter the signal and reject outlying points, recognize baseline segments and peaks, resolve overlapping peaks and finally calculate peak heights and areas (Kipiniak, 1981).

For dynamic function tests there is no evidence that better quantification of the response gives more information to clinicians than a simpler approach, and in current practice most dynamic tests are judged in terms of the presence or absence of a significant response. Thus the glucose tolerance test shown in Figure 6.4.2 is judged by whether any sample falls into the shaded area. This type of approach is probably used because the large variations in individual responses to many stimuli make more sophisticated judgements difficult.

At present, the application of mathematics to dynamic tests is in defining the optimum number and timing of samples needed to demonstrate the presence or absence of a significant change. This is a complex problem since both assay

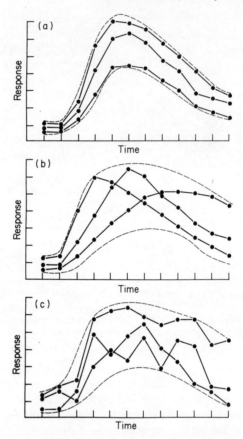

Figure 6.4.3 Responses in dynamic function tests. (a) This shows a response envelope and three typical responses for a test in which the precision is good and in which individuals differ little in their timing of response. To detect a response, only two samples are needed. (b) This shows responses for a test in which there is large individual variation in timing (e.g. a test where the initial step, such as gut absorption, can be slow). To detect the response, at least three samples are needed. Note that in this situation the areas under the response curves are likely to be more uniform than the timing of peak response. (c) This shows that a similar broad envelope can be generated by poor assay precision. Even in the absence of wide individual variation, at least three samples are needed to detect a response.

imprecision and individual variability of response affect the results. Empirical solutions can be found by plotting the detailed responses of a large number of individuals and calculating the position of the envelope which includes 95 per cent of the measured responses. If both assay imprecision and variability in individual response are small (Figure 6.4.3a) it is likely that only two samples will be needed. The timing of these should be chosen so as to maximize the probability of detecting a difference between them. If there is a large individual variation in timing of response (Figure 6.4.3b) or if assay imprecision is large (Figure 6.4.3c), more samples will be needed. The easiest way of interpreting these is still to look for a significant difference between the basal and the highest value. If there are both large individual variations and large assay imprecision, it is difficult to interpret the results of dynamic function tests with any confidence.

6.5 ANALYTICAL TECHNIQUES AND RESULT DERIVATION

To obtain a quantitative result, the response given by a sample must be compared with the responses given by one or more standards. There are three basic problems:

(a) How can results best be derived?
(b) How can the bias and imprecision of results be determined and minimized?
(c) How can analytical methods be compared?

6.5.1 The standard curve

The *standard curve* is the curve which relates the assay responses given by a range of standard solutions to their known concentrations. It permits the analyte concentration of an unknown solution to be inferred from its assay response by interpolation [see III, §2.3].

Assays exist in which the position of the standard curve can be inferred from the position of a single standard point or from a previously known value. Examples include gravimetric assays in which a product is weighed and spectrophotometric assays in which the absorbence of a standard solution is known or measured. In the latter, absorbence of an assay blank is internally compensated (so that the standard curve passes through the origin) and a linear relationship exists between absorbence and concentration over the assay range considered.

For this type of assay, there is no mathematical problem in the derivation of results. The error in results can be calculated from the formulae for combination of errors (see Table 6.4.1) or assessed empirically by using quality control techniques (see Section 6.6 below).

It is more common to set up several standard points and to draw a straight line or a curve through them in order to derive results. For this process, many mathematical techniques exist [see III, Chapter 6], of which the commonest is linear regression (see Section 1.3.13).

6.5.2 Linear standard curves

For many assays, a straight-line relationship can be constructed between the assay response y (the dependent variable) and the analyte concentration x (the independent variable). For some assays, the linear equation

$$y = a + bx$$

can be fitted directly to the data to determine constants a and b; however, it is more common to transform one or both variables in order to linearize the data, e.g. by using the equation [see IV, §2.11]

$$y = a + b \log x.$$

Although such standard curves can be drawn manually, regression techniques [see VI, §§3.5.2 and 6.5] are preferable, being more objective. These derive a best fit by calculating the gradient and intercept of a straight line so that errors in the dependent variable, y, are minimized (the method of least squares).

If the number of standard points used is the same as the number of constants in the equation being fitted (two in the example above), the fitted function will automatically pass through every standard point. It is better practice to use more standard points, since this allows the magnitude of the error to be identified. The larger the residual error [see VI, §8.2.4] associated with a standard point, the likelier it is to be associated with error. Calculation of the residuals associated with each standard point in turn permits a correction to be made to the position of the standard curve, either by omitting standard points which have un-characteristically large residuals (Hawker and Challand, 1981) or by weighting techniques. Typically, standard points are weighted [see III, §6.1.7, and VI, §8.1] according to the measured or the theoretical imprecision of the estimate at each analyte concentration (see for example, Rodbard and Hutt, 1974).

6.5.3 Non-linear standard curves

Some standard curves, particularly those from binding assays, are difficult to linearize (see Chapter 7 for a detailed discussion of ligand binding). It is then common practice in laboratory medicine to connect the standard points together manually, by drawing either a smooth curve or a series of straight lines through the points (Reekie, Marshall and Fleck, 1973; Challand, Goldie and Landon, 1974). These procedures are subjective and are likely to increase assay variability (Hawker and Challand, 1981). To fit an equation to such data, there are two main approaches.

The first is to fit more complex *non-linear models* of the data using regression techniques (see Section 2.1.5) (e.g. Healy, 1972; Malan *et al.*, 1978), computing model parameters by iterative procedures (e.g. Bates and McAllister, 1974) [see VI, §12.3.5]. The second is to fit a smooth curve to the data using *spline functions* (e.g. Reinsch, 1971; Marschner, Erhardt and Scriba, 1974; Mosley and Bevan, 1977) [see III, §6.5]. This is a mathematical procedure which mimics manual curve-fitting. It calculates trial functions between pairs of points on the standard curve and uses iterative techniques to minimize the overall oscillation in the fitted curve. The less the oscillation, the smoother the standard curve and the smaller the effect of inaccurate standard points. The smoothing function minimizes the area under the second derivative of the curve [see IV, §5.5] which is used as a measure of the oscillation of the whole function. The degree of smoothing depends both on the number of standard points and on the imprecision of the assay.

(a) Theoretical immunoassay optimization

Mathematical models, based, for example, on the law of mass action, have been developed to describe the behaviour of reagents in an assay. It is possible to use these model equations not only to fit non-linear standard curves to assay data (e.g. Malan *et al.*, 1978; Wilkins *et al.*, 1978) but also to predict the changes in assay performance which would be achieved by changing certain assay conditions such as the concentration of reagents. This approach has been applied particularly to saturation analysis such as radioimmunoassay (see, for example, Ekins, 1974, 1975, 1978; Chard, 1978).

(b) Optimization of continuous flow analysis

Continuous flow analysis, widely used in laboratory medicine, presents special problems of optimization (Henry, Cannon and Winkelman, 1974; Tietz, 1976). These are due primarily to the possibility of adjacent samples interacting with each other when inserted in a continuous stream of reagents (carryover). Comparatively simple correction factors can be applied to all results when the percentage carryover is low (Tietz, 1976). More rigorous mathematical approaches have considered the dynamics of continuous flow analysis, and general equations have been derived which describe the relative importance of analytical factors and the shape of the peak output (Thiers, Cole and Kirsche, 1967; Walker, Pennock and McGowan, 1970; Begg, 1971; Fleck *et al.*, 1971; Walker, 1971; Henry, Cannon and Winkelman, 1974; Tietz, 1976). These have permitted a better understanding of assay optimization and much higher sample throughput with the aid of computer-assisted response curve regeneration.

6.5.4 Analysis of bio-assay data

The results of a bio-assay may be assessed graphically and/or arithmetically. The statistical procedures normally used have been well described by Emmens (1948), Finney (1964) and Bliss (1967).

In most bio-assays, standards and samples are analysed in replicate at several dilutions. To analyse the results, regression techniques are used to relate the responses to dose. The *dose-response curve* is typically log-linear and is fitted separately for the standard solutions and for dilutions of each sample of unknown potency. The gradients of the regression lines obtained for the standards and for dilutions of unknown samples should not differ significantly. On the log-scale, horizontal distance between the two lines gives the ratio of concentrations of standard and unknown sample.

A range of mathematical operations can be carried out to assess results. The most useful of these is an *analysis of variance* (see Sections 2.1.1 to 2.1.4) (Bliss, 1967) from which can be derived the linearity of the standard curve, the degree of parallelism between the standard and unknown and the confidence limits (see Section 1.3.11) for each estimate of potency.

6.5.5 Validity of curve-fitting

Three distinct types of error occur in curve-fitting. These are:

(a) The equation used does not adequately fit the data (e.g. a straight line is fitted when a curve would be more appropriate).
(b) Outlying and aberrant standard points are used.
(c) Standard chemical solutions do not behave identically to samples.

The difficulty often encountered when assessing the validity of the equation used for curve-fitting is that the data are insufficiently reliable to distinguish the possibilities. A standard curve is associated with an envelope of uncertainty within which many equations can be fitted, and it is not easy to decide which is valid.

In comparing equations or methods of curve-fitting, it is usual to choose one method as valid and to describe other methods in terms of their deviations from this. Ideally, the method of choice should be the one with most theoretical justification, but alternatively the mean position of the standard curve after fitting by different techniques (Hawker and Challand, 1981) or the position of the standard curve as drawn manually by an experienced analyst have been used.

A variety of approaches have been employed to check whether a standard curve departs significantly from linearity. A simple approach is to test whether the observed position of a standard point is significantly different from its expected position (Emmens, 1948). For example, for three equally spaced standards giving responses S_1, S_2 and S_3, the index of curvature H is defined by

$$\frac{H}{2} = \frac{S_1 + S_3}{2} - S_2 . \tag{6.5.1}$$

The significance of the curvature is assessed by Student's t test. This is an insensitive test that may well fail to detect a real curvature.

It may therefore be better to use a more complex approach (Bliss, 1967). The data are fitted by the parabola

$$y = a + bx + cx^2$$

using least squares regression (Section 2.1.5) [see III, §6.1.3], and c is tested to see whether it differs significantly from zero (Bliss, 1967).

(a) The identification of outliers

An *outlier* is an individual response observed in an assay system which departs from expectations based upon the behaviour of other samples in the system (Ekins and Malan, 1978). Outliers among the standard points have a serious effect on curve-fitting (Cornbleet and Gochman, 1979; Hawker and Challand, 1981) and should be identified and eliminated. There are two alternative approaches. The first is to set up replicates of each standard point and to identify outliers by an essentially arbitrary choice of a maximum allowed difference of response between them; e.g. twice the mean difference (Ekins and Malan, 1978). The second is to examine the difference between observed and expected positions of the standard points. Where an appropriate equation has been used for the standard curve, this can be effective (Hawker and Challand, 1981). However, particularly for outlying standard points near the extremities of the standard curve, it is often not clear whether the point is an outlier or the position of the standard curve is inappropriate. This can best be decided by reference to the behaviour of previous assay runs.

(b) Differences between standards and samples

Pure preparations of some analytes are available and an appropriate solvent is available for dissolving standard material so that it behaves identically to a sample of unknown potency. However, for many analytes, pure preparations are not available and the material used for standardization may show some different properties from those of the analyte present in the unknown sample. It is usual to apply a test of parallelism to detect differences in behaviour (Bliss, 1967). This consists of analysing a series of dilutions of the standard and sample and calculating the slope of each dose-response line by regression analysis (see Section 1.3.13). A t test (Section 1.3.5) is then used to assess the significance of the observed difference in slope.

In practice, problems can occur. For example, in a sigmoid dose-response curve, the zero-dose and infinite-dose asymptotes and the slope factor (the gradient of the curve at its mid-point) should be the same for reference standard and sample. Solvent effects of the assay diluent may cause the asymptotes to be non-identical and valid slope comparisons are therefore difficult. In comparing dose-response curves for a range of standards and samples, it may be helpful to use the arithmetic means of all estimates of each asymptote as the basis of calculating the slope factor for each sample tested. This can be more reliable than ignoring differences between the estimated asymptotes, and more objective than a visual comparison of slopes (Gaines Das and Cotes, 1978).

6.5.6 Uncertainty of position of the standard curve

Regression techniques have been described for assessing the uncertainty of position of a standard curve and the confidence interval for an analyte concentration derived from the standard curve (e.g. Finney, 1964; Bliss, 1967; Freund, 1973). It is debatable how much value these are in laboratory medicine, since they make many assumptions which are seldom correct. For most users, predictions of the inaccuracy of analysis should be made on the basis of the observed variability in results, taking into account intra-assay variability and comparing results with those obtained by different analysts and by different techniques (see Section 6.6 below).

6.5.7 Assay bias

Bias is a systematic tendency to over- or under-estimate measurements. The main causes of *assay bias* are:

(a) Impurity or other defects in the standard material.
(b) Lack of specificity of method due to
 (i) direct interference and cross-reactivity,
 (ii) indirect interference and non-specific effects.

Evidence of bias is usually looked for in one of the following ways:

(a) By analysing samples in parallel in more than one laboratory or by more than one technique.
(b) By analysing dilutions of a sample or mixtures of samples of known concentrations and looking for differences from expected results.
(c) By adding known amounts of purified analyte to samples and looking for differences from expected results.

Where differences are found, it is often difficult to decide which assay is giving more accurate results. When a pure preparation of analyte is not available for reference purposes, it is usual to define bias in terms of deviation from the mean result obtained by laboratories. For some causes of bias (for example, parallel cross-reaction by a related analyte, the concentration of which can be measured) a simple correction can be applied to results (Finney, 1964; Bliss, 1967). More usually the cause of bias in an assay should be identified and eliminated.

6.5.8 Inherent variation

The imprecision of results is caused in part by the inherent variation of every step in the assay. The quality control procedures described in Section 6.6.1 should be used to check the imprecision of results produced by an assay (Figure 6.5.1). For example, an assay which performs counts (e.g. in detection of radioisotope decay or observing cells within a microscope field) has two main sources of inherent variation. The first is the variation in the sample preparation step (e.g. dilution). The variation in any pipetting step can easily be measured by, for example, repeatedly pipetting aliquots of distilled water and weighing each. The second source of variation is in the counts themselves. Poisson distributions [see II, §5.4] (Freund, 1973; Henry, Cannon and Winkelman, 1974) are found for variables such as these, which can only assume integer values. For the Poisson distribution, the standard deviation is equal to the square root of the mean. For any analytical process involving several independent steps, variances are additive [see II, §9.2.3]. That is, the variance of the result is equal to the sum of the variances of each step. In this example, the variance in results is equal to the variance due to sample preparation plus the variance due to counting. If any two are known, the third can be calculated.

The mathematics applicable to radioisotope-counting experiments is considered in more detail in Chapter 8 which covers diagnostic tracer techniques and nuclear medicine.

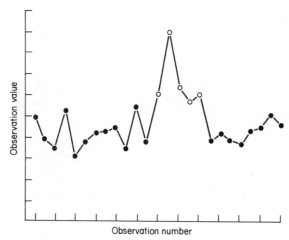

Figure 6.5.1 Causes of assay imprecision. The figure shows successive values recorded for a control sample. The inherent variation of the assay causes a small variation in results, shown by the closed circles. A change in bias (the open circles) causes results to shift, thus increasing the total variability. The highest result here was probably caused by gross error.

6.5.9 Imprecision and replicate analysis

In many assays, replicate assay tubes are set up for each standard and sample. This has the effect of reducing assay imprecision by a factor equal to the square root of the number of replicates [see II, §9.2.4]. The main justification for assaying replicates is, however, to detect gross error in assays in which mistakes occur frequently. For this purpose, duplicate assay tubes are almost as effective as higher order replication. The improvement in precision gained by higher order replication is not usually worth while, since the value of the increase

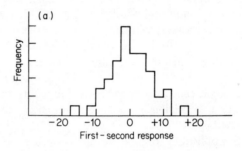

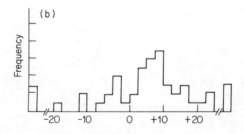

Figure 6.5.2 Histograms of replicate differences in an assay. (a) This shows the distribution of differences between the first and second response (in arbitrary units) of each duplicate pair in an assay set up by an experienced technician. (b) This shows the same data for the same assay set up by an inexperienced technician. The mean difference is not zero, indicating a systematic difference between duplicates; the range of spread of the distribution is larger, indicating a higher level of inherent error; and outliers exist, suggesting a high degree of gross error.

in precision is less than the increase in the cost of analysis (Challand, 1979).

When duplicate assay tubes are set up, the relative contributions to assay imprecision of different types of error can be identified (Challand, Ratcliffe and Ratcliffe, 1975; Challand, 1976). The difference in response between the individual tubes in a duplicate pair is recorded, corrected if necessary for variable error across the standard curve and values for a whole assay run are plotted (Figure 6.5.2). If the histogram is not centred on zero, there is a systematic difference between duplicate tubes. The incidence of outliers to the histogram is the incidence of gross error in the assay run. The standard deviation of the distribution (after excluding outliers) [see II, §9.2] is linearly related to the inherent error of the assay run. Thus, the errors in two types of assay, or made by two different analysts, can be rapidly compared.

A more sophisticated analysis of replicate values is possible in that the variation in the response given by replicates can be plotted directly against the corresponding analyte concentration (Figure 6.5.3a) and used to obtain the *response-error relationship* (Figure 6.5.3b). Although such data are always widely scattered, this relationship between error in the response and analyte concentration can be derived by methods such as grouping the data and taking the median [see II, §15.5] of each group (Finney, 1976). This can be used to yield weights in regression techniques for curve-fitting.

In assessing overall assay performance, it is very useful to estimate the imprecision of results at each point along the standard curve. To obtain this, it is necessary to use the errors shown in the response-error relationship to estimate measurement errors in analyte concentration. The analysis is complex but approximate values can easily be obtained; the error in analyte concentration is equal to the error in response divided by the slope of the standard curve at that response point (Ekins, Newman and O'Riordan, 1970). The plot of SD or CV of the result is called the *precision profile* of an assay (Figure 6.5.4) and is an effective method of summarizing assay performance (Ekins, Malan and Sufi, 1978).

6.5.10 Drift

Drift is the term used for a progressive change in assay results through an assay run. It is easy to recognize drift, either by analysing the same sample periodically through an assay run and demonstrating significant change in results or by setting up standard curves at the beginning and the end of the assay run and showing they are different (Figure 6.5.5).

Drift corrections tend to be based on rule-of-thumb adjustment of results, either multiplying by or adding a factor which changes through the assay run (McLelland and Fleck, 1978). However, in general, drift does not affect results in a simple arithmetic manner; nor does it occur at a constant rate through an assay run. As with bias, when possible it is better to identify and eliminate the causes of drift rather than to perform arithmetic corrections of dubious validity.

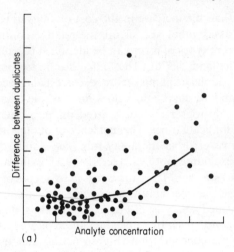

(a)

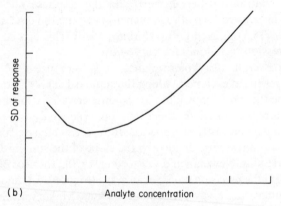

(b)

Figure 6.5.3 The response-error relationship. (a) The difference between the responses given by duplicates are plotted
against the analyte concentration derived
from the mean response of the duplicates. A
wide scatter exists; but by grouping ('bin-
ning') the data and taking medians the
underlying pattern can be seen. This is called
a response-error relationship. (b) A typical
response-error relationship is derived by
plotting the standard deviation of response
across a range of analyte concentrations.

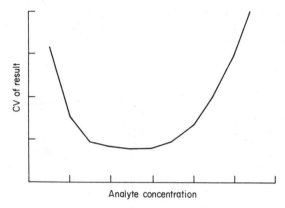

Figure 6.5.4 The precision profile. The response-error relationship is used to derive the precision profile – the relationship between the standard deviation (or coefficient of variation) of a result and the result itself.

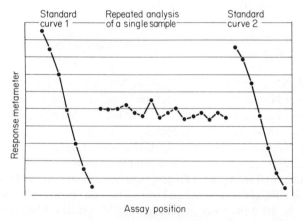

Figure 6.5.5 Drift. The responses plotted were obtained from an assay containing standard curves at the beginning and the end and a single sample analysed repetitively in the middle. A gradual decline of response occurred.

6.5.11 Comparison of analytical methods

When two methods are compared, it is usual to plot results using one method against results from the same samples using other methods. The two regression coefficients (the gradient and intercept of the regression line) are useful in estimating proportional and constant errors, but non-linearity and outlying points can seriously perturb results. The correlation coefficient, r [see VI, §2.5.7],

Table 6.5.1 Method of Deming for model II regression analysis

---

Assume that error exists in both x and y and a linear relationship exists between x and y of the form

$$y = a + bx.$$

Then

$$b = U + \sqrt{U^2 + (1/\lambda)},$$

where

$$U = \frac{\sum_{i=1}^{n} (y_i - \bar{y})^2 - (1/\lambda) \sum_{i=1}^{n} (x_i - \bar{x})^2}{2 \sum_{i=1}^{n} (y_i - \bar{y})(x_i - \bar{x})}$$

and

$$\lambda = \frac{\text{error variance of a single } x \text{ value}}{\text{error variance of a single } y \text{ value}},$$

$$a = \bar{y} - b\bar{x}.$$

From Deming (1943, p. 184).

is influenced by the scatter of points and in this context is not easily interpreted (Westgard and Hunt, 1973; Cornbleet and Gochman, 1979).

The slope and intercept are usually calculated by a least squares procedure in which the dependent variable y is regarded as being subject to error, error in the independent variable being ignored. In method-comparison studies, there is error in both variables and the regression analysis should therefore be modified (Cornbleet and Gochman, 1979). Deming's method (Deming, 1943) minimizes the sums of the squares of the residuals in both x and y directions (see Table 6.5.1) and seems to be the most useful regression method for method-comparison studies (Cornbleet and Gochman, 1979).

6.6 RESULT ASSESSMENT AND QUALITY CONTROL

The purpose of *quality control* of an assay is to ensure that results are as accurate as possible. Quality control techniques can be divided into internal and external programmes. Internal programmes include the assessment which a laboratory can make of its own performance, not necessarily influenced by data from outside. External programmes involve the comparison of assay performance between two or more laboratories. The main emphasis of internal programmes is usually on precision and error detection; for external programmes it is on bias and the identification of poor technique.

6.6.1 Internal quality control techniques

Internal quality control involves four separate steps:

(a) Derivation of statistics descriptive of an assay run.
(b) Comparison with statistics from previous assay runs.
(c) Decision on whether the assay run is in control.
(d) Appropriate action.

Ideally, quality control parameters should be sensitive enough to reveal trends in assay performance, so that corrective action can be taken before a trend is sufficiently serious to warrant rejection of an assay run.

(a) Quality control statistics

Quality control statistics fall into four groups: statistics descriptive of instrument performance, standard curve statistics, result statistics and replicate statistics (Challand *et al.*, 1981).

Statistics descriptive of instrument performance are usually the observed signals from a calibrating or reference material. Standard curve statistics fall into two groups: measurements of position, such as the position of the bottom of the standard curve (the response for a blank sample), the top of the standard curve and the result corresponding to half the difference between them (the curve midpoint); and measurements of curve-fitting (see Section 6.5.5), such as the slope and intercept after a linearizing transform and the correlation coefficient.

Result statistics are derived from results obtained from samples of known concentration analysed within the assay run (quality control samples) and from all results within an assay run (the assay mean). In any assay run, at least two quality control samples should be included, the results of which span the range of clinical importance. It may be more informative to use, as quality control statistics, the mean [see VI, §2.3.1] and range [see II, §15.5] of these sample results rather than the results themselves (Challand and Chard, 1973). The assay mean is of most value for quality control purposes when the population is homogenous. These conditions can be checked by inspection of results and by calculation of the variance of results from each assay run. When these conditions do not apply, it is possible to refine the calculation of a daily mean, either by including only results within a defined range (Whitehead and Morris, 1969) or results from patients in a defined category (Challand and Chard, 1973).

Finally, statistics derived from replicates include the statistics derived from duplicate assay tubes and the statistics derived from drift control values. These are described in Section 6.5.3 above.

(b) Use of quality control statistics

The aim of gathering quality control statistics is to monitor the performance of successive assay runs. Not all statistics are equally effective or sensitive. Thus those derived from results measure directly the quality of assay performance; those derived from checks of instrument performance or from standard curve analysis may reveal a reason for deteriorating quality, but are not of prime importance; those derived from within-assay replicates are sensitive to change in imprecision but insensitive to change in bias. It is best to choose which statistics are most useful in a given assay by trial and error; ideally, at least one from each of the four groups of statistics should be used routinely (Challand *et al.*, 1981).

Statistics from successive assay runs should be plotted on a simple graph, refined if possible by the addition of warning and action limits to give the familiar Levey–Jennings *control chart* (Levey and Jennings, 1950; see Figure 6.6.1). Traditionally, warning and action limits are derived by collecting statistics from assay runs believed to be in control. If the distribution of a statistic [see VI, §§2.1 and 2.2] is skewed [see II, §9.10], it should, if possible be transformed to give a Gaussian distribution [see II, §11.4] (e.g. by logarithmic transformation [see VI, §2.7.3]). The mean and standard deviation are calculated. The warning limits are then set to the mean plus or minus two standard deviations; the action limits are the mean plus or minus three standard deviations. By chance, one result in every

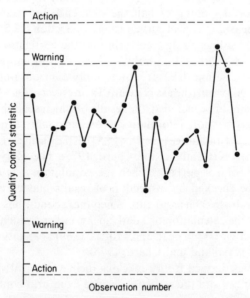

Figure 6.6.1 A Levey–Jennings control chart. Successive results obtained from a control sample are compared with warning and action limits which are based upon the previous known behaviour of the control sample.

twenty should fall outside warning limits, but any results outside the action limits should be treated as an indication of lack of control.

The aim of good quality control is to detect and remedy changes occurring within the assay before these become sufficiently serious to reject an assay run. To achieve this, methods of *trend detection* are needed. The commonest method for monitoring trends occurring in results from a clinical laboratory is the use of *cumulative sum techniques* (Woodward and Goldsmith, 1964). A grand mean for each quality control statistic is calculated from past data. The difference between each new result and the grand mean is calculated, and the cumulative sum of the differences is plotted. This procedure is summarized in Figure 6.6.2. Change within the assay is detected by a change in slope of the cumulative sum plot. For most purposes this can be done by eye, but to assess the proper significance of a

A	B	C
49	− 1	− 1
59	9	8
36	− 14	− 6
54	4	− 2
32	18	− 20
39	− 11	− 31
43	− 7	− 38
44	− 6	− 44
46	− 4	− 48
36	− 14	− 62
51	1	− 61
34	− 16	− 77
57	7	− 70
75	25	− 45
60	10	− 35
53	3	− 32
56	6	− 26
65	15	− 11
55	5	− 6
42	− 8	− 14
40	− 10	− 24
64	14	− 10
48	− 2	− 12
54	4	− 8
Grand mean = 50		

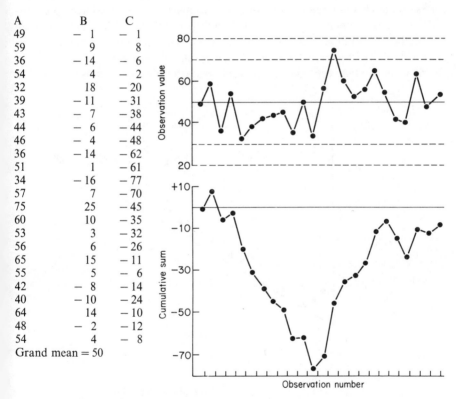

Figure 6.6.2 Derivation of the cumulative sum plot. Column A gives successive results obtained from a control sample. These are plotted on the Levey–Jennings control chart shown. Column B gives the successive differences of each result from a previously obtained grand mean of 50. Column C gives the cumulative sum of these differences, which are plotted. It is apparent that there was a change in bias halfway through the observations, the first twelve results being associated with a lower than normal mean.

trend, more rigorous techniques are needed. The most practical graphical solution is the use of a V-shaped mask, shown in Figure 6.6.3 (Woodward and Goldsmith, 1964; Kemp *et al.*, 1978; Edwards, 1980). This is superimposed on the cumulative sum chart with the vertex of the V pointing forward at a distance *d* ahead of the most recent point. If all previously plotted points lie within the limbs of the V, the process is likely to be in control, but if the cumulative sum path cuts one of the limbs of the V, the control mean has changed significantly. The parameter *d* and the slopes of the arms of the V-mask are selected depending on the length and magnitude of the trend to be detected (Woodward and Goldsmith, 1964).

Cumulative sum techniques are essentially graphical solutions to the problem of trend detection. Many alternative numerical solutions exist [see VI, Chapter 18]. Conceptually these are similar; they require the next element in a series (such as a set of quality control observations) to be predicted from previous data. The next element is then obtained and the residual (the difference between the predicted and observed values) is calculated. The accumulated magnitude of the residuals, taking into account their sign, is related to the size of the trend, and the relationship between this and the general scatter of observations is related to

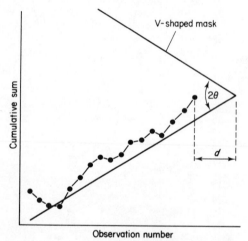

Figure 6.6.3 Assessing the significance of a cumulative sum trend. A V-shaped mask is placed on the cumulative sum plot with vertex at a distance *d* ahead of the most recent observation. The arms of the V are at an angle θ to the horizontal. The selection of θ and *d* depends on the length and magnitude of the trend to be detected. If the cumulative sum path cuts an arm of the V, a significant change in the control mean has occurred.

the significance of the trend. The whole process is summarized in the control loop shown in Figure 6.6.4.

An example is Trigg's technique (Trigg, 1964). The next result is predicted from an exponentially weighted running mean [see VI, §18.7.5]. The more weight that recent results are given in this calculation, the shorter the trend that is optimally detected. Residuals are also exponentially weighted, and *Trigg's tracking signal*, based on the accumulated residuals and the variability of the system, monitors the significance of the trend. This technique appears less useful than cumulative sum techniques in detecting step-wise changes in results (Cembrowski *et al.*, 1975), but is of value in monitoring drifting signals, which are characteristic of much analytical machinery (Challand and Cox, 1978).

A more sophisticated example is the use of linear Kalman filters (Kalman, 1960) [see VI, Chapter 20] which are used for general problems of estimating the state of a dynamic system when all observations within it are perturbed by noise

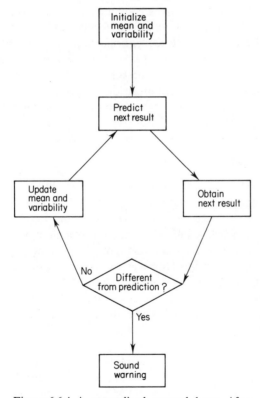

Figure 6.6.4 A generalized control loop. After initializing the process, arithmetic quality control follows a circular path until the process goes out of control.

[see VI, Chapter 20]. In this technique, the next state of the system is predicted from the last state of the system, perturbed by a stochastic variable with Gaussian distribution and zero mean. The Kalman gain is derived from the variances of the errors of estimates, which should attain a steady state value. To detect step-wise changes, individual residuals are monitored and compared with the steady state estimation errors; to detect a gradual trend, residuals are summed and compared with the steady state estimation errors. For a readable account see, for example, Lobdill (1981).

6.6.2 External quality assessment techniques

External quality assessment programmes monitor the performance of many different laboratories which may use different techniques to measure the same analyte. Typically, a range of samples is distributed to each participating laboratory every four weeks. Laboratories analyse the samples and return results to the organizer. Each then receives a summary of the results obtained by all laboratories together with assessments of performance (Brown, 1973; Whitehead, Browning and Gregory, 1973; Ratcliffe, Logue and Ratcliffe, 1978; Hunter and McKenzie, 1979; Challand *et al.*, 1981). A wide range of samples can be distributed in external programmes with the aim of answering specific questions concerning, for example, bias and imprecision. Assessments are made in a manner closely related to in-house methods for monitoring procedures (Lloyd, 1978; Percy-Robb *et al.*, 1980).

(a) The assessment of bias

The assessment of bias is difficult because of the problem of determining true values. Some analytes are available in pure form and a weighed amount can be used to prepare a reference solution. Even with this, it is difficult to find an appropriate solvent which mimics the behaviour of a biological fluid in the assay system. For other analytes, reference methods of known accuracy exist and may be used to define the true value. However, for many analytes, pure materials and reference methods do not exist. For these, the true result may be taken to be the mean result calculated either from the results of all laboratories participating in an external quality assessment scheme or from a sub-group of specialized laboratories. Where numbers are small, a single method may be defined as reference for the purpose of the study.

To determine bias, at least twenty samples spread over the analytical range are analysed by the in-house method. Results are plotted against the true results. The slope and intercept of the linear relationship are calculated (see Section 1.3.13). An intercept significantly different from zero (see Section 1.3.2) shows *constant bias*; a slope significantly different from unity shows *proportional bias*.

(b) *Imprecision*

The scatter of successive results from an individual laboratory around the true value gives one measurement of imprecision. A better measure is provided if the same sample is distributed anonymously at least three times in an external quality assessment programme. For an individual laboratory, the coefficient of variation of results [see II, §9.2.6] gives a good estimate of the imprecision of the assay at that sample concentration. However, it is important to recognize that the reliable measurement of imprecision over any time period involves storing samples for assay. Instability of the sample may therefore increase the measured imprecision.

In external quality assessment programmes, a running mean imprecision and bias over the present and previous results is often calculated. This is usually done by including a fixed number of results, each of which has equal weighting. An alternative possibility is to use exponential weighting [see IV, §2.11] to enhance the importance of more recent results [see VI, §18.7.5].

(c) *Linearity*

A linearity check can be included in an external quality assessment programme by distributing a series of samples at known dilutions from a sample of known high concentration. Where solvent effects are important, it is preferable to mix a high value and a low value sample in different proportions. Results should always be plotted graphically. As with analysis of bias, significant departure of slope from unity or intercept from zero are evidence of non-linearity. A curvilinear response may be identified by the methods in Section 6.5.5.

(d) *Sensitivity*

The sensitivity of a method is best defined in terms of the minimum amount of analyte which can be distinguished reliably from zero. It is therefore related directly to the precision of estimate of low analyte concentrations. It can be assessed empirically in an external quality assessment programme by distributing, anonymously, analyte-free samples for analysis. Provided that bias is absent, the sensitivity of the assay is likely to be close to the actual results which are obtained.

(e) *Performance rankings and the 'blunder index'*

Several ranking indices have been used for laboratories participating in external quality assessment schemes. Typically, each laboratory is allotted a score for accuracy which is based upon the absolute magnitude of its running bias and imprecision. There is now a tendency to exclude results likely to be caused by gross mistakes, which are clearly outliers, and to include these in a separate assessment called the 'blunder index'. The blunder index is, of course, directly related to gross error incidence in a laboratory.

All laboratories make blunders; it has been estimated that even with careful organization approximately 3 per cent of everything that one does is a mistake (McSwiney and Woodrow, 1969). When techniques are complex and organization and skill are lacking, the incidence of mistakes is far higher. The application of mathematical techniques is perhaps one of the more promising ways of rectifying a situation in which 'some laboratories... would be more usefully employed collecting random numbers' (Whitehead, 1977).

G.S.C

REFERENCES

Barber, B. (1978). An examination of some problems of evaluating the usefulness of computer systems in a health care environment—an operation analyst's viewpoint, in *Computing in Clinical Laboratories* (Ed. F. Siemaszko), pp. 126–136, Pitman Medical, London.

Bates, W. K., and McAllister, D. F. (1974). Some methods for non-linear regression using desk-top calculators with an application to the Lowry protein method, *Analyt. Biochem.*, **59**, 190–199.

Begg, R. D. (1971). Dynamics of continuous segmented flow analysis, *Analyt. Chem.*, **43**, 854–857.

Bliss, C. I. (1967). *Statistics in Biology*, Vol. I, McGraw-Hill New York.

Brown, S. S. (1973). Notes on the quality of performance of serum cholesterol assays, *Ann. Clin. Biochem.*, **10**, 146–154.

Carruthers, M. E. (1970). Computer analysis of routine pathology work schedules using a simulation program, *J. Clin. Path.*, **23**, 269–272.

Cembrowski, G. S., Westgard, J. O., Eggert, A. E., and Toren, E. C. (1975). Trend detection in control data: optimisation and interpretation of Trigg's technique for trend analysis, *Clin. Chem.*, **21**, 1396–1405.

Challand, G. S. (1976). The within-laboratory validation of radioimmunoassay results, in *Protides of the Biological Fluids* (Ed. H. Peeters), 24th Colloquium, pp. 731–734, Pergamon Press, Oxford.

Challand, G. S. (1979). Is replication worthwhile?, Abstract, Third European Congress of Clinical Chemistry, Brighton 1979, British Medical Association.

Challand, G. S., Cartledge, C., and Munro, A. (1981). Quality control in the immunoassay of drugs, in *Progress in the Quality Control of Medicines* (Ed. P. B. Deasy and R. F. Timoney), pp. 69–95, Elsevier-North Holland Biomedical Press, Amsterdam.

Challand, G. S., and Chard, T. (1973). Quality control in radioimmunoassay: observations on the operation of a semi-automated assay for human placental lactogen, *Clin. Chim. Acta*, **46**, 133–138.

Challand, G. S., and Cox, L. (1978). Identification of an unusual gamma counter fault using Trigg's technique for trend detection, *Ann. Clin. Biochem.*, **15**, 117–120.

Challand, G. S., Goldie, D., and Landon, J. (1974). Immunoassay in the diagnostic laboratory, *Brit. Med. Bull.*, **30**, 38–43.

Challand, G. S., Ratcliffe, W. A., and Ratcliffe, J. G. (1975). Semi-automated radioimmunoassays for total thyroxine and tri-iodothyronine, *Clin. Chim. Acta*, **60**, 25–32.

Chard, T. (1978). An introduction to radioimmunoassay and related techniques, Vol. 6, Part II of *Laboratory Techniques in Biochemistry and Molecular Biology* (Eds T. S. Work and E. Work), pp. 324–328, Elsevier-North Holland Biomedical Press, Amsterdam.

Cornbleet, P. J., and Gochman, N. (1979). Incorrect least-squares regression coefficients in method comparison analysis, *Clin. Chem.*, **25**, 432–438.

Cundy, A. D. (1972). A simulation study of the clinical laboratory office, in *Spectrum* 71, *a Conference on Medical Computing* (Ed. M. E. Abrams), pp. 124–138, Butterworths, London.

Dacie, J. V., and Lewis, S. M. (1975). *Practical Haematology*, 5th ed., Churchill Livingstone, Edinburgh.

Deming, W. E. (1943). *Statistical Adjustment of Data*, Wiley, New York.

Dickey, R. P., Besch, P. K., Vorys, N., and Ullery, J. C. (1966). Diurnal excretion of oestrogen and creatinine during pregnancy, *Amer. J. Obstet. Gynae*, **94**, 591–595.

Duguid, J. P., Marmion, B. P., and Swain, R. H. A. (Eds) (1975). *Mackie and McCartney Medical Microbiology*, Vol. 11: *The Practice of Medical Microbiology*, 12th ed., Churchill Livingstone, Edinburgh.

Dybkaer, R. (1972). Concepts and nomenclature in the theory of reference values, *Scand. J. Clin. Lab. Invest.*, **29**, Suppl. 126, 19.1.

Edwards, R. W. H. (1980). Internal analytical quality control using the cusum chart and truncated V-mask procedure, *Ann. Clin. Biochem.*, **17**, 205–211.

Ekins, R. P. (1974). Basic principles and theory, *Brit. Med. Bull.*, **30**, 3–11.

Ekins, R. P. (1975). Assay design, in *Radioimmunoassay in Clinical Biochemistry* (Ed. C. A. Pasternak), pp. 3–13, Heyden and Son Ltd, London.

Ekins, R. P. (1978). Quality control and assay design, in *Radioimmunoassay and Related Procedures in Medicine*, Vol. II, p. 39, International Atomic Energy Agency, Vienna.

Ekins, R. P., and Malan, P. G. (1978). Identification of outliers, *Ann. Clin. Biochem.*, **15**, 125–126.

Ekins, R. P., Malan, P. G., and Sufi, S. B. (1978). Making better use of scintillation counters, in *Computing in Clinical Laboratories* (Ed. F. Siemaszko), pp. 93–102, Pitman Medical, London.

Ekins, R. P., Newman, G. B., and O'Riordan, J. L. H. (1970). In *Statistics in Endocrinology* (Eds J. W. McArthur and T. Colton), pp. 345–378, MIT Press, Cambridge, Massachusetts.

Emmens, C. W. (1948). *Principles of Biological Assay*, Chapman and Hall, London.

Finney, D. J. (1964). *Statistical Methods in Biological Assay*, Charles Griffin, High Wycombe.

Finney, D. J. (1976). Radioligand assay, *Biometrics*, **32**, 721–740.

Fleck, A., Begg, R. D., Williams, P. I., and Racionzer, D. (1971). Some fundamental aspects of continuous flow analysis, *Ann. Clin. Biochem.*, **8**, 13–15.

Fleck, A., Robinson, R., Brown, S. S., and Hobbs, J. R. (1974). Definitions of some words and terms used in automated analysis, *Ann. Clin. Biochem.*, **11**, 242–257.

Freund, J. E. (1973). *Modern Elementary Statistics*, Prentice-Hall, Hemel Hempstead.

Gaines Das, R. E., and Cotes, P. M. (1978). Comparison of radioimmunoassay dose response curves: Calibration of standards, *Ann. Clin. Biochem.*, **15**, 126–127.

Galen, R. S., and Gambino, S. R. (1975). *Beyond Normality: The Predictive Value and Efficiency of Medical Diagnoses*, Wiley, New York.

Gove, P. B. (Ed.) (1966). *Webster's Third New International Dictionary of the English Language*, G. Bell and Sons, London.

Gowenlock, A. H. (1969). The influence of accuracy and precision on the normal range, *Ann. Clin. Biochem.*, **6**, 12.

Grasbeck, R. (1972). Types of reference groups, *Scand. J. Clin. Lab. Invest.*, **27**, Suppl. 126, 19.2.

Halberg, F., Engel, M., Hamburger, C., and Hillman, D. (1965). Spectral resolution of low-frequency small amplitude rhythms in excreted 17-ketosteroids: probable androgen-induced circaseptan desynchronisation, *Acta Endocrinol.* (*Copenhagen*), Suppl. 103, 1–54.

Halberg, F., Tong, Y. L., and Johnson, E. A. (1967). Circadian system phase: an aspect of temporal morphology. Procedures and illustrative examples, in *Cellular Aspects of Biorhythms* (Ed. H. Von Meyersbach), pp. 24–40, Springer-Verlag, Berlin Heidelberg, New York.

Hall, R. (1971). The clinical significance of the TRH-test, *Symposium, VII Acta Endocr. Congress*, Copenhagen.

Hawker, F. J., and Challand, G. S. (1981). The effect of outlying standard points on curve fitting in radioimmunoassay, *Clin. Chem.*, **27**, 14–19.

Healy, M. J. R. (1969). Normal values from a statistical viewpoint, *Ann. Clin. Biochem.*, **6**, 12.

Healy, M. J. R. (1972) Statistical analysis of radioimmunoassay data, *Biochem. J.*, **139**, 207–210.

Henry, R. J., Canon, D. C., Winkelman, J. W. (Eds) (1974). *Clinical Chemistry, Principles and Technics* 2nd ed., Harper and Row, Maryland.

Holland, M. R., and Jacobs, A. G. (1982). On the transportability of linear discriminant functions, *Ann. Clin. Biochem*, **19**, 47–51.

Hunter, W. M., and McKenzie, I. (1979). Quality control of radioimmunoassays for proteins: the first two and a half years of a national scheme for serum growth hormone measurements, *Ann. Clin. Biochem.*, **16**, 131–146.

Jusko, W. J., Slaunwhite, W. R., and Aceto, T. (1975). Partial pharmacodynamic model for the circadian-episodic secretion of cortisol in man, *J. Clin. Endocrinol. Metab.*, **40**, 278–289.

Kalman, R. E. (1960). A new approach to linear filtering and prediction problems, *J. Basic Eng.*, **82**, 35–46.

Kemp, K. W., Nix, A. B. J., Wilson, D. W., and Griffiths, K. (1978). Internal quality control of radioimmunoassays, *J. Endocrinol.*, **76**, 203–210.

Kipiniak, W. (1981). A basic problem: the measurement of height and area, *J. Chromatograph. Sci.*, **19**, 332–337.

Krause, R. D., Anand, V. D., Gruemer, H. D., and Willke, T. A. (1975). The impact of laboratory error on the normal range: a Bayesian model, *Clin. Chem.*, **21**, 321–324.

Kynch, G. J. (1955). *Mathematics for the Chemist*, Butterworth's Scientific Publications, London.

Levey, S., and Jennings, E. R. (1950). The use of control charts in the clinical laboratory, *Amer. J. Clin. Path.*, **20**, 1059–1066.

Lloyd, P. H. (1978). A scheme for the evaluation of diagnostic kits, *Ann. Clin. Biochem.*, **15**, 136–145.

Lobdill, J. (1981). Kalman mileage predictor monitor, *Byte*, **6**, 230–248.

McLelland, A. S., and Fleck A. (1978). Drift correction—a comparative evaluation of some alternatives, *Ann. Clin. Biochem.*, **15**, 281–290.

McSwiney, R. R., and Woodrow, D. A. (1969). Types of error within a clinical laboratory, *J. Med. Lab. Technol.*, **26**, 340–346.

Malan, P. G., Cox, M. G., Long, E. M. R., and Ekins, R. P. (1978). Development in curve fitting procedures for radioimmunoassay data using a multiple binding site model, in *Radioimmunoassay and Related Procedures in Medicine*, Vol. I, International Atomic Energy Agency, Vienna.

Marschner, I., Erhardt, F., and Scriba, P. C. (1974). Calculation of the radioimmunoassay standard curve by spline function, in *Radioimmunoassays and Related Procedures in Medicine*, Vol. I, Istanbul 1973, International Atomic Energy Agency, Vienna.

Mosley, J., and Bevan, B. R. (1977). Spline function analysis applied to a human placental lactogen assay, *Ann. Clin. Biochem.*, **14**, 16–21.

Percy-Robb, I. W., Broughton, P. M. G., Jennings, R. D., McCormack, J. J., Neill, D. W, Saunders, R. A., and Warner, Mary (1980). A recommended scheme for the evaluation of kits in the clinical chemistry laboratory, *Ann. Clin. Biochem.*, **17**, 217–226.

Peto, J., Whitby, L. G., and Finney, D. J. (1972). The role of operational research in clinical chemistry, *J. Clin. Path.*, **25**, 989–996.

Pickardt, C. R., Erhardt, F., Gruner, J., Horn, K., and Scriba, P. C. (1972). Stimulation der TSH-Sekretion Durch TRH bei blander Struma: Diagnostiche Bedeutung und pathophysiologische Folgerungen, *Klin. Wochenschr.*, **50**, 1134–1137.

Pryce, J. D., Haslam, R. M., and Wootton, I. D. P. (1969). Extraction of normal values from a mixed hospital population, *Ann. Clin. Biochem.*, **6**, 6–11.

Ratcliffe, W. A., Logue, F. C., and Ratcliffe, J. G. (1978). Scottish immunoassay support service quality control scheme for thyroxine, triiodothyronine and digoxin assays, *Ann. Clin. Biochem.*, **15**, 203–207.

Rath, G. J., Alvarez Balbas, J. M., Ikeda, T., and Kennedy, O. G. (1970). Simulation of a haematology department, *Health Serv. Res.*, **5**, 25–35.

Reed, A. H., Henry, R. J., and Mason, W. B. (1971). Influence of statistical method used on the resulting estimate of normal range, *Clin. Chem.*, **17**, 275–284.

Reekie, D., Marshall, R. B., and Fleck A. (1973). The use of calibration curves in biochemical analyses with particular reference to computer data processing, *Clin. Chim. Acta.*, **47**, 123–31.

Reinsch, C. H. (1971). Smoothing by spline functions II, *Numer. Math.*, **16**, 451–454.

Rodbard, D., and Hutt, D. M. (1974). Statistical analysis of radioimmunoassays and immunoradiometric (labelled antibody) assays, in *Radioimmunoassays and Related Procedures in Medicine*, Vol. I, Istanbul 1973, International Atomic Energy Agency, Vienna.

Sanders, P. G. (1980). *Evolution of Clinical Biochemistry in Relation to Clinical Practice*, PhD Thesis, University of Cambridge.

Sederberg-Olsen, P., Binder, C., Kehlet, H., Neville, A. M., and Nielsen, L. M. (1973). Variation in plasma corticosteroids in subjects with Cushing's Syndrome of different etiology, *J. Clin. Endocrinol. Metab.*, **36**, 906–910.

Shelley, T. F., Cummings, R. V., Bourke, J. E., and Marshall, L. D. (1970). Estrogen creatinine ratios. Clinical application and significance, *Obstet. Gynec.*, **35**, 184–188.

Simpson, H. W. (1976). A new perspective: chronobiochemistry, in *Essays in Medical Biochemistry* (Eds V. Marks and C. N. Hales) Vol. 2, pp. 115–187, The Biochemical Society and the Association of Clinical Biochemists, London.

Thiers, R. E., Cole, R. R., and Kirsche (1967). Kinetic parameters of continuous flow analysis, *Clin. Chem.*, **13**, 451–467.

Tietz, N. W. (Ed.) (1976). *The Fundamentals of Clinical Chemistry*, W. B. Saunders Co., Philadelphia.

Tocher, K. D. (1963). *The Art of Simulation*, English University Press.

Tonks, D. B. (1963). A study of the accuracy and precision of clinical chemistry determinations in 170 Canadian laboratories, *Clin. Chem.*, **9**, 217–233.

Tournaire, J., Orgaizy, J., Rivere, J. F., and Roussel, H. (1971). Repeated plasma cortisol determinations in Cushing's Syndrome due to adrenocortical adenoma, *J. Clin. Endocrinol. Metab.*, **32**, 66–68.

Trigg, D. W. (1964). Monitoring a forecasting system, *Oper. Res. Quart.*, **15**, 271–274.

Tyler, F. H., Migeon, D., Florentin, A. A., and Samuels, L. T. (1954). The diurnal variation of 17 hydroxycorticosteroid levels in plasma, *J. Clin. Endocrinol. Metab.*, **14**, 774.

Walker, W. H. C. (1971). Curve regeneration in continuous flow analysis, *Clin. Chim. Acta*, **32**, 305–306.

Walker, W. H. C., Pennock, C. A., and McGowan, G. K. (1970). Practical considerations in kinetics of continuous flow analysis, *Clin. Chim. Acta*, **27**, 421–435.

Weitzman, E. D., Fukushima, D., and Nogeire, C. (1971). Twenty-four hour pattern of the episodic secretion of cortisol in normal subjects, *J. Clin. Endocrinol. Metab.*, **33**, 14–22.

Westgard, J. O., and Hunt, M. R. (1973). Use and interpretation of common statistical tests in method comparison studies, *Clin. Chem.*, **19**, 48–57.

Whitehead, T. P. (1977). Advances in quality control, *Advances in Clinical Chemistry*, **19**, 175–205.

Whitehead, T. P., Browning, D. M., and Gregory, A. (1973). A comparative survey of the results of analyses of blood serum in clinical chemistry laboratories in the United Kingdom, *J. Clin. Path.*, **26**, 435–446.

Whitehead, T. P., and Morris, L. O. (1969). Methods of quality control, *Ann. Clin. Biochem.*, **6**, 94–103.

Wilkins, T. A., Chadney, D. C., Bryant, J., Palmstrom, S. H., and Winder, R. L. (1978). Non-linear least squares curve fitting of a simple statistical model to radioimmunoassay dose-response data using a mini-computer, in *Radioimmunoassay and Related Procedures in Medicine*, Vol. I, pp. 399–420, International Atomic Energy Agency, Vienna.

Woodward, R. H., and Goldsmith, P. L. (1964). *Cumulative Sum Techniques*, ICI Monograph no. 3, Oliver and Boyd, Edinburgh.

Mathematical Methods in Medicine
Edited by D. Ingram & R. F. Bloch
© 1984 John Wiley & Sons Ltd.

7

Mathematical Aspects of Pharmacokinetics and Protein–Ligand Binding

7.1 INTRODUCTION

In this chapter we will discuss two main areas of application of mathematics in pharmacology and pharmacy, pharmacokinetics and protein–ligand binding. These two areas are of clinical importance and the mathematics involved is common to many other areas, e.g. in the description of saturable processes such as drug–receptor interactions and in many rate processes such as descriptions of enzyme kinetics. In each case we have concentrated on the development, validation and limitations of the basic mathematical models used. It is hoped that, with the aid of this chapter and others in the Guidebook, the inexperienced worker will be able to avoid the pitfalls of ignoring the mathematical foundation and only using the final equation from a publication to interpret data, without appreciating the assumptions implicit in the derivation.

In introducing the mathematical techniques used in pharmacokinetics—the study of drug absorption, distribution and elimination—we are concerned mainly with the topic of compartmental modelling, the most widely used (and abused) technique. Some widely used models are described and solutions derived using both direct and Laplace transform techniques for integration of the systems of linear differential equations [see IV, §§7.9 and 13.4.6]. The problems of fitting such models to experimental data are reviewed, covering both graphical methods and techniques of numerical analysis. Other widely used concepts such as bioavailability and clearance are only briefly introduced. These are mainly concerned with clinical interpretation of data and more detailed discussions can be found in standard texts such as Jusko (1972), Wagner (1975) and Rowland and Tozer (1980).

In the discussion of protein–ligand binding we consider models to describe a system where, on a given protein, there may be several binding sites, each with its specific mass action equilibrium coefficient and where, moreover, because of cooperative effects, the equilibrium coefficient at one site may be affected by the occupancy of other sites. The models described vary in the simplifying assumptions made. We consider once more both graphical and numerical techniques for analysing the experimental data and problems of interpretation of the derived binding coefficients. A fully worked example is given to illustrate the methods.

7.2   COMPARTMENTAL ANALYSIS

7.2.1   Introduction

Following its administration a drug can pass through some or all of the stages of absorption, distribution, metabolism and elimination. Compartmental analysis, also widely used in tracer kinetic studies (see Chapter 8 of this Guidebook), is a convenient method of studying the time course of the drug through these stages. A compartment is defined as follows (Riggs, 1963): 'If a substance, S, is present in a biological system in several distinguishable forms or locations, and if S passes from one form or location to another form or location at a measurable rate, then each form or location constitutes a separate compartment for S.' Thus the definition encompasses both transfer between compartments and chemical transformation of the substance.

There are usually three fundamental assumptions in linear compartmental analysis:

(a) The size of the compartment remains constant.
(b) Distribution of the substance throughout the compartment is considered to occur instantaneously.
(c) Transfer between compartments is a first-order process; i.e. proportional to drug concentrations and not other or higher order functions, the system thus being linear (non-linear mechanisms are considered in Section 7.2.6).

The object of the analysis is to describe the time course of the drug by a set of n differential equations, where n is the number of compartments (Atkins, 1969).

A compartment system can be open, where substances can be exchanged with the environment, or closed, where no substances can enter or leave the system. Only open models are considered in this chapter. Transfer between compartments is traditionally described by the first-order equations

$$\frac{dc_i}{dt} = -c_i \sum_i k_{ij} + \frac{1}{V_i} \sum_j c_j V_j k_{ji}, \qquad i,j = 1,2,\ldots,n \tag{7.2.1}$$

[see IV, §7.2 and (1.7.1)]. Here c_i is the drug concentration in compartment i, which is related to the compartmental volume V_i and mass of drug x_i, where

$$x_i = c_i V_i \tag{7.2.2}$$

and k_{ij} are rate coefficients. The first subscript, i, denotes the compartment from which the drug is coming and the second subscript, j, the compartment to which it is going. Thus in (7.2.1) the first term represents transfer from compartment i and the second to compartment i, where the volume ratio is needed because, for a given amount of drug transferred, the associated changes in concentration are inversely related to compartmental volume.

Riegelman, Loo and Rowland (1968) have established that in general a one-compartment model is inadequate to describe pharmacokinetic data and at least one additional peripheral compartment is required. For this reason the next two sections present detailed analyses of the two-compartment open model following intravenous injection and first-order absorption respectively. In each case the analysis is carried out by direct methods and using Laplace transforms; this latter method is preferred to allow the general method for any linear model developed in Section 7.2.4 to be used. (See also Chapter 10 of this guidebook for a useful graphical technique to aid solution of linear compartmental models.)

The technique for solving the pharmacokinetic models is independent of the complexity of the model and involves four stages:

(a) Write down the rate equations for the compartments.
(b) Transform the variables in the equations to those you require and can measure.
(c) Solve the equations, either analytically or by numerical integration [see III, Chapter 7].
(d) Verify that the model describes the data.

7.2.2 Rapid intravenous injection in a two-compartment open model

The compartmental model and associated nomenclature is shown in Figure 7.2.1. A bolus amount of drug, D_0, is administered to the central compartment 1 at time $t = 0$, and it is only eliminated from this compartment. There is reversible

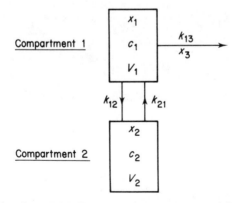

Figure 7.2.1 Two-compartment open model used to describe drug kinetics after rapid intravenous injection.

disposition to the peripheral compartment 2. The amount of drug eliminated is denoted by x_3.

The rate equations for the concentration time course in each compartment are, following (7.2.1),

$$\frac{dc_1}{dt} = -(k_{12} + k_{13})c_1 + \frac{V_2}{V_1}k_{21}c_2, \tag{7.2.3}$$

$$\frac{dc_2}{dt} = \frac{V_1}{V_2}k_{12}c_1 - k_{21}c_2, \tag{7.2.4}$$

where the volume ratio allows for the different, but unknown, volumes of the compartments. In terms of amounts these may be written, using (7.2.2), as

$$\frac{dx_1}{dt} = -k_{12}x_1 - k_{13}x_1 + k_{21}x_2,$$

$$\frac{dx_2}{dt} = k_{12}x_1 - k_{21}x_2.$$

In general, we can only make measurements of the central compartment, e.g. plasma, so we will solve (7.2.3)—it being necessary to eliminate the unknown terms involving the peripheral compartment. Differentiating (7.2.3) with respect to t,

$$\frac{d^2c_1}{dt^2} = -(k_{12} + k_{13})\frac{dc_1}{dt} + \frac{V_2}{V_1}k_{21}\frac{dc_2}{dt}.$$

Substituting from (7.2.4) we have

$$\frac{d^2c_1}{dt^2} = -(k_{12} + k_{13})\frac{dc_1}{dt} + \frac{V_2}{V_1}k_{21}\left(\frac{V_1}{V_2}k_{12}c_1 - k_{21}c_2\right)$$

$$= -(k_{12} + k_{13})\frac{dc_1}{dt} + k_{21}k_{12}c_1 - \frac{V_2}{V_1}k_{21}^2c_2.$$

Finally, we eliminate c_2 by using its value as given by (7.2.3), viz.

$$\frac{V_2}{V_1}k_{21}c_2 = \frac{dc_1}{dt} + (k_{12} + k_{13})c_1.$$

Thus,

$$\frac{d^2c_1}{dt^2} = -(k_{12} + k_{13} + k_{21})\frac{dc_1}{dt} - k_{21}k_{13}c_1. \tag{7.2.5}$$

This is a homogeneous linear second-order differential equation with constant coefficients. The general solution of an equation of this form is

$$c_1(t) = A_1 \exp(m_1 t) + A_2 \exp(m_2 t), \tag{7.2.6}$$

where A_1 and A_2 are constants to be determined by the initial conditions and m_1, m_2 are the (distinct) roots of the quadratic characteristic equation

$$m^2 + (k_{12} + k_{21} + k_{13})m + k_{21}k_{13} = 0. \tag{7.2.7}$$

[see IV, §7.4.1.] Here the roots are known to be real, negative and distinct; in fact they are given by

$$m = \{ -(k_{12} + k_{21} + k_{13}) \pm \sqrt{(k_{12} + k_{21} + k_{13})^2 - 4k_{21}k_{13}} \}/2.$$

Denoting $(k_{12} + k_{21} + k_{13})$ by K and the term within the square root by L, a little algebra shows that $L \geq 0$ for real positive values of the rate constants k_{ij}. Also $L \leq K^2$ and hence m_1 and m_2 are both negative (or zero). The solution (7.2.6) is a bi-exponential curve traditionally written in the form

$$c_1(t) = A \exp(-\alpha t) + B \exp(-\beta t), \tag{7.2.8}$$

where α and β are measured experimentally in terms of the elimination time constants or half lives of elimination of the drug.

Note that (7.2.7) may be written in the form

$$(m + \alpha)(m + \beta) = 0,$$

and thus equating coefficients we have

$$\alpha + \beta = k_{12} + k_{21} + k_{13},$$
$$\alpha\beta = k_{13}k_{21}. \tag{7.2.9}$$

The values of A and B are determined by the initial boundary conditions for c_1 and dc_1/dt. These are that the drug dose D_0 is distributed in compartment 1 with concentration $c_1(0) = D_0/V_1$ and that compartment 2 is empty.

Remembering that $\exp(0) = 1$ and that $(d/dt)(e^{-kt}) = -ke^{-kt}$, where k is constant, we have, from (7.2.8) and (7.2.3) respectively,

$$A + B = c_1(0),$$
$$\alpha A + \beta B = (k_{12} + k_{13})c_1(0). \tag{7.2.10}$$

Making use of (7.2.9), the solution to this pair of simultaneous equations is

$$A = \frac{c_1(0)(k_{21} - \alpha)}{\beta - \alpha},$$
$$B = \frac{c_1(0)(k_{21} - \beta)}{\alpha - \beta}. \tag{7.2.11}$$

The general solution for $c_2(t)$ is of the form

$$c_2(t) = C \exp(-\alpha t) + D \exp(-\beta t)$$

where C and D are determined by the same boundary conditions applied to c_2 and dc_2/dt. We find

$$C = c_1(0) \frac{V_1}{V_2} \frac{k_{12}}{\beta - \alpha},$$

$$D = -C. \tag{7.2.12}$$

We will now use the more general technique of Laplace transforms [see IV, §13.4.6] to solve the pair of equations (7.2.3) and (7.2.4). The Laplace transform (LT) of a function $c(t)$ will be denoted by $\bar{c}(s)$, where

$$\bar{c}(s) = \int_0^\infty \exp(-st) c(t) dt \tag{7.2.13}$$

[see IV, §13.4]. The most important properties, for the application we have in mind, are that the LT of $B_1 c_1(t) + B_2 c_2(t)$ is $B_1 \bar{c}_1(s) + B_2 \bar{c}_2(s)$, if B_1 and B_2 are constants. If, then, we take the Laplace transform of (7.2.3) and (7.2.4), we obtain the equations

$$s\bar{c}_1(s) - c_1(0) = -(k_{12} + k_{13})\bar{c}_1(s) + \frac{V_2}{V_1} k_{21} \bar{c}_2(s), \tag{7.2.14}$$

$$s\bar{c}_2(s) - c_2(0) = \frac{V_1}{V_2} k_{12} \bar{c}_1(s) - k_{21} \bar{c}_2(s). \tag{7.2.15}$$

These are not differential equations, they are linear algebraic equations which may easily be solved for $\bar{c}_1(s)$ and $\bar{c}_2(s)$. In the following manipulations, we abbreviate $\bar{c}_1(s)$ and $\bar{c}_2(s)$ to $\bar{c}_1$ and $\bar{c}_2$, respectively, for convenience.

Noting that $c_2(0) = 0$ and substituting c_2 from (7.2.15) into (7.2.14) we obtain

$$\bar{c}_1 = \frac{c_1(0)(s + k_{21})}{s^2 + (k_{12} + k_{13} + k_{21})s + k_{13}k_{21}}.$$

Note that the quadratic in s in the denominator is identical to that in m of (7.2.7). Denoting the roots by $-\alpha$, $-\beta$ as before, it may be written in the form $(s + \alpha)(s + \beta)$.

All that now remains is to derive the function $c_1(t)$ from its LT, $\bar{c}_1(s)$. The simplest way of performing this inverse transform is to express $\bar{c}_1$ in partial fraction form and then use standard tables of inverse Laplace transforms. If we write

$$\bar{c}_1 = \frac{c_1(0)(s + k_{21})}{(s + \alpha)(s + \beta)} = \frac{A}{s + \alpha} + \frac{B}{s + \beta}, \tag{7.2.16}$$

the terms on the right-hand side being the partial fractions in which A and B are to be determined, and then recombine the partial fractions as

$$\frac{A(s+\beta)+B(s+\alpha)}{(s+\alpha)(s+\beta)},$$

we are led to the identity

$$c_1(0)(s+k_{21}) \equiv A(s+\beta)+B(s+\alpha).$$

It is true for all s, in particular for $s = -\alpha$, whence

$$A = \frac{c_1(0)(k_{21}-\alpha)}{\beta-\alpha},$$

and for $s = -\beta$, whence

$$B = \frac{c_1(0)(k_{21}-\beta)}{\alpha-\beta}.$$

Hence

$$\bar{c}_1 = \frac{c_1(0)(k_{21}-\alpha)}{\beta-\alpha}\frac{1}{s+\alpha} + \frac{c_1(0)(k_{21}-\beta)}{\alpha-\beta}\frac{1}{s+\beta}.$$

We now have an expression for $\bar{c}_1(s)$ in terms of s. We invert the LT to regain $c(t)$ on the left. The inverse LT of $1/(s+k)$ is e^{-kt}, where k is constant, as can readily be demonstrated by applying the LT (7.2.13) to the function e^{-kt}. Using this result we have the general solution

$$c_1(t) = \frac{c_1(0)(k_{21}-\alpha)}{\beta-\alpha}e^{-\alpha t} + \frac{c_1(0)(k_{21}-\beta)}{\alpha-\beta}e^{-\beta t}, \tag{7.2.17}$$

which is the same result as before. The solution for $c_2(t)$ can be arrived at by an indentical procedure and is

$$c_2(t) = c_1(0)\frac{V_1}{V_2}\frac{k_{12}}{\beta-\alpha}e^{-\alpha t} - c_1(0)\frac{V_1}{V_2}\frac{k_{12}}{\beta-\alpha}e^{-\beta t}. \tag{7.2.18}$$

Note that this expression, unlike that for $c_1(t)$, contains the ratio of the two unknown volumes of the compartments.

We have now established that the time course of the drug in the central compartment can be described by a bi-exponential equation

$$c_1 = A\exp(-\alpha t) + B\exp(-\beta t).$$

This contains four model-fitting parameters A, α, B, β, and the final task is to relate these to the three rate coefficients k_{12}, k_{21} and k_{13}.

The amount of drug eliminated from the beginning up to time t is given by

$$x_3(t) = k_{13} V_1 \int_0^t c_1 \, dt$$

$$= k_{13} V_1 \int_0^t [A \exp(-\alpha t) + B \exp(-\beta t)] \, dt.$$

In the limit as $t \to \infty$, all drug will be eliminated and therefore

$$D_0 = k_{13} V_1 \int_0^\infty [A \exp(-\alpha t) + B \exp(-\beta t)] \, dt.$$

Recalling that $\exp(0) = 1$ and $\exp(-\infty) = 0$ [see IV, §2.11], this leads to the result

$$c_1(0) = \frac{D_0}{V_1} = k_{13} \left(\frac{A}{\alpha} + \frac{B}{\beta} \right).$$

Also, from (7.2.8) at time $t = 0$,

$$c_1(0) = A + B.$$

Hence,

$$k_{13} = \alpha\beta \left(\frac{A + B}{A\beta + \alpha B} \right). \tag{7.2.19}$$

Finally, using (7.2.9), we have

$$k_{21} = \frac{\alpha\beta}{k_{13}} \tag{7.2.20}$$

and

$$k_{12} = \alpha + \beta - k_{13} - k_{21}. \tag{7.2.21}$$

It is the accepted convention when describing data with (7.2.8) to describe α as the fast disposition coefficient and β as the slow disposition coefficient. These are determined from the measurements of plasma concentration over time. Examples of this procedure are given in Section 7.3 and in Chapter 8.

7.2.3 First-order absorption in a two-compartment open model

This model is used when the drug has to be absorbed prior to distribution, as, for example, following oral or intra-muscular administration (Figure 7.2.2). The rate equations describing this model are the same as those for the model described in Section 7.2.2 but for the addition of a term to describe the rate of absorption of the drug (dose D_0 as before) from its site of administration (in a new compartment a) into the central compartment. Drug is taken to be absorbed from this site

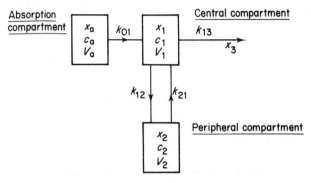

Figure 7.2.2 Compartmental model used to describe absorption of drug, then distribution and elimination. The subscript 'a' denotes a third compartment representing unabsorbed drug.

according to the first-order rate equation

$$\frac{dx_a}{dt} = -k_{01}x_a,$$

which has the solution

$$x_a = c_a V_a = D_0 e^{-k_{01}t}. \tag{7.2.22}$$

The equations for the central and peripheral compartments are:

$$\frac{dc_1}{dt} = -(k_{13} + k_{12})c_1 + \frac{V_2}{V_1}k_{21}c_2 + k_{01}\frac{c_a V_a}{V_1}, \tag{7.2.23}$$

$$\frac{dc_2}{dt} = \frac{V_1}{V_2}k_{12}c_1 - k_{21}c_2. \tag{7.2.24}$$

Differentiating (7.2.23), substituting from (7.2.24) to eliminate c_2 and using (7.2.22), we are led to the second-order linear inhomogeneous differential equation [see IV, §7.6]

$$\frac{d^2c_1}{dt^2} + (k_{12} + k_{21} + k_{13})\frac{dc_1}{dt} + k_{21}k_{13}c_1$$

$$= -k_{01}(k_{01} - k_{21})\frac{D_0}{V_1}e^{-k_{01}t}. \tag{7.2.25}$$

The general solution of (7.2.25) is given by the linear combination of the general solution of the homogeneous equation (7.2.8) and a particular solution of the inhomogeneous equation.

To obtain a particular solution we can use the method of undetermined coefficients [see IV, §7.6.1] and assume a solution of the form

$$c_1 = E \exp(-k_{01}t). \tag{7.2.26}$$

Then

$$\frac{dc_1}{dt} = -k_{01}E \exp(-k_{01}t),$$

$$\frac{d^2c_1}{dt^2} = k_{01}^2 E \exp(-k_{01}t).$$

Substituting these expressions in (7.2.25) and rearranging,

$$E(k_{01}^2 - (k_{12} + k_{21} + k_{13})k_{01} + k_{21}k_{13}) = -k_{01}(k_{01} - k_{21})\frac{D_0}{V_1},$$

and using the relationships (7.2.9),

$$E = \frac{-k_{01}(k_{01} - k_{21})}{(k_{01} - \alpha)(k_{01} - \beta)}\frac{D_0}{V_1}.$$

we thus have the general solution

$$c_1 = A \exp(-\alpha t) + B \exp(-\beta t) + E \exp(-k_{01}t) \tag{7.2.27}$$

where A and B are determined by the initial boundary conditions as before.

We will now solve the rate equations using Laplace transforms. Taking transforms of (7.2.23) and (7.2.24),

$$s\bar{c}_1 - c_1(0) = -(k_{13} + k_{12})\bar{c}_1 + k_{21}\frac{V_2}{V_1}\bar{c}_2 + \frac{k_{01}D_0}{V_1(s + k_{01})}, \tag{7.2.28}$$

$$s\bar{c}_2 - c_2(0) = k_{12}\frac{V_1}{V_2}\bar{c}_1 - k_{21}\bar{c}_2. \tag{7.2.29}$$

Using the initial conditions $c_1(0) = c_2(0) = 0$, we have

$$s\bar{c}_1 + (k_{13} + k_{12})\bar{c}_1 - k_{21}\frac{V_2}{V_1}\bar{c}_2 = \frac{k_{01}D_0}{V_1(s + k_{01})}, \tag{7.2.30}$$

$$-k_{12}\frac{V_1}{V_2}\bar{c}_1 + (s + k_{21})\bar{c}_2 = 0. \tag{7.2.31}$$

Substituting from (7.2.31) into (7.2.30) and rearranging,

$$\bar{c}_1(s) = \frac{k_{01}D_0(s + k_{21})}{(s + k_{01})(s + \alpha)(s + \beta)V_1}. \tag{7.2.32}$$

To obtain the inverse Laplace transform and hence $c_1(t)$, we expand in partial fractions [see I, §14.10] in the form

$$\frac{k_{01}D_0(s+k_{21})}{(s+k_{01})(s+\alpha)(s+\beta)V_1} = \frac{A}{s+\alpha} + \frac{B}{s+\beta} + \frac{C}{s+k_{01}}.$$

Recombining and equating coefficients as before we find

$$A = \frac{k_{01}D_0(k_{21}-\alpha)}{V_1(\beta-\alpha)(k_{01}-\alpha)},$$

$$B = \frac{k_{01}D_0(k_{21}-\beta)}{V_1(\alpha-\beta)(k_{01}-\beta)}, \qquad (7.2.33)$$

$$E = \frac{k_{01}D_0(k_{21}-k_{01})}{V_1(\alpha-k_{01})(\beta-k_{01})}.$$

Thus, taking the inverse transform [see IV, §13.4.2],

$$c_1 = A\exp(-\alpha t) + B\exp(-\beta t) + E\exp(-k_{01}t). \qquad (7.2.34)$$

The concise nature of the Laplace transform technique for the solution of differential equations should be apparent from these examples, and it is to be recommended as the method of choice. Further justification for its use is given in the next section where a general method of solving compartmental systems of equations is described.

7.2.4 A general input and output model

The derivation of integrated rate equations for more complicated systems uses the methods of the previous sections, but, even allowing for the concise nature of the Laplace transform, this can involve some complicated and tedious mathematical manipulation. A comparison of the previous two systems reveals considerable similarity between the solutions, and this is not surprising as they have the same output system, a two-compartment open model, and differ only in the method of drug input. This leads to a simple method of solving general linear models by isolating the input and output or disposition functions (Benet, 1972).

Consider an input function $i(t)$ describing the rate of arrival of the drug into the central compartment and a distribution function $d(t)$ describing the concentration in the central compartment as a function of time following a bolus input at time $t=0$. The function $d(t)$ reflects the processes of distribution, metabolism and elimination of the drug; $i(t)$ reflects absorption. The function $i(t)$ could be considered as a continuous succession of bolus inputs. Then the concentration in the central compartment $c_1(t)$ may be written as a convolution integral

$$c_1(t) = \int_0^t i(\tau)d(t-\tau)\,d\tau, \qquad (7.2.35)$$

where drug entry at time τ is multiplied by the distribution function for time $t - \tau$ after entry to give the concentration due to the bolus at time t. The integration over entry times τ between 0 and t, valid for a linear system, enables us to calculate the overall concentration at time t; only drugs entering before time t can affect this! Units of $i(t)$ will be in units of milligrams per hour or if we are dealing immediately in terms of concentrations in the central compartment, milligrams per litre per hour. In the Laplace notation, (7.2.35) can be expressed as

$$\bar{c}(s) = \bar{i}(s)\bar{d}(s), \tag{7.2.36}$$

convolution in the time domain being equivalent to multiplication in the Laplace domain (see Section 5.A.2 of this Guidebook).

Let us now look again at the expressions for $\bar{c}_1(s)$ derived for the models of Sections 7.2.2 and 7.2.3. These were

Bolus injection: $\displaystyle \bar{c}_1(s) = \frac{c_1(0)(s + k_{21})}{(s + \alpha)(s + \beta)}.$

First-order absorption: $\displaystyle \bar{c}_1(s) = \frac{k_{01} D_0 (s + k_{21})}{V_1(s + k_{01})(s + \alpha)(s + \beta)}.$

For a bolus injection of mass D_0 of drug occurring at time $t = 0$ the function $i(t)$ will take the form

$$D_0 \delta(t) \quad \text{or} \quad \frac{D_0}{V_1}\delta(t),$$

where $\delta(t)$ is the Dirac delta function and the form chosen depends on whether we are dealing in terms of mass or concentration of drug in the central compartment. If we chose concentration, $i(t) = c_1(0)\delta(t)$, and, using the standard result $LT[f(t)\delta(t)] = f(o)$

$$\bar{i}(s) = c_1(0). \tag{7.2.37}$$

The distribution function is then identified with the response when the bolus gives rise to unit initial concentration of drug, That is,

$$\bar{d}(s) = \frac{(s + k_{21})}{(s + \alpha)(s + \beta)}. \tag{7.2.38}$$

For the first-order absorption model, the rate of entry of drug into the central compartment is found from (7.2.22) to be

$$i(t) = -\frac{dx_a}{dt} = k_{01}\frac{D_0}{V_1}e^{-k_{01}t},$$

where again we use units of milligrams per litre per hour and relate it to central compartment concentration. Hence in this case

$$\bar{i}(s) = \frac{k_{01}c_1(0)}{s + k_{01}}. \tag{7.2.39}$$

The distribution function is the same as that for the bolus injection model.

For the case of the central compartment, concentration c_1, communicating directly with $n-1$ peripheral compartments, $c_2, \ldots, c_n$, Benet (1972) has derived the expression

$$\bar{d}(s) = \frac{\prod\limits_{i=2}^{n} (s + E_i)}{\prod\limits_{i=1}^{n} (s + E_i) - \sum\limits_{j=2}^{n} k_{1j} k_{j1} \prod\limits_{\substack{m=2 \\ m \neq j}}^{n} (s + E_m)},$$

which is equivalent to

$$\bar{d}(s) = \frac{1}{(s + E_1) - \sum\limits_{j=2}^{n} [k_{1j} k_{j1}/(s + E_j)]}, \tag{7.2.40}$$

where n is the number of compartments, k_{ij} the first-order rate coefficient from compartment i to j and E_i the sum of the exit rate coefficients from compartment i.

We will demonstrate the simplicity of this method by again considering first-order absorption in a two-compartment model. Referring to Figure 7.2.2 we have $n = 2$, $E_1 = k_{12} + k_{13}$ and $E_2 = k_{21}$. Hence, from (7.2.40),

$$\bar{d}(s) = \frac{1}{(s + k_{12} + k_{13}) - k_{12}k_{21}/(s + k_{21})}$$

$$= \frac{s + k_{21}}{s^2 + s(k_{12} + k_{21} + k_{13}) + k_{12}k_{21} + k_{21}k_{13} - k_{12}k_{21}}$$

$$= \frac{s + k_{21}}{(s + \alpha)(s + \beta)},$$

where α and β are defined by (7.2.9). This is the result we obtained previously in (7.2.38), but by a much simpler method.

If the concentration in a compartment other than the central (e.g. the peripheral) is required, we can still use (7.2.40) in the following manner:

(a) Solve for $\bar{c}_1(s)$.
(b) Write down the rate equation for the required compartment and take the Laplace transform. Thus, for example, looking at compartment 2 as in (7.2.24),

$$\frac{dc_2}{dt} = k_{12}c_1 \frac{V_1}{V_2} - k_{21}c_2$$

$$\bar{c}_2(s) = \frac{V_1}{V_2} \frac{k_{12}}{s + k_{21}} \bar{c}_1(s).$$

(c) Substitute for $\bar{c}_1(s)$ from (a) and take the inverse Laplace transform of the result.

The input functions for an intravenous IV bolus and first-order absorption have been derived and, for completeness, we note that the function for an IV infusion commencing at time a and terminating at time b is

$$\bar{i}(s) = \frac{k_0[\exp(-as) - \exp(-bs)]}{s} \tag{7.2.41}$$

where k_0 is the zero-order (constant) infusion rate. This arises as the difference between the input functions for in fusions starting (step function input) at time a and at time b. For further examples of this very powerful general technique the reader should consult Benet's (1972) paper, cited above.

7.2.5 Multiple dosing

It is a simple matter to modify the single-dose equations derived in the preceding sections to describe the multiple-dosing situation commonly encountered in practice. To illustrate this we will first derive a general multiple-dose function.

Let D be the dose administered at a dosing interval τ and let $\theta(t)$ be a decay function such that at time t the concentration will be

$$c(t) = D\theta(t),$$

At the end of the dosage period τ the concentration will be

$$c(\tau) = D\theta(\tau)$$

and, if a further dose D is administered, this will rise to

$$D\theta(\tau) + D.$$

At the end of this dosage period the concentration will have decayed to

$$[D\theta(\tau) + D]\theta(\tau)$$

and the next dose will cause this to rise to

$$[D\theta(\tau) + D]\theta(\tau) + D.$$

This process will continue until all n doses have been administered and the concentration will decay according to $\theta(t)$, the expression for the concentration being given by

$$c = D[\theta(\tau)^{n-1} + \theta(\tau)^{n-2} + \cdots + \theta(\tau) + 1]\theta(t) \tag{7.2.42}$$

and the total time course by

$$T = (n-1)\tau + t. \tag{7.2.43}$$

The expression in square brackets in (7.2.42) is a finite geometric series [see IV, (1.7.4)] with the sum

$$g = \frac{1 - \theta(\tau)^n}{1 - \theta(\tau)},$$

(7.2.44)

and so from (7.2.42) and (7.2.44) the concentration at any time after the final dose can be written as

$$c = D\left[\frac{1 - \theta(\tau)^n}{1 - \theta(\tau)}\right]\theta(t).$$

(7.2.45)

Applying this procedure to the solutions of Sections 7.2.2 and 7.2.3, we find the following multi-dose expressions:

$$c = A\left[\frac{1 - \exp(-n\alpha\tau)}{1 - \exp(-\alpha\tau)}\right]\exp(-\alpha t) + B\left[\frac{1 - \exp(-n\beta\tau)}{1 - \exp(-\beta\tau)}\right]\exp(-\beta t)$$

and

(7.2.46)

$$c = A\left[\frac{1 - \exp(-n\alpha\tau)}{1 - \exp(-\alpha\tau)}\right]\exp(-\alpha t) + B\left[\frac{1 - \exp(-n\beta\tau)}{1 - \exp(-\beta\tau)}\right]\exp(-\beta t)$$
$$+ E\left[\frac{1 - \exp(-nk_{01}\tau)}{1 - \exp(-k_{01}\tau)}\right]\exp(-k_{01}t).$$

(7.2.47)

The multiple-dose input function, using the approach of Section 7.2.4, is

$$\bar{i}(s) = \left[\frac{1 - \exp(-n\tau k_i)}{1 - \exp(-\tau k_i)}\right]\exp(-k_i t)$$

(7.2.48)

where, as defined in (7.2.43), t is the time after the last dose was administered.

7.2.6 Non-linear systems

The models derived in the preceding sections are only applicable to linear systems, in which an n-fold increase in dose results in an n-fold increase in c. Few drugs exhibit this linear response over the entire dosage range, it often being observed that the rate of elimination tends to a limiting value with increased dose. Although there are several reasons for this non-linearity, the two major causes are:

(a) The drug is metabolized prior to elimination, and elimination is described by a Michaelis–Menten or similar enzyme mechanism where

$$-\frac{dc}{dt} = \frac{V_m c}{k_m + c},$$

(7.2.49)

k_m being the Michaelis–Menten coefficient and V_m the maximum rate of the enzyme reaction.

(b) The drug binds to plasma proteins by a saturable mechanism which can be described by an absorption isotherm (e.g. Langmuir) where

$$c_2 = \frac{c_m c_1}{c_1 + k_1}. \tag{7.2.50}$$

Here c_2 is the concentration of the bound drug, c_1 that of the free drug and c_m is the saturation concentration in the binding compartment (2).

It is an unfortunate fact that while drugs exhibit non-linearity to a greater or lesser extent, very few pharmacokinetic investigations are designed to detect non-linearity. A typical investigation involves the administration of a single dose to a set of volunteers or patients and then the determination of the appropriate pharmacokinetic model; it is extremely unlikely that this type of experiment would detect non-linearity. The detection of non-linearity is, in principle, very simple and requires the determination of the plasma concentration–time profiles at a series of doses, followed by:

(a) Normalizing the data by dividing the concentration by the dose and plotting these normalized curves for each dose on the same graph. If the curves are not superimposable, a non-linear mechanism is operating.

(b) Determining the area under the concentration–time curve [see IV, §4.2]. For a linear system this should exhibit a linear dependence on dose.

(c) Fitting the data to the 'appropriate' pharmacokinetic model [see IV, Chapter 14]. If the rate coefficients exhibit a dose dependence, then a non-linear mechanism is operating.

Numerical examples of the above tests are given by Wagner (1975). Chau (1976) has extended (b) above not only to detect but to identify the type of non-linearity. The area under the concentration curve (AUC) is determined and plotted against c^0, the initial concentration. If a Michaelis–Menten mechanism is operating, the curve will be convex; if a Langmuir binding isotherm is operating, the curve will be concave [see IV, §15.2.6]. If both mechanisms are operating then the curve can include both convex and concave portions. The original paper should be consulted for the underlying theory and techniques for calculating AUC and c.

Non-linear models are derived in a similar manner to linear models except that the general method of Section 7.2.4 cannot be applied. The rate equations corresponding to the model of Section 7.2.2, with elimination from compartment 1 by a Michaelis–Menten mechanism, can be written directly as

$$\frac{dc_1}{dt} = -k_{12}c_1 - \frac{V_m c_1}{k_m + c_1} + k_{21}c_2 \frac{V_2}{V_1}, \tag{7.2.51}$$

$$\frac{dc_2}{dt} = \frac{V_1}{V_2} k_{12} c_1 - k_{21} c_2, \tag{7.2.52}$$

and solution involves direct numerical integration of these differential rate equations. The usual technique is the Runge–Kutta procedure [see III, §8.2.2], although the more sophisticated predictor–corrector methods due to Adams, Merson and Gear [see III, §8.3.1] usually provide a more stable solution but involve an increase in computer time (Walsh, 1974; Shampine and Gordon, 1975). The form of the Michaelis–Menten expression can lead to severe numerical instability in the solution, as discussed by Tong and Metzler (1980).

7.3 EVALUATION OF PHARMACOKINETIC PARAMETERS

In the preceding section mathematical models for various dosage forms were derived. In this section the problem of fitting these models to clinical data is considered.

7.3.1 Graphical technique

This technique is commonly known as 'feathering', 'back-stripping' or the 'method of residuals', and makes use of the limit

$$\lim_{x \to \infty} \exp(-x) = 0. \tag{7.3.1}$$

Consider the bi-exponential expression for IV bolus administration (7.2.8):

$$c_1 = A \exp(-\alpha t) + B \exp(-\beta t),$$

where by convention $\alpha > \beta$. At long times, $A \exp(-\alpha t)$ will be effectively zero and the expression reduces to

$$c_1 = B \exp(-\beta t), \tag{7.3.2}$$

which can be linearized by taking logarithms [see IV, §2.11] to give

$$\log c_1 = \log B - \beta t. \tag{7.3.3}$$

To use the method we first plot the c_1, t data on semi-logarithmic graph paper and determine B and β from the terminal linear portion of the curve. We then extrapolate this line to the ordinate [see III, §2.4] and calculate the 'residuals', the difference between the observed and extrapolated concentrations. These residuals correspond to the α-phase, and A and α are determined by plotting the residuals on the semi-logarithmic paper as above. Complete numerical examples are given by Wagner (1975). See also the worked example in Section 8.5.5, using a tracer to determine effective renal plasma flow.

A similar approach is used for oral data except that we must now take into account the lag-time (t_{lag}) before the drug appears in the plasma. Recalling that the boundary condition for the oral absorption model of Section 7.2.3 is $c_1 = 0$ at

$t = 0$, the real time scale must be adjusted for the lag-time in order to satisfy this condition. The simplest way to determine t_{lag} is to plot the data for the absorption phase and extrapolate it back to the abscissa. Although more accurate methods are available (Wagner, 1975) it is doubtful whether their use is justified due to errors inherent in the graphical procedure.

The critical step in feathering is the extrapolation through the late time data region, a region where errors in the data are liable to be high, and any errors in this extrapolation are propagated through the parameter estimates. For this reason, and the fact that it is not possible to calculate meaningful statistics from the graphical estimates, we do not favour this procedure for model-fitting.

7.3.2 Numerical technique

The method of choice is that of non-linear optimization as discussed in Section 7.8.2 on ligand–protein interactions. The main problem in the analysis is deciding on the appropriate model, a problem complicated both by the inherent scatter in biological data and the flexibility in the general exponential solution of ordinary linear differential equations (7.2.6). Several attempts have been made to produce computer programs which automatically select the 'best' model to describe the data (Pilo and Mancine, 1970; Sedman and Wagner, 1974), as opposed to fitting a specific model to the data.

Typical of these decision-making programs is AUTOAN (Sedman and Wagner, 1974), which is based on the NONLIN optimization program of Metzler, Elpring and McEwan (1974) and has a library of eight linear and four non-linear pharmacokinetic models. Given a set of concentration–time data and the route of administration, the program tests for Michaelis–Menten kinetics and determines the number of exponentials which best describe the data using a modified Foss technique (Foss, 1971) to generate initial estimates for the optimization of (7.2.8). The optimum number of exponentials is selected by sequentially fitting one to five exponentials to the data and calculating a goodness-of-fit parameter r^2, where

$$1 - r^2 = \frac{\sum_{1}^{n} (c_j - \hat{c}_j)^2}{\sum_{1}^{n} c_j^2 - \left(\sum_{1}^{n} c_j \right)^2 \Big/ n} \tag{7.3.4}$$

and c_j is the observed and $\hat{c}_j$ the predicted concentration for the jth of n observations. In the program, the optimum number of exponentials is considered to be found when one of the following criteria is satisfied:

(a) $r^2 \geq 0.98$.
(b) The percentage improvement in r^2 is not significant.

(c) The number of exponentials equals 5.

(d) There are too many exponentials for a given class of model.

Having determined the number of exponentials, the appropriate model is selected and the individual pharmacokinetic coefficients determined by optimization techniques.

When using this method, it is important to appreciate that the decision to select a model is made numerically on the criteria indicated above and that these criteria may not necessarily be appropriate to the experimental data being analysed. It is essential to check that the model does adequately describe the data using the usual verification procedures (see, for example, Berman, 1963).

7.3.3 Examination of the fitted model

In mathematical modelling in general, a theoretical model is proposed and the experiment carried out to test the model. In pharmacokinetics the analysis is usually different in that the experiment is carried out, i.e. plasma concentration–time data obtained, and then choice of the model is determined *a posteriori* from the number of exponentials required to describe the data. Although this has the advantage of determining compartmental order (Smith and Mohler, 1976) within the range of the data, it has the disadvantage that it can lead to a model which does not reflect the physiological structure of the system (Godfrey, Jones and Brown, 1980). The exponential fitting process has already been described, and Boxenbaum, Riegelman and Elashoff (1974) have given an excellent summary of the statistical requirements for the satisfactory estimation of pharmacokinetic parameters. In addition to performing a statistical analysis of the type indicated by Boxenbaum and colleagues it is also necessary to appreciate the effect of (a) the paucity of data in most clinical investigations, (b) the error inherent in such data and (c) the characteristics of the numerical procedures used with the fitted model. The effects of these on the fitting process have been established by many authors, but their results appear to have been largely unappreciated by authors of many clinical publications.

Westlake (1971) simulated fourteen data points from the two-compartment open model with first-order absorption using realistic values for the pharmacokinetic parameters. He applied a low level of random noise to the data and then estimated the parameters using a standard program. In all cases the parameter estimates were significantly different from the known values. Typical results for k_{01} were an initial value of 2.389 per hour, a least squares estimate of 1.774 per hour with approximate 95 per cent confidence limits of -0.54 to 4.09 per hour— the estimate being ill defined in parameter space and having no predictive power. Similar results have been obtained by Saunders and Natunen (1972) and Fell and Stevens (1975). Despite these parameter discrepancies, the fitted model was still an adequate predictor of the plasma curve, and this leads one to question why modelling was carried out.

If the reason was to represent the data set then the modelling was successful, although it would have been more satisfactory to use the general exponential solution rather than the full pharmacokinetic model, as the former requires fewer parameters to be estimated. If, however, the reason was to obtain 'meaningful pharmacokinetic parameters' for subsequent use in predicting concentrations in inaccessible compartments or developing dosage regimes, then the modelling has failed. Indeed, any pharmacokinetic parameter that is published without the associated statistics must be treated with extreme scepticism as most clinical investigations will have more inherent noise than the simulation studies mentioned above. It is for this reason that the calculation of dosage regimes has not been considered in this chapter. Although the mathematics is straightforward (Wagner, 1975) the errors in the available pharmacokinetic parameters are such that the predictions will have little clinical relevance and empirical methods are to be preferred (Westlake, 1971).

The uncertainty in published parameter estimates, which reduces their clinical relevance, has been recognized by Sheiner, Benet and Pagliaro (1981) in their compilation of clinical pharmacokinetic data. To allow for the variations between K different studies, they suggest that the parameter P be assigned a concensus value P which is also weighted for the number of patients N within each study and for the quality of experimental methodology Q (ranked 1, poor to 3, good). They used

$$P = \frac{\sum\limits_{i=1}^{K} N_i Q_i p_i}{\sum\limits_{i=1}^{K} N_i Q_i}, \tag{7.3.5}$$

where p_i is the value obtained in the ith study containing N_i subjects and quality of study rated to be Q_i. They gave examples of this technique for a selection of cardiovascular drugs.

Godfrey, Jones and Brown (1980) considered the problem of parameter identifiability: i.e. given an input and the experimental response, can the parameters of a compartmental model be determined uniquely or is additional information required. They showed that for any general two-compartment model (i.e. the addition of an elimination pathway from the peripheral compartments in the models of Sections 7.2.2 and 7.2.3), the model is non-identifiable from a classical single-input–single-output experiment, the analysis resulting in the four rate coefficients being defined by three equations. The additional information required to make the model uniquely identifiable is either *a priori* assumptions concerning the rate coefficients (usually $k_{23} = 0$, as in the solutions given in Section 7.2.2 and 7.2.3) or the use of a second input, simultaneous with the first, into the second compartment but still only measuring the first compartment. It was established that this technique will make the model identifiable only if the two inputs have a different shape, e.g. infusion into compartment 1 with a simultaneous bolus into compartment 2. They further showed that measurement of urine concentrations is only of use in improving identifiability if all the rate coefficients from the central compartment are known.

The final problem concerns the use of the Michaelis–Menten expression in non-linear models. The mathematical properties of this expression have been investigated by Tong and Metzler (1979) with respect to parameter estimation. They established error bounds on the expression and showed that the parameter estimates are very sensitive to minor changes in the data and choice of initial parameter values for optimization. A simulation with $V_m = 3$ and $k_m = 1$ was performed and, using initial estimates of $V_m = 3.9$ and $k_m = 0.7$, the optimized values were 3.004 and 1.001 respectively. However, a slight change in the initial estimates to 3.95 and 0.7 produced final estimates of 40.66 and 14.63. Obviously great care must be taken when examining the results from compartmental models involving non-linear mechanisms of this type.

7.4 SIMULATION PHARMACOKINETICS

The methods of the preceding sections have been concerned with the development of mathematical models and then fitting the relevant model to a data set. In simulation techniques, a model structure, which may be of any degree of complexity, is assumed and a data set generated. This approach may be used as an educational aid ('What is the effect of changing various parameters?') or, by matching the simulated data set with the observed data set, to investigate the system structure.

The simplest simulation models are those designed to investigate dosage regimes; these are purely kinetic in nature in that a particular drug is assigned a particular compartmental model. Typical of this class of simulation are the programs GENT, THEOT and PHENYT which describe the pharmacokinetics of gentamycin, theophylline and phenytoin by one-compartment, two-compartment and one-compartment with Michaelis–Menten kinetics respectively (Sullivan and Wunderley, 1980). To make simulations unique, the mean pharmacokinetic parameters in the models are modified by a random number multiplier each time the program is executed to simulate different patients. Although this approach is useful in testing dosage regimes it has the disadvantage of assuming that each drug is described by a specific compartmental model.

The alternative class of simulations are based on physiological as well as kinetic considerations, the most sophisticated of these models being MacDope (Ingram *et al.*, 1979— Bloch *et al.*, 1980a, 1980b). The model consists of eight interacting compartments described by a set of eight coupled differential equations. The program consists of three independent modules which:

(a) Allow a variety of prescription routines and dosage regimes,
(b) Define the physical, chemical and pharmacological properties of drugs available to the program,
(c) Describe the patho-physiology of the patient.

First-order equations are used to describe equilibration between the eight compartments [see IV, §7.2], while the law of mass action is used to describe hepatic drug metabolism, drug transport by the kidney tubules and protein binding of the drug. This formulation enables the simulation to cope with a maximum of six drugs and their metabolites and also with drug interactions. For n drugs or metabolites in the system, in the mathematical model there is a set of $8 \times n$ coupled non-linear differential equations which, for computational convenience, are linearized over short time periods and solved by a standard Runge–Kutta procedure [see III, §8.2.2].

The advantages of this approach include: (i) a patient can be represented in a variety of disease states, (ii) no prior compartmental model is built into the system as in the first class of simulations and (iii) a variety of dosage regimes can be investigated. After selecting a patient, drug(s) and dosage regime, the drug is administered via a prescribing routine, and the drug–patient factors interact in the body model to give the drug concentrations in various body compartments. At the end of a simulation the compartmental concentrations (e.g. plasma and urine) are available for analysis by conventional compartmental or clearance techniques, and by varying the patient and drug factors it is possible to gain an insight into the physiological significance (if any) of the model parameters.

7.5 AVAILABILITY AND CLEARANCE

Availability, F, is a useful concept for comparing different formulations of the same drug. The amount of drug absorbed may be obtained from the area under a concentration–time curve (AUC) by application of the trapezoidal rule [see III, §7.1.3]. It is assumed that absorption following IV administration is instantaneous and that this AUC may be used as a reference for comparison with test administration routes having delayed absorption, e.g. an oral dose. F is given by

$$F = \frac{\text{AUC}_{\text{test}}}{\text{AUC}_{\text{IV}}}. \tag{7.5.1}$$

It may alternatively be obtained from the total recovery of unchanged drug in the urine denoted by X_u^∞, where

$$F = \frac{X_{u\,\text{test}}^\infty}{X_{u\,\text{IV}}^\infty}. \tag{7.5.2}$$

Availability provides a combined measure of the effects of formulation and route of administration.

Bio-equivalence is concerned with the application of the availability concept to supposedly equivalent formulations of the same drug. Chodos and Disanto (1973) have indicated that the determination of F is inadequate for this purpose. The same AUC may be obtained from high concentrations over a short time or low concentrations over a long time, but in this latter case the therapeutic concentration may not be obtained. These authors suggest that the peak concentration and time for this concentration should also be determined. Their monograph should be consulted for details of the protocol for a single-dose bio-availability/bio-equivalence study and the statistics necessary for comparing several formulations.

An alternative approach to pharmacokinetics, and one that is favoured by many clinicians and clinical pharmacists, is through the concept of *clearance*, $\mathscr{C}$ (Wilkinson and Shand, 1975; Rowland and Tozer, 1980). This is a very simple and useful concept in that it provides a method of specifying the overall effectiveness of a process in removing a drug from a particular compartment by a particular route. Clearance is defined as the volume of the eliminating compartment from which a drug is completely removed per unit time by a specified pathway. It follows from this definition that $\mathscr{C}$ has the dimensions of flow, and it has sometimes been referred to as 'virtual flow' (Riggs, 1963).

It is common practice to refer clearance values to a particular eliminating organ rather than to an empirical compartment, e.g. hepatic, renal or total body clearance. A convenient method of representing clearance across an eliminating organ is in terms of organ blood flow $\dot{Q}$ and extraction ratio E of the drug by the organ, where

$$\mathscr{C} = \dot{Q}E. \tag{7.5.3}$$

If E is unity then all drug (free and bound) passing through the organ will be removed, but if E is reduced, e.g. with renal dysfunction, then less drug will be cleared and a toxic level may result.

It is not particularly easy to model protein binding and its effects using traditional pharmacokinetics, but Wilkinson and Shand (1975) obtained simple relationships using clearance.

The rate of elimination R is, by definition, the product of the clearance and the free drug plasma concentration, c_f. This clearance, $\mathscr{C}$, has been termed the intrinsic clearance, and it is a characteristic of both the drug and the eliminating environment:

$$R = \mathscr{C}c_f \tag{7.5.4}$$

The hepatic clearance, $\mathscr{C}_H$, is obtained from this expression by dividing by the total plasma concentration of drug, c_p. Hence

$$\mathscr{C}_H = \frac{R}{c_p} = \frac{\mathscr{C}c_f}{c_p} = \mathscr{C}f_f \tag{7.5.5}$$

where f_f is the fraction of free drug. Then also, from (7.5.3),

$$\mathscr{C}_H = \dot{Q} E f_f. \tag{7.5.6}$$

If the drug has a low extraction ratio, e.g. theophylline with $E < 0.3$, the degree of binding will have a marked effect on $\mathscr{C}_H$, the magnitude of the effect depending on $\mathscr{C}$. If, however, the extraction ratio is high, e.g. lignocaine with $E > 0.7$, the drug will be cleared, and $\mathscr{C}_H$ will be controlled by the flow rate $\dot{Q}$ with f_f having only a minor effect (flow limited conditions).

The complete and detailed analysis of this model including the effects of binding, metabolism and disease states on $\mathscr{C}_H$ is given by Wilkinson and Shand (1975). A full description of the use of clearance in clinical pharmacokinetics is given in the text by Rowland and Tozer (1980).

7.6 INTRODUCTION TO LIGAND BINDING

Proteins are capable of binding ligands in a reversible manner. If the protein is a plasma protein and the ligand a drug, this is of considerable therapeutic importance as it is generally accepted that only free drug is capable of therapeutic action. A knowledge of binding is important when designing a dosage regime because:

(a) Many patients have multiple-drug therapy and some drugs are capable of displacing an already bound drug which may then exceed its toxic concentration.

(b) Many disease states are capable of altering drug binding.

For the purposes of this chapter it will be assumed that the experimenter has a knowledge of the amount of drug bound by the protein, as expressed by the binding ratio r, when

$$r = \frac{\text{moles of bound drug}}{\text{total protein concentration}},$$

and the concentration of free drug, $[A]$. All concentrations are molar. Methods for the determination of r and $[A]$ are given in standard texts such as Anton and Solomons (1973).

We will consider a simple approach to the quantification of binding data and then develop a rigorous mathematical model that is generally applicable. Consider the reversible binding of ligand A to protein P

$$P + A \rightleftharpoons PA,$$

where we can write the association constant k for the reaction as

$$k = \frac{[PA]}{[P][A]}, \tag{7.6.1}$$

and the binding ratio r as

$$r = \frac{[PA]}{[P] + [PA]}.$$

Now from (7.6.1)

$$[PA] = k[P][A]$$

and thus

$$r = \frac{k[P][A]}{[P] + k[P][A]} = \frac{k[A]}{1 + k[A]}. \tag{7.6.2}$$

This can be rearranged to give

$$\frac{r}{[A]} = k - kr \tag{7.6.3}$$

and so a plot of $r/[A]$ versus r (r and $[A]$ both being measured at various levels of total drug concentration) will be linear of slope $-k$, and one can, in principle, use this value of k to predict the required dose to maintain a therapeutic concentration of drug.

This model is too simple for most purposes and we can extend it to the protein with n identical binding sites and obtain

$$r = \frac{nk[A]}{1 + k[A]} \tag{7.6.4}$$

and, rearranging,

$$\frac{r}{[A]} = kn - kr, \tag{7.6.5}$$

which enables estimates to be made of both n and k.

As will be shown later, many researchers use this simple model to obtain binding parameters without considering or appreciating the assumptions underlying the model, with the result that an incorrect analysis is made. In the next section these assumptions will be discussed and a rigorous model described.

7.7 MATHEMATICAL MODELS

There are two models commonly used to relate the molar binding ratio r to the concentration of free ligand $[A]$. Although they are both based on the law of mass action they are fundamentally different in concept. One considers the stoichiometry of the binding reaction whereas the other is concerned with individual binding sites.

7.7.1 The stoichiometric model

In this model (Klotz, 1946, 1953, 1974), the concentrations of sequential stoichiometric species PA_1, $PA_2, \ldots, PA_i, \ldots, PA_n$ are calculated, where the subscript denotes the number of bound ligands and n is the total number of binding sites per protein molecule. It is important to note that PA_i is the total concentration of species with i bound ligands and no distinction is made between individual binding sites with i bound ligands. Thus we can write a series of multiple equilibria:

$$P + A \rightleftharpoons PA_1,$$

$$PA_1 + A \rightleftharpoons PA_2,$$

$$PA_{i-1} + A \rightleftharpoons PA_i,$$

and for each binding step we can define a stoichiometric equilibrium coefficient K_i. Thus,

$$K_1 = \frac{[PA_1]}{[P][A]}$$

or

$$[PA_1] = [P][A]K_1,$$

$$K_2 = \frac{[PA_2]}{[PA_1][A]} = \frac{[PA_2]}{[P][A]^2 K_1}$$

or

$$[PA_2] = K_1 K_2 [P][A]^2,$$

and for the ith binding step

$$[PA_i] = (K_1 K_2 \ldots K_i)[P][A]^i. \tag{7.7.1}$$

The parameter of interest, the molar binding ratio r, is defined by

$$r = \frac{[A]_b}{[P]_t}, \tag{7.7.2}$$

where $[P]_t$ is the total concentration of protein and $[A]_b$ the number of moles of bound ligand. Since one mole of PA_i binds i moles of A we can write

$$[A]_b = [PA_1] + 2[PA_2] + \cdots + i[PA_i] + \cdots + n[PA_n]$$

and

$$[P]_t = [P] + [PA_1] + [PA_2] + \cdots + [PA_i] + \cdots + [PA_n].$$

Therefore,

$$r = \frac{[PA_1] + 2[PA_2] + \cdots + i[PA_i] + \cdots + n[PA_n]}{[P] + [PA_1] + [PA_2] + \cdots + [PA_i] + \cdots + [PA_n]}.$$

On substituting (7.7.1) for $[PA_i]$ and cancelling $[P]$ we obtain

$$r = \frac{K_1[A] + 2(K_1 K_2)[A]^2 + \cdots + n(K_1 K_2 \ldots K_n)[A]^n}{1 + K_1[A] + K_1 K_2[A]^2 + \cdots + (K_1 K_2 \ldots K_n)[A]^n}, \tag{7.7.3}$$

which can be written concisely as

$$r = \frac{\displaystyle\sum_{i=1}^{n} i\left(\prod_{j=1}^{i} K_j\right)[A]^i}{1 + \displaystyle\sum_{i=1}^{n} \left(\prod_{j=1}^{i} K_j\right)[A]^i}. \tag{7.7.4}$$

If we denote the denominator of (7.7.4) by Z and its first derivative with respect to $[A]$ by $\dot{Z}$ [see IV, §3.2.1], we have an alternative expression

$$r = \frac{[A]\dot{Z}}{Z}. \tag{7.7.5}$$

It is important to note that in this derivation the states of the bound system are defined only in terms of overall occupancy of sites; no assumptions have been made concerning the nature of the binding sites or any antagonistic or cooperative interactions among occupied sites.

7.7.2 The site-binding model

This model, due to Scatchard (1949), is concerned with individual binding sites and involves the important assumption that each binding site on the protein has a fixed affinity for the ligand and that this affinity is unaffected by occupancy of other sites, i.e. antagonistic or cooperative binding is forbidden. Following the method used for the stoichiometric model we can write the series of multiple equilibria as

$$_1P + A \rightleftharpoons {}_1PA,$$

$$_2P + A \rightleftharpoons {}_2PA,$$

$$_jP + A \rightleftharpoons {}_jPA,$$

where the subscript j refers to the jth binding site and for each binding site we can define a site equilibrium coefficient k_j. Thus,

$$k_1 = \frac{[_1PA]}{[_1P][A]},$$

$$k_2 = \frac{[_2PA]}{[_2P][A]}, \tag{7.7.6}$$

$$k_j = \frac{[_jPA]}{[_jP][A]}$$

or

$$[_jPA] = k_j[_jP][A].$$

Considering the jth binding site, the number of moles of bound ligand is $[_jPA]$ and the protein concentration is $[_jP] + [_jPA]$. On substituting these expressions into (7.7.2),

$$
\begin{aligned}
r_j &= \frac{[_jPA]}{[_jP] + [_jPA]} \\
&= \frac{k_j[_jP][A]}{[_jP] + k_j[_jP][A]} \\
&= \frac{k_j[A]}{1 + k_j[A]}.
\end{aligned}
\tag{7.7.7}
$$

The molar binding ratio r is now found by summing r_j over all n binding sites which, because they are equivalent, have the same site equilibrium coefficient k_j:

$$
\begin{aligned}
r &= \sum_{j=1}^{n} r_j \\
&= \sum_{j=1}^{n} \frac{k_j[A]}{1 + k_j[A]} \\
&= \frac{nk_j[A]}{1 + k_j[A]}.
\end{aligned}
\tag{7.7.8}
$$

The assumption of equal affinity of all binding sites is extremely limiting and has been shown experimentally to be incorrect. For this reason it is common to modify (7.7.8) by defining m classes of binding with n_j sites in each class having the same site equilibrium coefficient k_j and here

$$
r = \sum_{j=1}^{m} \frac{n_j k_j[A]}{1 + k_j[A]},
$$

$$
n = \sum_{j=1}^{m} n_j.
\tag{7.7.9}
$$

7.7.3 Applicability of the models

The stoichiometric or step-wise model (7.7.4) is a general thermodynamic model which is always applicable to the data. The site-binding or Scatchard model (7.7.9) is only applicable when there are independent and non-interacting sites. Failure to appreciate the implications of this restriction can, and often does, result in an erroneous data analysis.

When considering a non-interacting system, (7.7.4) and (7.7.9) both define r

under the same conditions and there is a formal relationship between the sets K and k. The nature of this relationship has been established by several authors (e.g. Fletcher, Spector and Ashbrook, 1970; Klotz, 1974) by a variety of techniques.

Using the nomenclature

$$C_1 = \sum_{j_1 = 1}^{n} k_{j_1},$$

$$C_2 = \sum_{j_1 = 1}^{n-1} \sum_{j_2 = j_1 + 1}^{n} k_{j_1} k_{j_2},$$

$$C_p = \sum_{j_1 = 1}^{n-p+1} \cdots \sum_{j_p = j_{p-1} + 1}^{n} k_{j_1} k_{j_2} \ldots k_{j_p} \qquad (1 \leq p \leq n), \tag{7.7.10}$$

we have

$$K_1 = C_1,$$

$$K_{p+1} = \frac{C_{p+1}}{C_p} \qquad (p = 1, 2, \ldots, n - 1). \tag{7.7.11}$$

It can be seen that whilst the K values can be readily calculated from the k values, the reverse is not true.

We now consider the general situation with no restrictions on affinities or interactions as typified by a simple two-binding site system, illustrated in Figure 7.7.1. Scheme (a) is uniquely described by the step-wise model with two stoichiometric coefficients K_1 and K_2. Scheme (b) is more complicated in that there are four site coefficients and there are problems in describing the scheme by

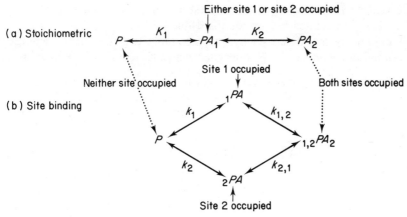

Figure 7.7.1 Stoichiometric and site-binding representations of a simple two-binding site model.

the Scatchard model. In particular, if a two-class Scatchard model is used, how are the coefficients from the scheme to be assigned to the model? If, however, the data are fitted to this model to give two arbitrary coefficients k_α and k_β these coefficients are just data-fitting coefficients which in general do not uniquely define the site-binding coefficients. This fundamental mistake of identifying the data-fitting coefficients directly with the site-binding coefficients is, unfortunately, all too common in published data.

Problems associated with uniqueness in the Scatchard model are compounded by the fact that not all the site-binding coefficients are independent.

The bound complex $_{1,2}PA_2$ can be formed either from $_1PA$ or $_2PA$ and this effectively applies a constraint on the system. We have

$$[_{1,2}PA_2] = k_{1,2}[_1PA][A] \tag{7.7.12}$$

and

$$[_{1,2}PA_2] = k_{2,1}[_2PA][A]. \tag{7.7.13}$$

Also, from (7.7.6),

$$[_1PA] = k_1[P][A],$$

$$[_2PA] = k_2[P][A]. \tag{7.7.14}$$

On substituting (7.7.14) back into (7.7.12) and (7.7.13) and equating the expressions,

$$k_1 k_{1,2} = k_2 k_{2,1}, \tag{7.7.15}$$

a constraint which must be satisfied by parameters of the system.

In general, Klotz and Hunston (1975) have shown that if there are n binding sites then there are a total of $n \times 2^{n-1}$ site-binding coefficients, of which $2^n - 1$ are independent. There are, of course, only n stoichiometric coefficients. The effect of this is best appreciated by considering Table 7.7.1.

A binding system described by four stoichiometric coefficients requires the determination of fifteen site-binding coefficients. If these K_j's are known then the

Table 7.7.1 Relationship between the number of stoichiometric and site-binding coefficients.

Stoichiometric	Site	
	Total	Independent
1	1	1
2	4	3
3	12	7
4	32	15
5	80	31

corresponding k_j's can be calculated, but the reverse is again not true. It follows from this discussion that, unless there is incontrovertible experimental evidence for non-interacting independent binding sites or only an empirical equation to describe the binding data is required (in which case a spline [see III, §6.5] or polynomial [see I, §14.1] is to be preferred), a Scatchard model analysis should be avoided.

In the ideal situation of non-interacting independent binding sites the n binding coefficients k_j of (7.7.6) can be related to a single coefficient k. Consider the simple example of three binding sites. From (7.7.10) we have

$$C_1 = k_1 + k_2 + k_3 = 3k,$$
$$C_2 = k_1 k_2 + k_1 k_3 + k_2 k_3 = 3k^2,$$
$$C_3 = k_1 k_2 k_3 = k^3,$$

and

$$K_1 = C_1 = 3k,$$
$$K_2 = \frac{C_2}{C_1} = k,$$
$$K_3 = \frac{C_3}{C_2} = \frac{k}{3}.$$

This result can be generalised to

$$K_i = \frac{(n - i + 1)k}{i}.$$

Rearranging this expression,

$$iK_i = k(n + 1) - ki, \tag{7.7.16}$$

which is linear in i. A plot of iK_i versus i has been termed an 'affinity profile' and its use will be discussed in Section 7.9.1.

7.8 ANALYSIS OF BINDING DATA

7.8.1 Graphical techniques

In most binding studies the range of $[A]$ covers several orders of magnitude and this can present problems when plotting the data—an essential precursor to the analysis.

Linear plots tend to compress data at the low concentration range of the scale, making interpretation difficult, and, for this reason, an r versus $\log [A]$ plot is to be preferred. In an ideal situation this plot will be sigmoidal in shape [see V, Chapter 3] with a plateau corresponding to occupation of all the sites and a point of inflexion at half-maximum occupation. If this plateau is not observed then any estimates of the total number binding sites n must be treated with extreme caution as long extrapolations may be involved.

Transforms are usually applied to the site-binding data and the underlying philosophy is to transform the model to produce a linear or series of linear plots. The Scatchard model for an ideal situation (7.7.8) has the form of a rectangular hyperbola [see V, §1.3.4] and there are numerous linearizing transforms available (Daniel and Wood, 1971); two widely used ones being due to Scatchard (1949),

$$\frac{r}{[A]} = kn - kr, \tag{7.8.1}$$

and Klotz (1946),

$$\frac{1}{r} = \frac{1}{nk[A]} + \frac{1}{n}. \tag{7.8.2}$$

The relevant plots are shown in Figure 7.8.1.

Unfortunately, very few real systems exhibit this ideal behaviour and the above transformations lead to non-linear plots. Although it is possible to analyse these curved plots by considering the limiting slopes and intercepts there is a folklore which interprets these values as the site-binding coefficients and number of binding sites within each class. This is incorrect, as can be seen by considering the behaviour of the models, as the variables tend to the limiting values of 0 and ∞. The relevant parameters for the general Scatchard model (7.7.9) are shown in Figure 7.8.2 (Klotz and Hunston, 1971).

The slope S as a function of r is given by [see IV, §3.1.1]

$$S = \frac{d(r/[A])}{dr} \tag{7.8.3}$$

$$= -\frac{\sum_{i=1}^{m} n_i k_i^2 /(1 + k_i[A])^2}{\sum_{i=1}^{m} n_i k_i /(1 + k_i[A])^2}, \tag{7.8.4}$$

which can also be written as

$$S = -\frac{\sum_{i=1}^{m} n_i k_i^2 /(1/[A] + k_i)^2}{\sum_{i=1}^{m} n_i k_i /(1/[A] + k_i)^2} \tag{7.8.5}$$

As $[A] \to 0$, from (7.8.4), the limiting slope is given by

$$S_1 = \lim_{A \to 0} \frac{d(r/[A])}{dr} = -\frac{n_i k_i^2}{n_i k_i}. \tag{7.8.6}$$

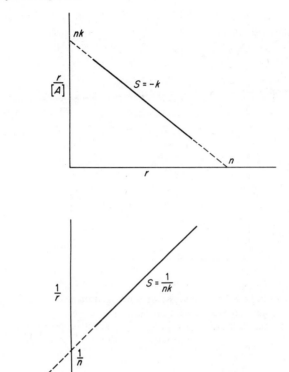

Figure 7.8.1 The Scatchard plot (7.8.1) and the Klotz plot (7.8.2) for graphical analysis of binding studies.

As $A \to \infty$, $1/[A] \to 0$ and thus, from (7.8.5), the limiting slope in the other direction is given by

$$S_2 = \lim_{A \to \infty} \frac{d(r/[A])}{dr} = -\frac{n_i}{n_i/k_i}. \tag{7.8.7}$$

Rearranging (7.7.9) in the form

$$\frac{r}{[A]} = \sum \frac{n_i k_i}{1 + k_i[A]} \tag{7.8.8}$$

as $[A] \to 0$, we define

$$I_1 = \lim_{A \to 0} \frac{r}{[A]} = \sum n_i k_i. \tag{7.8.9}$$

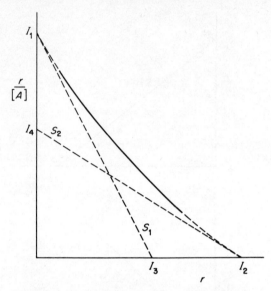

Figure 7.8.2 Analysis of binding data using the general Scatchard model (7.7.9). The meanings of the limiting slopes (S_1 and S_2) and intercepts (I_1–I_4) are discussed in the text.

Similarly, rearranging (7.7.9) as

$$r = \sum \frac{n_i k_i}{1/[A] + k_i},$$

(7.8.10)

as $A \to \infty$, $1/[A] \to 0$ and we define

$$I_2 = \lim_{A \to \infty} r = \frac{\sum n_i k_i}{\sum n_i} = \sum n_i = n.$$

(7.8.11)

By geometrical considerations it can be shown that

$$S_1 = \frac{-I_1}{I_3}$$

(7.8.12)

and

$$S_2 = \frac{-I_4}{I_2}.$$

(7.8.13)

Hence

$$I_3 = \frac{(\sum n_i k_i)^2}{\sum n_i k_i^2}$$

(7.8.14)

and

$$I_4 = \frac{(\sum n_i)^2}{\sum (n_i/k_i)}.$$ (7.8.15)

A study of these equations shows that the only parameter that can be determined directly from these limiting slopes and intercepts is the total number of binding sites $\sum n_i$, and even this may require a substantial extrapolation [see III, §2.4].

To demonstrate the implications of these limiting expressions we consider as an example a system of two independent classes of binding site with binding coefficients k_1, k_2 and numbers of sites $n_1 = n_2 = 3$. Then we have:

$$S_1 = -\frac{3k_1^2 + 3k_2^2}{3k_1 + 3k_2},$$

$$S_2 = \frac{-6}{3/k_1 + 3/k_2},$$

$$I_1 = 3k_1 + 3k_2,$$

$$I_2 = 6,$$

$$I_3 = \frac{(3k_1 + 3k_2)^2}{3k_1^2 + 3k_2^2},$$

$$I_4 = \frac{36}{3/k_1 + 3/k_2}.$$

Knowing the structure of the system, a reasonable amount of algebraic manipulation is required to recover the binding parameter from the slopes and intercepts, but if the structure is unknown—as it is in most experiments—the recovery of the parameters is extremely complicated, if not impossible.

To achieve a successful analysis of a Scatchard or similar plot it is necessary to have experimental data over a wide range of concentration of A. Unfortunately, most experiments do not provide these data and, to overcome this, Thompson and Klotz (1971) developed a double logarithmic plot of $\log r$ against $\log [A]$ to maximize the information obtainable from data over a limited range. Assuming the non-interacting equivalent site model (7.7.8) we can write the slope σ of the double logarithmic plot as

$$\sigma = \frac{d(\log r)}{d(\log [A])} = \frac{1}{1 + k[A]},$$ (7.8.16)

which has limiting values of 1, as $A \to 0$, and 0, as $A \to \infty$. If $[A_{0.5}]$, $r_{0.5}$ are the coordinates for $\sigma = 0.5$,

$$n = 0.5 r_{0.5},$$ (7.8.17)

$$k = \frac{1}{[A_{0.5}]}.$$

(7.8.18)

To obtain a better estimate of n we rearrange (7.7.8) as

$$\frac{1}{1 + k[A]} = \frac{n - r}{n}.$$

(7.8.19)

Hence, using (7.8.16),

$$\sigma = \frac{d(\log r)}{d(\log [A])} = 1 - \frac{r}{n}$$

(7.8.20)

and a plot of σ against r should be linear with an extrapolated intercept of n on the abscissa at $\sigma = 0$. Values of σ are best obtained by a numerical differentiation procedure [see III, §6.1.8], but it may be necessary to smooth the data prior to differentiation to prevent oscillations in the σ values. If the data points deviate from linearity, this may be an indication of cooperativity or non-equivalent sites. In particular, if the initial slope of the double logarithmic plot is less than unity, it is an indication of negative cooperativity and if the slope is greater than unity, the indication is positive cooperativity.

Let us now consider a situation where cooperative interactions occur to such an extent that as soon as one site is occupied the remaining $n - 1$ sites are immediately occupied. The stoichiometry of this reaction can be represented by

$$P + nA \rightleftharpoons PA_n,$$

$$K = \frac{[PA_n]}{[P][A]^n}.$$

The only species present in significant concentrations are P and PA_n and thus the step-wise model (7.7.3) reduces to

$$r = \frac{nk[A]^n}{1 + k[A]^n},$$

(7.8.21)

where k is defined by equation (7.8.16). The molar binding ratio r is related to the fraction of occupied sites, θ, by

$$r = n\theta.$$

Substituting for r in (7.8.21),

$$\frac{r}{n - r} = \frac{\theta}{1 - \theta} = k[A]^n$$

and, taking logarithms,

$$\log \frac{\theta}{1 - \theta} = \log k + n \log [A].$$

(7.8.22)

A plot of $\log[\theta/(1-\theta)]$ versus $\log[A]$ should then be linear of slope n. This is known as a *Hill plot* and has a slope of unity for independent sites and greater than unity for cooperative interactions. In general the interactions are not strong enough to fulfil the requirements of (7.8.21) and the plot is only linear over a limited range of $\log[A]$. This effect is, for example, demonstrated in the binding of oxygen to myoglobin and haemoglobin. The myoglobin plot shows independent binding, whereas the haemoglobin plot shows cooperative effects which change with concentration. Cook and Koshland (1970) have shown both Scatchard and Hill plots for the binding of nicotinamide-adenine dinucleotide to yeast glyceraldehyde 3-phosphate dehydrogenase which exhibit positive and negative cooperativity.

Although only two graphical procedures have been discussed, a large number have been published, some of which are given in the references. If the experimenter chooses to analyse the data by graphical methods, the following factors should be noted: (a) they can only cope with simple systems, (b) the interpretation of slopes and intercepts is often complicated and (c) it is difficult to discriminate between possible models. In general, the problems associated with graphical analysis are such that it should be avoided.

7.8.2 Numerical techniques

The disadvantages of graphical methods including difficulties in parameter estimation, lack of knowledge of parameter errors, problems in model discrimination and the inability to cope with interacting sites in a satisfactory manner are largely overcome by the use of computer procedures, although these do introduce problems of a different nature. A large number of such procedures have been published, most of which are based on some form of non-linear optimization to estimate the parameters which minimize the residual sum of squares (RSS) given by

$$\text{RSS} = \sum_{i=1}^{l} w_i(\hat{r}_i - r_i)^2 \tag{7.8.23}$$

where r_i is the observed molar binding ratio, $\hat{r}_i$ that predicted from the model, w_i a weighting function and l is the number of data points [see III, Chapter 11, and IV, Chapter 15]. The assumptions underlying the method are:

(a) The independent variable, $[A]$, is error-free.
(b) The errors in the dependent variable, r, follow a normal distribution; they are not auto-correlated or correlated with the independent variable.
(c) The errors are homoscedastic i.e. they have constant variance; all observations are equally liable to error.

The significance of these assumptions is discussed below.

We will first consider the analysis of the generalized site-binding model,

$$r = \sum_{j=1}^{m} \frac{n_j k_j [A]}{1 + k_j [A]},$$ (7.8.24)

for which Fletcher and Spector (1968) have published an elegant program. The object is to obtain estimates of m, n_j and k_j, together with their associated errors, which minimize RSS in (7.8.23). In this model n_j is an integer whereas k_j is real, and this combination of integer and real optimization within the same program is difficult. To overcome this they define two new variables.

$$P_j = n_j k_j,$$
$$P_{j+1} = k_j,$$ (7.8.25)

and the model is transformed to

$$\hat{r} = \sum_{j=1}^{m} \frac{P_j [A]}{1 + P_{j+1} [A]},$$ (7.8.26)

which can be satisfactorily minimized. At the minimum, the integer estimates of n_j are obtained from

$$n_j = \frac{P_j}{P_{j+1}}$$ (7.8.27)

with rounding of the result. The optimization is now repeated holding n_j as a constant in (7.7.9) and fitting the k_j only. To allow for possible errors in the rounding step (7.8.27), the optimization must be repeated for $n_j - 1$ and $n_j + 1$ to give a total of 3^m possible models which must be examined to choose the 'best' model.

No definite rules for selecting this model can be laid down but the following points of procedure should be considered with reference, for example, to one of the standard computer programs available for the tests, as discussed below:

(a) Plot the observed and predicted data and check for any deviations.
(b) Plot the residuals against both the dependent and independent variable. (The residuals should be Normally distributed.)
(c) The 'best' model should have the minimum residual sum of squares (RSS).
(d) Investigate the standard deviations of the estimates; as a 'rule of thumb', if these approach half the magnitude of the parameter then the parameter is ill-determined and should be held as a constant or the model rejected.
(e) The parameter correlation matrix should be investigated for evidence of significant correlations which may affect the result and the eigenvector decomposition of this matrix checked for indications of ill-conditioning [see III, Chapter 4].

If the choice of model is still uncertain there are a range of powerful discriminatory techniques (e.g. Atkinson, 1980) but one should bear in mind the general level of accuracy in this type of experiment.

The optimization procedure is an iterative process which requires initial estimates of parameters as starting values. These can be obtained from an initial graphical analysis as described above or from prior knowledge of the system. However, it is essential that a range of initial estimates be investigated to try to ensure that the program optimizes to a global and not a local minimum.

Fitting of the step-wise model is best accomplished by rewriting the model as

$$\hat{r} = \frac{C_1[A] + 2C_2[A]^2 + \cdots + nC_n[A]^n}{1 + C_1[A] + C_2[A]^2 + \cdots + C_n[A]^n},\tag{7.8.28}$$

where the C_n are defined by (7.7.10). Once again, a non-linear optimization procedure is used with the stoichiometric coefficients being calculated from the C_n at the minimum RSS. In this situation there is no problem with integer/real optimization, but it is advisable to use a constrained optimization technique to prevent the parameters becoming negative (the optimization algorithm does not respect the physical requirements of the system unless constrained to do so) [see IV, §15.10]. As previously indicated, estimates of stoichiometric coefficients cannot be obtained graphically and these must be obtained by first carrying out a Scatchard analysis and then using the estimates of the site-binding coefficients to calculate the C_n from (7.7.10). An example of this analysis is given by Fletcher, Spector and Ashbrook (1970) and by Cornish-Bowden and Koshland (1970).

The remaining problem is the selection of the optimization procedure to be used, and, unless the user is experienced in optimization theory, numerical analysis and programming, it is recommended that no attempt is made to write a program (Chambers, 1973). There are a large number of programs available, some of which have been described by Jennrich and Ralston (1979), together with discussion of the theory and philosophy of fitting non-linear models to experimental data. It is not yet possible to make a general stipulation as to which particular program should be used, but programs which have been shown to perform in a satisfactory manner with binding data are NONLIN (Metzler, Elfring and McEwan, 1974) and NIHH22/23 (Fletcher and Shrager, 1968), which are both modified Gauss–Newton programs and the modified Newton method due to Gill and Murray (1976) [see IV, §15.9.6]. Whichever program is chosen, it is advantageous for it to be able to cope with both constrained and unconstrained optimizations, and before attempting to analyse data it must be thoroughly tested with synthetic data to determine its characteristics such as sensitivity to initial estimates, practical rate of convergence and effect of noisy data.

We must now consider whether or not the analyses described above conform to the requirements for least squares regression [see VI, §6.5.1]; we conclude that in general they do not. The observations are generally heteroscedastic, but this can be accommodated by a suitable choice of weighting function (Ottaway, 1973). More serious is the fact that the independent variable A is not error-free (Rodbard and Hutt, 1974; Perrin, Vallner and Wold, 1974). As the latter paper points out, in a typical binding experiment the total ligand concentration C_t is accurately known, with the bound B and free ligand concentration A measured to a lower accuracy. As these concentrations are related by

$$C_t = A + B,$$

any error in A (or B) will be correlated with B (or A) and r, giving rise to biased parameter estimates. To circumvent this problem, Perrin, Vallner and Wold (1974) reformulated the regression model in terms of C_t and B, and Plumbridge, Aarons and Brown (1977) suggested that the model be expressed in terms of the actual experimental variables measured. Although the intentions of such modifications are sound it must be realized that it is not possible to measure any experimental variable in an error-free manner (the competent experimenter will of course minimize the errors and know their magnitude!) and the assumptions of least squares minimization will always be violated to some extent. Whether this will seriously bias the results is difficult to decide, but a simple test is to apply random noise to the independent variable and observe the effect on the parameter estimates.

Of interest is the question as to why least squares fitting has become the 'method of choice'. The answer is quite simple: the mathematics of the method are straightforward, its numerical properties well established and any computer centre can offer several 'off the shelf' packages which implement it. These obvious advantages lead most investigators to conveniently ignore violations of assumptions discussed above. This is not a satisfactory state of affairs, but the solution is no easy matter. The analogous problem in simple linear systems has been satisfactorily solved but the extension to non-linear systems is complicated. A possible approach, and one that should prove very useful, is to use the technique of 'robust regression' which is able to cope with noisy data and outliers. An example of a program for robust regression is given by Jennrich and Ralston (1979). Whilst these alternative methods are more complicated than the least squares method, there is no doubt that they produce more statistically satisfactory results, and any further developments in analysis of binding data should be in this area.

7.8.3 A strategem for the analysis of binding data

Although it is not possible to provide a strategem that will work for every binding analysis, the following approach, which is essentially that of Fletcher, Ashbrook and Spector (1973), has been found to be extremely successful. It is assumed that the experimenter has access to both a computer and optimization programs, as it has already been shown that a graphical analysis is extremely limited.

(a) Plot the data on single and double logarithmic axes. This will give an indication of whether or not the data range is adequate for further analysis, any outliers in the data, the total number of binding sites and whether or not cooperative effects are occurring.
(b) Fit the data to a Scatchard model. If the slope of the Scatchard plot is negative for all r then the model is applicable to the data, but it is most unlikely that the model-fitting coefficients will be the binding coefficients.
(c) Estimate the step-wise coefficients from the Scatchard coefficients.
(d) Fit the data to the step-wise model using initial estimates from (c). If (b) has failed then it may be necessary to use random initial estimates for this stage.

At all stages it is essential to check the fitting procedure carefully and not let the computer choose the best model. Remember that (a) and (b) will indicate a total of n binding sites, giving rise to n step-wise coefficients, but the data may be adequately described by less than n step-wise coefficients. An example of this is given by Fletcher, Ashbrook and Spector (1973).

At the conclusion of the analysis it is important to remember that the data can always be represented by the general step-wise model whereas the Scatchard model is subject to severe restrictions.

7.9 INTERPRETATION OF BINDING COEFFICIENTS

7.9.1 The affinity profile

A step-wise analysis allows for inter-site interactions and a site-binding analysis does not. But how are we to know from the data whether interactions are occurring or not? The Hill plot described in Section 7.8.1 may give some indication, but a more powerful technique is based on (7.7.16):

$$ik_i = k(n + 1) - ki.$$

A plot of ik_i versus i is known as an affinity profile, and for ideal binding it is linear with the intercept on the abscissa being $n + 1$. No knowledge of n is required for this plot. If, however, interactions occur then there will be deviations from linearity. To quantify these deviations in terms of positive or negative cooperativity it is necessary to define both a reference state, e.g. the binding of the first ligand, and an interaction parameter. The choice of these is beyond the scope of this chapter, and the reader should consult Klotz and Hunston (1975) for full details.

It is, however, possible to carry out a preliminary, yet informative, analysis of the profile by noting that (a) any binding step can be taken as the reference state and (b) in the absence of interactions two or more binding points will lie on the same straight line with an intercept at $n + 1$. Thus the first m occupied sites may exhibit interactions after which the sites behave independently, and the profile would show the last $n - m$ sites to fall on a straight line with reference to the nth site.

7.9.2 Drug Distribution

It is the free drug concentration in the plasma that is of clinical significance, as this is the drug that is available for distribution and elimination. Both the site-binding and step-wise coefficients contain the necessary information to compute the free drug concentration, the distribution between sites and complexes, and how this distribution changes with the total drug concentration. The solution to this problem is essentially the reverse of the parameter estimation described in Section 7.8 as we wish to find the free drug concentration A which satisfies the binding model, given the protein concentration, the total drug concentration and the binding coefficients. Techniques for computing these distributions from Scatchard (Mais *et al.*, 1974) and step-wise coefficients (Wosilait and Nagy, 1976a) are available, but we shall only discuss the latter as it is more general. It has been shown by Wosilait and Nagy (1976b) that the results from the two sets of coefficients are comparable.

Given the model of (7.7.4),

$$r = \frac{\sum_{i=1}^{n} i \left(\prod_{j=1}^{i} K_j \right) [A]^i}{1 + \sum_{i=1}^{n} \left(\prod_{j=1}^{i} K_j \right) [A]^i},$$

a linear search, using ten intervals in the range $[A] = 0$ to $[A] = C_t$, is used to find an approximate root $[A^0]$ which is then refined by a Newton–Raphson procedure [see III, §5.4.1]. Once this root has been obtained to the required accuracy, the free protein concentration P_f and concentration of drug bound in the mth complex B_m are given in terms of total protein concentration P_t by

$$[P_f] = \frac{[P_t]}{1 + \sum_{i=1}^{n} \left(\prod_{j=1}^{i} K_j \right) [A^0]^i}, \tag{7.9.1}$$

$$[B_m] = \frac{m [P_t] [A^0]^m \prod_{1}^{m} K_j}{1 + \sum_{i=1}^{n} [A^0]^i \prod_{j=1}^{i} K_j}. \tag{7.9.2}$$

This calculation is repeated for each total drug concentration to give the distribution of drug between the complexes as a function of the total drug to protein ratio. These data can then be used to study the effects of clearance on distribution and redistribution within the complexes, the significance of various complexes and, possibly more important, how the free drug and protein concentrations vary with the total drug concentration.

7.10 A WORKED EXAMPLE OF DRUG–PROTEIN BINDING

Many techniques are available to study the binding of drugs to proteins; these include dialysis, high-pressure liquid chromatograpy, fluorescence and visible spectroscopy. Dialysis is the most commonly used method but it is time-consuming. Spectroscopic techniques are quicker but suffer from the disadvantage that the probe and the drug must bind to the same site on the protein. In this worked example, we analyse data obtained using the fluorescence technique.

For the binding of a drug to a single site we can write

$$\phi = \frac{k[A]}{1 + k[A]}, \tag{7.10.1}$$

where ϕ is the fractional coverage of the binding site by the drug whose free concentration is $[A]$. If there are n independent sites, all having the same association constant k, the above equation becomes

$$r = \frac{nk[A]}{1 + k[A]}, \tag{7.10.2}$$

where r is the number of moles of drug (or probe) bound per mole of protein.

When performing binding studies the first titration should be a 'stoichiometric' titration to determine n. In this titration the protein concentration is kept high, at least ten times higher than the value of the dissociation constant of the probe for the site, and the added probe concentration should cover at least two decades of concentration. The value of n is obtained from a plot of r against $[A_0]/[P_0]$ (see Figure 7.10.1), where $[A_0]$ is the total ligand concentration and $[P_0]$ the total protein concentration at any point in the titration.

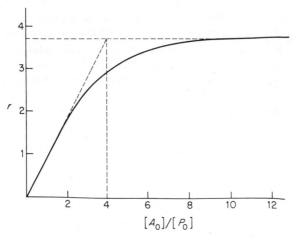

Figure 7.10.1 'Stoichiometric' plot.

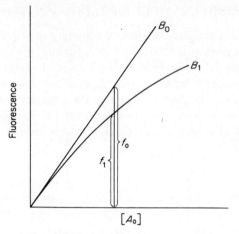

Figure 7.10.2 'Equilibrium' plot. Titration of the protein with the probe.

The next step in the procedure is to determine the association constant for the probe. In this titration the protein concentration should be similar to the dissociation constant for the probe so that there is not enough protein to bind all probe molecules and therefore measurable equilibrium concentrations $[PA]$, $[A]$ and $[P]$ exist throughout the titration. The results of such a titration are shown in Figure 7.10.2. The curve B_0 represents the titration of the protein against the probe when there is sufficient protein to bind all the probe molecules. When the protein concentration is reduced by a factor of ten, a curve similar to B_1 is obtained f_0; represents the fluorescence intensity when there is excess protein and f_1 the intensity when the protein concentration is reduced. The fraction of probe bound will be given by the ratio f_1/f_0 and the number of moles of probe bound $[PA]$ will be equal to $(f_1/f_0)[A_0]$, where A_0 is the total amount of probe added at that point in the titration. The free ligand concentration is equal to $[A] = [A_0](1 - f_1/f_0)$. A Scatchard plot of $r/[A]$ versus r will yield a value of n, the total number of binding sites, from the intercept on the x axis, and the association constant for the probe can be calculated from the slope of the curve.

The protein is then titrated with the probe in the presence of a competitor, e.g. a drug such as warfarin or tolbutamide, the protein concentration being kept the same as in titration B_1. The binding of the drug molecules to the protein will result in the displacement of the probe molecules from the protein and as a consequence the fluorescence intensity will be reduced and the titration curve B_2 will lie below the B_1 curve. This is shown in Figure 7.10.3. The concentration of the free probe in the presence of the competitor can be calculated from the equation $[A] = [A_0](1 - f_2/f_0)$. Scatchard plots for curves B_1 and B_2 should

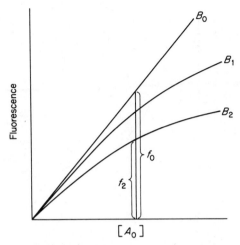

Figure 7.10.3 Titration of the protein with the probe in the presence of the competitor.

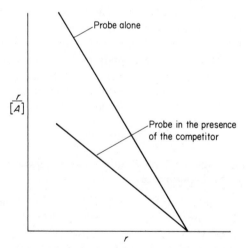

Figure 7.10.4 Scatchard plot for the probe and for the probe in the presence of the competitor.

have a common intercept on the x axis, as is shown in Figure 7.10.4. This indicates that the competitor and the probe are competing for the same sites on the protein molecule.

If the Scatchard plot is curved, as illustrated in Figure 7.10.5, it may indicate that there is more than one class of site on the protein molecule. Each class will

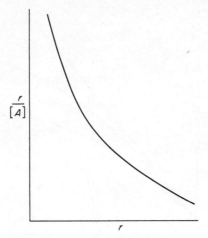

Figure 7.10.5 Curved Scatchard plot.

have its own n_i and k_i and the data are analysed using equations (7.7.9) and a non-linear least squares program.

The step-wise equilibrium model of Klotz (1953) incorporates many of the newer concepts in ligand macromolecule interactions and is the most satisfactory model for the analysis of binding data. Using the values for the Scatchard association constants obtained above (equations 7.7.9), approximate values of the step-wise coefficients can be obtained using equations (7.7.10). These approximate values are then refined using a non-linear optimization procedure [see IV, Chapter 15], the stoichiometric coefficients being calculated from the C_p values at the minimum residual sum of squares.

The binding of 1-anilino-8-naphthalene sulphonate to bovine plasma albumin and its displacement by Tolbutamide

The data given in Table 7.10.1 are the results of a fluorimetric titration experiment. In order to obtain the A_0 values, a 9.9554×10^{-5} M solution of bovine plasma albumin (BPA) was titrated against a 9.5320×10^{-4} M solution of 1-anilino-8-naphthalene sulphonate (ANS). Then 5 cm³ of the BPA solution was pipetted into a 10 cm³ beaker and this solution was fed continuously, using a peristaltic pump, to a length of quartz capillary tubing held in a position normally occupied by the 1 cm cuvette and then returned to the beaker. Additions of 30 µl of ANS were added to the beaker, and after allowing sufficient time for the solutions to mix, fluorescence readings were taken on a Perkin-Elmer LS-5 spectrometer. The first part of the curve was linear and this was extrapolated to obtain the A_0 values at the higher concentrations of ANS.

A portion of the BPA solution was diluted five times and a 5 cm³ aliquot of this

Table 7.10.1 Titration data.

ANS, μl	Fluorimeter readings		
	f_0	f_1	f_2
30	42.89	40.17	33.83
60	84.60	79.94	64.16
90	125.20	120.30	94.60
120	165.40	158.70	122.50
150	204.50	194.40	151.10
180	244.30	228.70	177.70
210	283.10	262.40	202.60
250	335.00	305.00	235.00
275	370.00	325.00	255.00
310	420.00	360.70	276.50
350	470.00	390.00	305.00
375	500.00	410.00	315.00
410	550.00	425.40	331.10
450	600.00	440.00	325.00
510	685.00	457.10	368.50

diluted solution was titrated against ANS to obtain the A_1 curve. Another portion of the original BPA solution was diluted five times and to it was added Tolbutamide such that the concentration of Tolbutamide was $5.2930 \times 10^{-4} M$. Then $5 \, cm^3$ of this solution was titrated against ANS to obtain the A_2 curve.

Using the data in Table 7.10.2 for the probe alone, a plot of $r/[A]$ against r had a slope of -3.4036×10^5 and an intercept on the x axis of 3.69, which is approximately equivalent to four binding sites. Starting values for the multi-class Scatchard NIHH computer program were therefore chosen to be three sites with an association constant of $3.404 \times 10^5 \, M^{-1}$ and one site with an association constant of $1 \times 10^4 \, M^{-1}$. The program processed the data to give the results shown in Table 7.10.3.

For this particular set of data, it would appear that the multiple Scatchard model with four sites with an association constant of 2.95×10^5 and two sites with an association constant of 3.05×10^4 best fitted the data since this particular model has the lowest sum of squares and residual mean square. Using these coefficients, approximate step-wise coefficients were calculated using equations (7.7.10) and refined using the non-linear least squares program of Fletcher, Ashbrook and Spector (1973). The step-wise coefficients $k(1)$ to $k(6)$ are shown in Table 7.10.4.

The value of the association constant for Tolbutamide can be calculated using the data for the binding of the probe in the presence of Tolbutamide and was found to be $2.65 \times 10^5 M^{-1}$.

The data analysed were taken from a student experiment. The data points were deliberately chosen so that ϕ lay between 0.1 and 0.9, thus ensuring that the

Table 7.10.2 Analysis of the titration data.

(a) Binding of the probe

ANS, μl	$[A_0], 10^{-6}M$	$[A], 10^{-6}M$	r	$r/[A], 10^6 M^{-1}$
30	5.68	0.360	0.2687	0.7462
60	11.29	0.622	0.5424	0.8719
90	16.84	0.659	0.8273	1.255
120	22.32	0.904	1.101	1.218
150	27.74	1.370	1.364	0.9957
180	33.09	2.113	1.612	0.7628
210	38.39	2.807	1.862	0.6634
250	45.35	4.061	2.177	0.5362
275	49.65	6.038	2.311	0.3827
310	55.60	7.850	2.547	0.3244
350	62.30	10.61	2.778	0.2620
375	66.44	11.96	2.942	0.2460
410	72.17	16.35	3.034	0.1855
450	78.63	20.97	3.157	0.1506
510	88.14	29.33	3.256	0.1110

(b) Binding of the probe in the presence of the competitor

ANS, μl	$[A_0], 10^{-6}M$	$[A], 10^{-6}M$	r	$r/[A], 10^6 M^{-1}$
30	5.68	1.20	0.2246	0.1887
60	11.29	2.728	0.4353	0.1596
90	16.84	4.115	0.6505	0.1581
120	22.32	5.789	0.8502	0.1469
150	27.74	7.243	1.060	0.1464
180	33.09	9.021	1.253	0.1388
210	38.39	10.92	1.438	0.1317
250	45.35	13.54	1.678	0.1239
275	49.65	15.43	1.813	0.1175
310	55.60	19.00	1.952	0.1028
350	62.30	21.87	2.173	0.0934
375	66.44	24.58	2.260	0.0919
410	72.17	28.72	2.361	0.0822
450	78.67	36.04	2.332	0.0642
510	88.14	40.73	2.625	0.0644

quantity $(A_0 - A)$ was not too small. If the number of data points was increased, particularly when ϕ exceeds 0.9, it was found that n lay between 3 and 4. The literature quotes values of 3 and 5. It was also found that the order of $k(1)$ and $k(2)$ changed in the step-wise analysis.

7.11 FURTHER APPLICATIONS

Although the expressions and techniques developed in this section have been concerned specifically with aspects of ligand–protein interactions, i.e. the evaluation of binding coefficients and the number of binding sites, they are

Table 7.10.3 Multi-class association constants.

n	k/M^{-1}	Sum of squares	Residual mean square
3	432114.2	2.4317	0.43
1	383192.0		
4	288631.0	0.6811	0.23
1	95795.7		
5	215671.6	0.5985	0.21
1	9851.2		
3	361018.0	0.6684	0.23
2	121313.0		
4	294453.0	0.4400	0.18
2	30486.1		
5	214445.4	0.5867	0.20
2	4989.5		

Table 7.10.4 Step-wise coefficients.

	Initial value	Refined value
$k(1)$	1238784.0	776519.0
$k(2)$	478661.0	1252720.0
$k(3)$	227558.2	157771.0
$k(4)$	105439.6	58144.0
$k(5)$	38887.1	41321.0
$k(6)$	12628.1	51614.0

Sum of squares   0.09708
Residual mean square   0.1

applicable to any saturable process, e.g. adsorption at an interface as described by Langmuir or Freundlich-type adsorption isotherms, enzyme-catalysed reactions and drug–receptor interactions.

Consider a simple enzyme-catalysed reaction between an enzyme E and substrate S:

$$\mathrm{E + S} \underset{k_{21}}{\overset{k_{12}}{\rightleftarrows}} \mathrm{ES} \overset{k_{23}}{\longrightarrow} \mathrm{E + products}$$

Using various assumptions, such as the steady state hypothesis, an expression for the overall rate of reaction v may be obtained in terms of the maximum rate of reaction, V, substrate concentration $[S]$ and the Michaelis–Menten coefficient K in the form

$$v = \frac{KV[S]}{1 + K[S]},$$
(7.11.1)

which has the same mathematical form as the site-binding expression (7.6.4) where we substitute symbols as shown below:

Ligand binding	Enzyme catalysed
r	v
n	V
k	K
A	S

The classical analysis of this type of expression, including the modifications for enzyme inhibition, to determine K and V has been by the use of linearizing transforms of the type described in Section 7.8, although the plots are given different names: Eadie and Hofstee for Scatchard and Lineweaver–Burke for Klotz (Piszkiewicz, 1977).

The comments of Section 7.8 concerning graphical analysis, i.e. that it should not be used for serious data analysis, are still applicable, as is the advocacy of numerical analysis. However, it is necessary to consider the numerical instability of the Michaelis–Menten type of expression, as previously mentioned and discussed in detail by Tong and Metzler (1980).

White and Neal (1976) and Neal and White (1978) have clearly demonstrated the limitations of graphical methods and the necessity for a non-linear regression analysis in their investigation of the uptake of L-glutamate in the isolated rat retina.

M.S.
R.F.

REFERENCES

Anton, A. H., and Solomons, H. M. (Eds) (1973). Drug protein binding, *Ann. N.Y. Acad. Sci.*, Suppl. 226.

Atkins, G. L. (1969). *Multicompartment Models in Biological Systems*, Science Paperbacks, Chapman and Hall, London.

Atkinson, A. C. (1980). A note on the generalized information criterion for choice of a model, *Biometrika*, **67**, 413–418.

Benet, L. Z. (1972). General treatment of linear mammillary models with elimination from any compartment as used in pharmacokinetics, *J. Pharm. Sci.*, **61**, 536–541.

Berman, M. (1963). The formulation and testing of models, *Ann. N. Y. Acad. Sci.*, **108**, 182–194.

Bloch, R., Ingram, D., Sweeney, G. D., Ahmed, K., and Dickinson, C. J. (1980a). MacDope: A simulation of drug disposition in the human body. Mathematical considerations, *J. theor. Biol.*, **87**, 211–236.

Bloch, R., Sweeney, G., Ahmed, K., Dickinson, C. J., and Ingram, D. (1980b). MacDope: A simulation of drug disposition in the human body: Applications in clinical pharmacokinetics, *Br. J. clin. Pharmac.*, **10**, 591–602.

Boxenbaum, H. G., Riegelman, S., and Elashoff, R. M. (1973). Statistical estimations in pharmacokinetics, *J. Pharmaco. Biopharm.*, **2**, 123–148.

Chambers, J. M. (1973). Fitting nonlinear models: numerical techniques, *Biometrika*, **60**, 1–13.

Chau, N. P. (1976). Area–dose relationships in nonlinear models, *J. Pharmaco. Biopharm.*, **4**, 537–551.

Chodos, D. J., and Disanto, A. R. (1973). *Basics of Bioavailability*, The Upjohn Company, Kalamazoo, Michigan.

Cook, R. A., and Koshland, D. E. (1970). Positive and negative cooperativity in yeast glyceraldehyde 3-phosphate dehydrogenase, *Biochemistry*, **9**, 3337–3342.

Cornish–Bowden, A., and Koshland, D. E. (1970). A general method for the quantitative determination of saturation curves for multisubunit proteins, *Biochemistry*, **9**, 3325–3336.

Daniel, C., and Wood, F. S. (1971). *Fitting Equations to Data*, Wiley–Interscience.

Fell, P. J., and Stevens, M. T. (1975). Pharmacokinetics–Uses and abuses. *Europ. J. Clin. Pharmacol.*, **8**, 241–248.

Fletcher, J. E., and Shrager, R. I. (1968). *Technol. Rep. No.* 1, DCRT, Bethesda, Md., NIH.

Fletcher, J. E., Spector, A. A., and Ashbrook, J. D., (1970). Analysis of macromolecule-ligand binding by determination of stepwise equilibrium constants, *Biochemistry*, **9**, 4580–4587.

Fletcher, J. E., and Spector, A. A. (1968). A procedure for computer analysis of data from macromolecule-ligand binding studies, *Comput. Biomed. Res.*, **2**, 164–175.

Fletcher, J. E., Ashbrook, J. D. and Spector, A. A. (1973). In *Drug Protein Binding*, (Eds A. H. Anton and H. M. Solomons) pp. 69–81, Ann. N.Y. Acad. Sci., Suppl. 226.

Foss, S. D. (1971). Estimates of chemical kinetic rate constants by numerical integration. *Chem. Eng. Sci.*, **26**, 485–486.

Gill, P. E., and Murray, W. (1976). Minimization of a nonlinear function subject to bounds on the variables, National Physical Laboratory *NAC Report No.* 72.

Godfrey, K. R., Jones, R. P., and Brown, R. F. (1980). Identifiable pharmacokinetic models: The role of extra inputs and measurements, *J. Pharmaco, Biopharm.*, **8**, 633–649.

Ingram, D., Dickinson, C. J., Saunders, L., Sherriff, M., Bloch, R., Sweeney, G., and Ahmed, K. (1979). Application of a pharmacokinetic simulation program in pharmacy courses, *Comput. and Educ.*, **3**, 335–345.

Jennrich, R. I., and Ralston, M. L. (1979). Fitting nonlinear models to data, *Ann. Rev. Biophys. Bioeng.*, **8**, 195–239.

Jusko, W. J. (1972). Pharmacokinetic principles in pediatric pharmacology, *Pediatric Clinics of North America*, **19**, 81–100.

Kendall, M. G., and Stuart, A. (1969, 1967, 1968). *The Advanced Theory of Statistics*, Volumes 1, 2, 3, Charles Griffin, London.

Klotz, I. M. (1946). The application of the law of mass action to binding by proteins. Interactions with calcium, *Arch. Biochem.*, **9**, 109–117.

Klotz, I. M. (1953). In *The proteins* (Eds. Neurath, H., and Bailey, K.) 1B, pp. 728–806, Academic Press, New York.

Klotz, I. M. (1974). Protein interactions with small molecules, *Accts. Chem. Res.*, **7**, 162–168.

Klotz, I. M., and Hunston, D. L. (1971). Properties of graphical representations of multiple classes of binding sites, *Biochemistry*, **10**, 3065–3069.
Klotz, I. M., and Hunston, D. L. (1975). Protein interactions with small molecules. Relationships between stoichiometric binding constants, site binding constants, and empirical binding parameters, *J. Biol. Chem.*, **25**, 3001–3009.
Mais, R. F., Keresztes-Nagy, S., Zaroslinski, J. F., and Oester, Y. T. (1974). Interpretation of protein–drug interaction through fraction bound and relative contribution of secondary sites, *J. Pharm. Sci.*, **63**, 1423–1427.
Metzler, C. M., Elfring, G. L., and McEwen, A. J. (1974). A package of computer programs for pharmacokinetic modeling, *Biometrics*, **30**, 562.
Neal, M. J., and White, R. D. (1978). Discrimination between descriptive models of L-glutamate uptake by the retina using non-linear regression analysis, *J. Physiol.*, **277**, 387–394.
Ottaway, J. H. (1973). Normalisation in the fitting of data by iterative methods. Application to tracer kinetics and enyzme kinetics, *Biochem. J.*, **134**, 729–736.
Perrin, J. H., Vallner, J. J., and Wold, S. (1974). An unbiased method for estimating binding parameters in a non-cooperative binding process, *Biochim. Biophys. Acta*, **371**, 482–490.
Pilo, A., and Mancini, P. (1970). A computer program for multiexponential fitting by the peeling method, *Comput. Biomed. Res.*, **3**, 1–14.
Piszkiewick, D. (1977). *Kinetics of Enzyme-Catalyzed Reactions*, Oxford University Press.
Plumbridge, T. W., Aarons, L. J., and Brown, J. R. (1978). Problems associated with analysis and interpretation of small molecule/macromolecule binding data, *J. Pharm. Pharmac*, **30**, 69–74.
Riegelman, S., Loo, J. C. K., and Rowland, M. (1968). Shortcomings in pharmacokinetic analysis by conceiving the body to exhibit properties of a single compartment, *J. Pharm. Sci.*, **57**, 117–123.
Riggs, D. S. (1963). *The Mathematical Approach to Physiological Problems*, The Williams and Wilkins Company, Baltimore.
Rodbard, D., and Hutt, D. M. (1974). In *Symposium on RIA and Related Procedures in Medicine*, Vol. 1, pp. 165–192, International Atomic Energy Agency, Vienna, Austria.
Rowland, M., (1980). Plasma protein binding and therapeutic drug monitoring, *Therapeutic Drug Monitoring*, **2**, 29–37.
Rowland, M., and Tozer, T. N. (1980). *Clinical Pharmacokinetics Concepts and Applications*, Lea and Febiger, Philadelphia.
Saunders, L., and Natunen, T. (1972). A statistical approach to pharmacokinetic calculations, *J. Pharm. Pharmac.*, **24**, 94P–99P.
Scatchard, G. (1949). The attractions of proteins for small molecules and ions, *Ann. N.Y. Acad. Sci.*, **51**, 660–673.
Sedman, A. J., and Wagner, J. G. (1976). *AUTOAN, A Decision Making Pharmacokinetic Computer Program*, Publication Distribution Service, Ann Arbor, Michigan.
Shampine, L. F., and Gordon, M. K. (1975). *Computer Solution of Ordinary Differential Equations. The Initial Value Problem*, W. H. Freeman, San Francisco.
Sheiner, L. B., Benet, L. Z., and Pagliaro, L. A. (1981). A standard approach to compiling clinical pharmacokinetic data, *J. Pharmaco. Biopharm.*, **9**, 59–127.
Smith, W. D., and Mohler, R. R. (1976). Necessary and sufficient conditions in the tracer determination of compartmental system order, *J. Theor. Biol.*, **57**, 1–21.
Stephenson, G. (1973). *Mathematical Methods for Science Students*, Second Edition, Longman, London.
Stround, K. A. (1973). *Laplace Transforms, Programmes and Problems*, Stanley Thornes, London.

Sullivan, T. J., and Wunderley, D. J. (1980). A package of computer programs designed to simulate pharmacokinetic monitoring of drug therapy, *Comput. Prog. Biomed.*, **12**, 85–95.

Thompson, C. J., and Klotz, I. M. (1971). Macromolecule–small molecule interactions: Analytical and graphical reexamination, *Arch. Biochem. Biophys.*, **147**, 178–185.

Tong, D. D. M., and Metzler, C. J. (1980). Mathematical properties of compartment models with Michaelis–Menten type elimination, *Math. Biosci.*, **48**, 293–306.

Wagner, J. G. (1975). *Fundamentals of Clinical Pharmacokinetics*, Drug Intelligence, Hamilton, Illinois.

Walsh, J. E. (1974). In *Software for Numerical Mathematics* (Ed. D. J. Evans), Academic Press.

Westlake, W. J. (1971). Problems associated with analysis of pharmacokinetic models, *J. Pharm. Sci.*, **60**, 882–885.

White, R. D., and Neal, M. J. (1976). The uptake of L-glutamate by the retina, *Brain Res.*, **111**, 79–93.

Wilkinson, G. R., and Shand, D. G. (1975). A physiological approach to hepatic drug clearance, *Clin. Pharmacol. Ther.*, **18**, 377–390.

Wosilait, W. D., and Nagy, P. (1976a). A method of computing drug distribution in plasma using stepwise association constants: Clofibrate acid as an illustrative example, *Comp. Prog. Biomed.*, **6**, 142–148.

Wosilait, W. D. and Nagy, P. (1976b). The distribution of halofenate in plasma: A comparative analysis using Scatchard vs. stepwise association constants, *Res. Comm. Chem. Path. and Pharmac.*, **14**, 75–81.

Mathematical Methods in Medicine
Edited by D. Ingram & R. F. Bloch
© 1984 John Wiley & Sons Ltd.

8

Tracer Techniques and Nuclear Medicine

8.1 INTRODUCTION

The use of tracer techniques has widespread application in the biological and medical field. Measurement of physiological parameters plays a crucial role in diagnostic medicine as well as in research. It is, of course, essential that such measurements are made without interfering with the normal function of the body, and tracer methods provide an ideal way of doing this.

The tracer technique is used to follow the passage of a substance, sometimes called the *tracee*, within a particular system by the addition of a small amount of *tracer*. The tracer must move within the system in a manner identical to the tracee and the amount of tracer added must be sufficiently small not to disturb the system significantly. Although the tracer must be indistinguishable from the tracee as far as the system under study is concerned, it must be identifiable in some way to the observer. Many different substances can be used as tracers in particular applications; e.g. ringed birds to study migration or coloured dye to investigate water flow in drains. In medicine chemical labelling or types of dye can be used in certain circumstances but by far the most convenient and widespread technique is the use of *radioactive isotopes* as tracers. *Diagnostic nuclear medicine* is the assessment of physiological function by the use of radioactive tracers, either by forming images showing the distribution of organ function (this aspect is dealt with in Chapter 3 of Part II) or by measuring the changing concentration of tracer (dealt with in this chapter).

Radioisotopes make ideal biological tracers because chemically they are virtually indistinguishable from the natural stable isotopes but, because of their radioactive emissions, they are easily distinguished physically, even in minute quantities (down to 10^{-15}g). Moreover, the strength of the radioactivity can be used to measure the quantity of tracer present.

The rest of this chapter will deal with some of the mathematical methods that are used in the application of the tracer technique in nuclear medicine. Examples are taken from some of the most common situations but the same methods can be extended to a wide range of investigations. Because almost all applications involve the measurement of radioactivity, Sections 8.2 and 8.3 will deal with the mathematics involved in radioactive sample-counting.

8.2 RADIOACTIVE DECAY

8.2.1 Exponential decay

Nuclear decay is a random process: if we take any individual atom we cannot predict exactly when it will disintegrate. All we can do is to say that there is a certain probability that it will disintegrate in any given time interval. If we call this probability λ (in units of, say, per second) and we take a large number of atoms, N, then the number of disintegrations that we expect will be λN. The rate of disintegration is just a measure of the stength or *activity* of the source and is measured in *becquerels* (1 Bq = 1 disintegration per second) or *curies* (1 Ci = 3.7×10^{10} disintegrations per second). Since the activity, A, is the rate of loss of atoms we can write

$$A = -\frac{dN}{dt} = \lambda N. \tag{8.2.1}$$

The solution of this differential equation is an exponential decay [see IV, §7.1]:

$$A(t) = A_0 e^{-\lambda t}, \tag{8.2.2}$$

where A_0 is the activity present at some reference time and $A(t)$ is the activity remaining after a time interval t. When t has the value $t_{1/2}$, where

$$t_{1/2} = \frac{0.693}{\lambda}, \tag{8.2.3}$$

the activity will have decayed to half its original value, so $t_{1/2}$ is called the *half-life* of the decay.

8.2.2 Parent–daughter relationship

When a radioactive atom decays it often happens that the new atom formed in the decay is also radioactive. Atoms of the original type, called the *parent*, may in fact decay to more than one different type of *daughter* atom. The *branching ratio*, f, is the fraction of the parent atoms which decays into the particular daughter in which we are interested. By extension of (8.2.1) we can write for the parent,

$$\dot{N}_p = -\lambda_p N_p, \tag{8.2.4}$$

and for the daughter,

$$\dot{N}_d = -\lambda_d N_d + f \lambda_p N_p, \tag{8.2.5}$$

where the additional term in the daughter's equation represents the number of new daughter atoms produced by decay of the parent. If we assume that initially (when $t = 0$) there are no daughter atoms present, this set of linear differential equations may be solved [see IV, §7.9] to give

$$N_p(t) = N_p(0)e^{-\lambda_p t},$$

$$N_d(t) = N_p(0)\frac{f\lambda_p}{\lambda_d - \lambda_p}\{e^{-\lambda_p t} - e^{-\lambda_d t}\}. \tag{8.2.6}$$

The activity of each radionuclide is given by

$$A_p(t) = \lambda_p N_p(t)$$

and

$$A_d(t) = \lambda_d N_d(t), \tag{8.2.7}$$

so the ratio of daughter to parent activity at any time is

$$\frac{A_d(t)}{A_p(t)} = \frac{f\lambda_d}{\lambda_d - \lambda_p}\{1 - e^{-(\lambda_d - \lambda_p)t}\}. \tag{8.2.8}$$

8.2.3 Example—The ^{99m}Tc generator

The radionuclide ^{99}Mo decays with a half-life of 67 hours to ^{99m}Tc which has a half-life of 6 hours. The branching ratio of this decay is 0.86. The process is used in the 99m-technetium generator; when saline is passed over a column containing ^{99}Mo all the ^{99m}Tc is eluted with the saline.

If a 99m-technetium generator contains 10 GBq of ^{99}Mo at the reference time: (a) What activity of ^{99}Mo is left 5 days after reference? (b) What activity of ^{99m}Tc can be eluted if the generator was last eluted 8 hours previously? (c) How much of this ^{99m}Tc is left 6 hours later and 24 hours later?

(a) For ^{99}Mo, $t_{1/2} = 67$ h and from (8.2.3)

$$\lambda_p = 0.693/t_{1/2} = 0.010 \text{ per hour.}$$

Thus at $t = 5$ days $= 120$ h, from (8.2.2)

$$^{99}\text{Mo activity} = 10 \times \exp(-0.01 \times 120)$$
$$= 3.0 \text{ GBq.}$$

(b) For ^{99m}Tc, $t_{1/2} = 6$ h and

$$\lambda_d = 0.693/t_{1/2} = 0.116 \text{ per hour.}$$

Eight hours previously ^{99m}Tc activity was zero because it was all eluted out. We use (8.2.8) to determine the ^{99m}Tc/^{99}Mo ratio for which

$$\frac{f\lambda_d}{\lambda_d - \lambda_p} = \frac{0.86 \times 0.116}{0.116 - 0.010} = 0.94,$$

$$\exp[-(0.116 - 0.010) \times 8] = 0.43.$$

Hence ^{99m}Tc/^{99}Mo $= 0.94 \times (1 - 0.43) = 0.54$, and therefore available ^{99m}Tc $= 3.0 \times 0.54$

$$= 1.6 \text{ GBq.}$$

(c) After   6 h ^{99m}Tc has decayed for 1 half-life to 0.8 GBq.
     After 12 h ^{99m}Tc has decayed for 2 half-lives to 0.4 GBq.
     After 18 h ^{99m}Tc has decayed for 3 half-lives to 0.2 GBq.
     After 24 h ^{99m}Tc has decayed for 4 half-lives to 0.1 GBq.

8.3 RADIOACTIVE SAMPLE COUNTING

8.3.1 Counting statistics

The activity of a radioactive sample is often assessed by counting the number of disintegrations detected in a given time by a suitable device. However, since radioactive decay is a random process, the count will not be exactly the same each time the measurement is repeated, even if the sample activity remains constant. The actual count obtained is due to a very large number of atoms, each with a very small probability of decaying. The total count, C, in a given time is therefore a measure of the activity, but the probability of obtaining any particular count will follow a Poisson distribution [see II, §5.4]. If a large number of separate counts were to be taken their mean, $\bar{C}$, would give the true activity but it follows from the properties of the Poisson distribution that the individual counts would be spread around the mean with a standard deviation estimated as $\sqrt{\bar{C}}$. Therefore, if we only take one count, C, it is reasonable to use this as our best estimate of the activity and assign to it a standard error [see VI, §2.1.2(c)] of $\sqrt{C}$; i.e. there is a 60 per cent probability that the 'true' count lies in the range $C \pm \sqrt{C}$ [see VI, Example 4.7.2]. The coefficient of variation, v, expresses this error as a percentage of C where

$$v = \frac{\sqrt{C}}{C} \times 100\% = \frac{100}{\sqrt{C}}\% \tag{8.3.1}$$

[see II, §9.2.6]. It is clear that the more counts that are acquired the more precise is the result, in the sense that the lower the value of v, the more precisely is C known. For example, a measurement of 100 counts would have a precision of 10 per cent whilst 10,000 counts would be required for a precision of 1 per cent.

8.3.2 Combination of counting measurements

When combining measurements representing radioactive counts the usual rules regarding combination of independent errors apply [see II, §9.2.3]. When taking the sum or the difference of two counts,

$$X = A + B \quad \text{or} \quad X = A - B,$$
$$\sigma_X^2 = \sigma_A^2 + \sigma_B^2. \tag{8.3.2}$$

When taking the product or the ratio of two counts,

$$X = AB \quad \text{or} \quad X = A/B,$$

$$\left(\frac{\sigma_X}{X}\right)^2 = \left(\frac{\sigma_A}{A}\right)^2 + \left(\frac{\sigma_B}{B}\right)^2, \tag{8.3.3}$$

approximately, where σ represents the standard error of the various quantities and the coefficients of variation of A and B are small [see VI, §2.7.1(b)]. For example, if a detector registers a count rate R_A (C_A counts in a time t_A) from a radioactive sample and a background rate R_B (C_B counts in a time t_B) when no sample is present, the count rate, R, from the sample is clearly the difference of the two rates; i.e.

$$R = R_A - R_B = \frac{C_A}{t_A} - \frac{C_B}{t_B}. \tag{8.3.4}$$

Since the error on C_A is $\sqrt{C_A}$ and the error on C_B is $\sqrt{C_B}$ (Section 8.3.1) and since also the error in the product of a constant and C is that constant times the error in C, using (8.3.2) we have

$$\sigma_R = \left(\frac{C_A}{t_A^2} + \frac{C_B}{t_B^2}\right)^{1/2} = \left(\frac{R_A}{t_A} + \frac{R_B}{t_B}\right)^{1/2} \tag{8.3.5}$$

In practice it is often convenient to make t_A and t_B equal, but if the total time available $(t_A + t_B)$ is limited, σ_R can be minimized [see IV, §5.15] by counting the sample for longer than the background such that

$$\frac{t_A}{t_B} = \left(\frac{R_A}{R_B}\right)^{1/2}. \tag{8.3.6}$$

For a product of counts, $X = C_A C_B$, on the other hand, from (8.3.3),

$$\left(\frac{\sigma_X}{X}\right)^2 = \left(\frac{\sigma_{C_A}}{C_A}\right)^2 + \left(\frac{\sigma_{C_B}}{C_B}\right)^2$$

$$= \frac{1}{C_A} + \frac{1}{C_B}$$

$$= \frac{1}{t_A R_A} + \frac{1}{t_B R_B} \tag{8.3.7}$$

If $t_A + t_B$ is held constant, σ_X will be a minimum if

$$\frac{t_A}{t_B} = \left(\frac{R_B}{R_A}\right)^{1/2} \tag{8.3.8}$$

This condition applies also to a ratio of counts.

8.3.3 Dual isotope counting

When counting samples containing more than one radionuclide it is sometimes possible to distinguish between them by their different energies and types of emission. Several counting conditions can be chosen so that each condition favours one of the nuclides in preference to the others. For example, gamma emissions of different energies may be separated by selecting two energy channels on a scintillation counter and gamma-emitting nuclides can be separated from beta emitters using two different types of counter. Although it is not usually possible to have perfect separation of the nuclides in the two counting conditions, by calibrating the apparatus it is still possible to calculate the actual activity of each nuclide.

Suppose that conditions 1 and 2 are selected to favour nuclides A and B respectively and we have available standard sources of both nuclides with known activities S_A and S_B. For standard A we obtain count rates under conditions 1 and 2 of $R_A(1)$ and $R_A(2)$ and for standard B we obtain $R_B(1)$ and $R_B(2)$. We now define the following calibration factors for the detector system:

$$\alpha = R_A(1)/S_A \qquad \text{(nuclide A sensitivity under condition 1)},$$
$$\beta = R_B(2)/S_B \qquad \text{(nuclide B sensitivity under condition 2)},$$
$$a = R_A(2)/R_A(1) \qquad \text{(nuclide A cross-talk from condition 1 to 2)}, \qquad (8.3.9)$$
$$b = R_B(1)/R_B(2) \qquad \text{(nuclide B cross-talk from condition 2 to 1)}.$$

The factors α and β are sensitivities which can be expressed in units of counts per second per becquerel (count/(sec Bq)), which is a measure of absolute efficiency since 1 Bq = 1 disintegration per second. The factors a and b are cross-talk ratios and have no units.

If we now count a mixture X containing unknown activities X_A and X_B of nuclides A and B we obtain count rates $R_X(1)$ and $R_X(2)$ in the two conditions where

$$R_X(1) = \alpha X_A + \beta b X_B,$$
$$R_X(2) = \alpha a X_A + \beta X_B. \qquad (8.3.10)$$

Solving these two simultaneous linear equations [see I, §5.7] gives

$$X_A = \frac{R_X(1) - b R_X(2)}{\alpha(1 - ab)}, \qquad (8.3.11)$$

$$X_B = \frac{R_X(2) - a R_X(1)}{\beta(1 - ab)}.$$

The significance of each term in this solution can be explained as follows. In the equation for X_A the numerator is the count rate from nuclide A in the mixture corrected for cross-talk from nuclide B. Dividing by α converts this to an activity and the factor $(1 - ab)$, which is unity unless both a and b are non-zero, allows for simultaneous cross-talk in both directions.

8.3.4 Example—Dual isotope vitamin B12 absorption test

Differential diagnosis of vitamin B12 malabsorption can be achieved using cyanocobalamin with and without the intrinsic factor, labelled with two different isotopes of cobalt (Bayley, Bell and Waters, 1971). This is the basis of the 'Dicopac' test (The Radiochemical Centre, Amersham). The patient is given an oral dose of ^{58}Co cyanocobalamin and ^{57}Co cyanocobalamin bound to the intrinsic factor. All urine is collected for the next 24 hours. The percentage of each isotope appearing in the urine will indicate whether absorption of vitamin B12 is impaired and, if so, whether this is improved by the addition of the intrinsic factor.

^{57}Co emits gamma rays of energy 122 keV whilst ^{58}Co gives gamma rays of 511 and 810 keV. Counts from the two isotopes can therefore be separated in a scintillation counter by setting the ^{57}Co channel to count gamma rays near to 122 keV and the ^{58}Co channel to count only gamma rays above 300 keV. The counter is calibrated using standard sources of ^{57}Co and ^{58}Co with known activities relative to the dose. Some sample results are as follows:

Dose administration: 20 kBq ^{57}Co

                                      30 kBq ^{58}Co

Standard sources: 0.8 kBq ^{57}Co

                                        1.2 kBq ^{58}Co

Total 24 h urine volume = 1,600 ml
Volume of urine counted = 200 ml

Sample	Counting time, sec	Counts in ^{57}Co channel	Counts in ^{58}Co channel
0.8 kBq ^{57}Co standard	300	12,172	312
1.2 kBq ^{58}Co standard	300	2,247	11,084
200 ml urine sample	300	9,752	7,392
Background	60	39	56

We use (8.3.4) and (8.3.5) to calculate the background corrected count rates and their errors:

	Rate in ^{57}Co channel, count/sec	Rate in ^{58}Co channel, count/sec
0.8 kBq ^{57}Co standard	39.9 ± 0.4	0.1 ± 0.1
1.2 kBq ^{58}Co standard	6.8 ± 0.2	36.0 ± 0.4
200 ml urine sample	31.9 ± 0.3	23.7 ± 0.3

From the standard measurements we can calculate the sensitivities and cross-talk factors using (8.3.9). The errors on the cross-talk factors are determined using (8.3.3):

$$^{57}\text{Co sensitivity} = \alpha = \frac{39.9 \pm 0.4}{0.8} = 50 \pm 0.5 \text{ count/(sec kBq)},$$

$$^{58}\text{Co sensitivity} = \beta = \frac{36.0 \pm 0.4}{1.2} = 30 \pm 0.3 \text{ count/(sec kBq)},$$

$$^{57}\text{Co cross-talk} = a = \frac{0.1 \pm 0.1}{39.9 \pm 0.4} = 0.002 \pm 0.002,$$

$$^{58}\text{Co cross-talk} = b = \frac{6.8 \pm 0.2}{36.0 \pm 0.4} = 0.19 \pm 0.006.$$

We can now use (8.3.11) to calculate the activity of the urine sample. The ^{57}Co cross-talk, a, is not significantly different from zero so we can replace the factor $(1 - ab)$ with 1 without significant error and there is no correction to make to the count rate in the ^{58}Co channel. The count rate in the ^{57}Co channel must be corrected for cross-talk from ^{58}Co, however, so the true count rates from the urine sample are

$$^{57}\text{Co} = (31.9 \pm 0.3) - (0.19 \pm 0.006)(23.7 \pm 0.3)$$
$$= (31.9 \pm 0.3) - (4.5 \pm 0.2)$$
$$= 27.4 \pm 0.4 \text{ count/sec},$$
$$^{58}\text{Co} = 23.7 \pm 0.3 \text{ count/sec},$$

where we have combined the errors according to (8.3.2) and (8.3.3). The corresponding activities in the urine sample are

$$^{57}\text{Co} = \frac{27.4 \pm 0.4}{50 \pm 0.5} = 0.55 \pm 0.01 \text{ kBq},$$

$$^{58}\text{Co} = \frac{23.7 \pm 0.3}{30 \pm 0.3} = 0.79 \pm 0.01 \text{ kBq}.$$

The urine sample constituted only 200 ml out of the 1600 ml passed so the total activity excreted in the urine in 24 hours was

$$^{57}\text{Co} = 4.4 \pm 0.1 \text{ kBq} = (22.0 \pm 0.5)\% \text{ of dose},$$
$$^{58}\text{Co} = 6.3 \pm 0.1 \text{ kBq} = (21.0 \pm 0.3)\% \text{ of dose}.$$

Note that the errors quoted on this result are those due to the random statistical error in the radioactive counting only. There may well be additional errors due to experimental technique or to biases in the method itself but these have been ignored for the purposes of this example. In practice it is not necessary to know the absolute activity of the dose or the standard, provided the dose to standard ratio is known, but activities have been assumed to be known in this example in order to illustrate the principles used. Use of the standard also obviates the necessity to apply any explicit correction for radioactive decay (see Section 8.4.1).

8.4 CURVE PROCESSING [see III, Chapter 6]

The results of tracer studies often appear in the form of serial measurements of a particular quantity taken at different times. These data can be represented by points on a graph of the measured quantity versus time. The data points may fall at equal time intervals (e.g. data from a dynamic gamma camera study) or at arbitrary times (e.g. blood samples) but in either case they form a curve, the shape of which embodies the essential results of the measurement.

Some form of processing of the curve data is often required. This may be because statistical errors on the individual data points obscure the underlying shape of the curve, in which case some form of curve-smoothing may be applied [see, for example, III, §6.5] or, if the theoretical shape of the curve is known, a least squares fit may be performed [see III, §6.1]. Sometimes when the shape of the curve can be described by a theoretical model (e.g. a compartmental model; see Section 8.5) it may be necessary to perform a fit in order to measure some parameter of the curve, such as the half-time of an exponential, in order to relate this to a value predicted by the model. Sometimes a fit is performed in order to extrapolate the data [see III, §2.4] beyond the range for which measurements were actually taken; commonly this is used to determine a hypothetical measurement at 'time zero' when this is not obtainable directly. Sometimes the data must be interpolated [see III, §2.3] in order to obtain a value of the measured quantity for times between the actual data points and then smoothing or fitting can provide a solution.

Other aspects of curve processing may also involve correction of the data for known effects such as radioactive decay and background activity as well as the correction of a measured response for the form of input applied, as in deconvolution. This section will describe some of these curve-processing techniques that are commonly employed in tracer studies.

8.4.1 Radioactive decay correction

Unless measurements representing activity of a radioactive tracer extend over a time interval very much less than the half-life of the radionuclide, it is necessary to allow for decay of the activity. This can be done in several ways.

If the measurements are activities of samples obtained at different times, then it is only necessary to save all the samples and count them at the same time so that they will have all decayed by the same factor since administration. It is often convenient to prepare a standard of the same radionuclide which is related to the patient dose by a known ratio and to count this standard along with the batch of samples. Then activity can be determined relative to the standard and no further decay correction is necessary.

When the measurements represent a variation of activity obtained in real-time (e.g. a dynamic gamma camera study) then the exponential decay formula (8.2.2) can be used to correct counts at any given time. However, in many studies the duration of the test is short compared with the half-life of the radionuclide and the correction may not be necessary.

8.4.2 Background corrections

There are three main sources of background counts in a tracer study using radionuclides. Room background is due to inevitable natural radioactivity and to system noise, and this will remain constant during a test. There is also a possibility that the patient may exhibit a significant background activity from previous tests, but this will also usually remain constant. These two sources of background may be allowed for by taking an appropriate background measurement before the test starts; then, provided the background does not swamp the actual data, it may be subtracted as a constant from all subsequent measurements.

Sometimes the test itself introduces a background of counts from activity in unwanted places and this may well vary during the test. The contribution of this source of background must then be determined for each measurement. This effect commonly occurs in dynamic gamma camera studies where curves are obtained representing counts within a defined region of interest on the images. If a suitable background region of interest is also defined, the counts in this region can be subtracted for each curve point. Unless the two regions are the same size, however, it will be necessary to scale the background counts to allow for the different sizes of the regions and then

$$C'(t) = C(t) - \frac{A_C}{A_B} B(t), \tag{8.4.1}$$

where $C(t)$ is the count from a region of size A_C, $B(t)$ the count from a background region of size A_B and $C'(t)$ is the background corrected count. The accuracy of this technique depends on the suitability of the background region chosen.

If the measurement represents counts from an external scintillation probe, contributions from unwanted tissues within the field of view are inevitable. Although the background may be sampled by another suitably placed detector the appropriate scaling factor will have to be determined by a separate calibration measurement for each test. A technique for performing direct background subtraction in this way for probe renography has been described by Britton and Brown (1971).

8.4.3 Linear least squares fit

If we make observations of a quantity, y, whose value varies with another quantity, x, then it is often desirable to determine the relationship between y and

x. In general, we can write this as

$$y = f(x), \tag{8.4.2}$$

where f is some function whose general form (e.g. linear, quadratic, exponential, etc.) may be known, or can be guessed, but where the coefficients remain to be determined. Suppose that the observations consist of a set of measurements of the dependent variable, y_i, at known values of the independent variable, x_i, for $i = 1$ to n. The values of x_i are assumed to be accurately known but we let each value of y_i be subject to a random error with standard deviation σ_i. If we plot a graph of y_i against x_i we would expect the points to be scattered randomly above and below the line given by (8.4.2). Provided the general form of $f(x)$ is known we can use the least squares principle [see VI, Example 4.5.3] to determine the most likely or 'best fit' line. The technique can be used for any form of $f(x)$ but most commonly it is applied to a linear function.

The following discussion is intended only to summarize the principal results used in the analysis of tracer measurements. (Section 1.3.13 and the core volume reference above should be consulted for a full explanation.) In the simplest case the form of $f(x)$ may be known to be a straight line passing through the origin. We therefore wish to find the value of m such that the line

$$y = mx \tag{8.4.3}$$

gives a best fit to the data. The goodness of the fit is quantified by χ^2, the weighted sum of the squared deviations of the data from the fitted line

$$\chi^2 = \sum_{i=1}^{n} \frac{(y_i - mx_i)^2}{\sigma_i^2}. \tag{8.4.4}$$

Good fits will have small χ^2 values and it can be shown by standard differential calculus [see IV, §5.6] that χ^2 is a minimum when

$$m = \frac{\sum w_i x_i y_i}{\sum w_i x_i^2}, \tag{8.4.5}$$

where the weights w_i are inversely proportional to the variance of the y_i:

$$w_i = 1/\sigma_i^2, \tag{8.4.6}$$

and the sums are taken over all measurements $i = 1$ to n. The precision of m is given by its standard error σ_m where

$$\sigma_m^2 = \frac{1}{\sum x_i^2/\sigma_i^2}. \tag{8.4.7}$$

If all the measurements have the same precision then all the σ_i are the same and equal to σ say, so (8.4.5) and (8.4.7) simplify to

$$m = \frac{\sum x_i y_i}{\sum x_i^2},$$ (8.4.8)

$$\sigma_m^2 = \frac{\sigma^2}{\sum x_i^2}.$$ (8.4.9)

In practice, σ is not actually known and in this case it can be replaced in (8.4.9) by the best estimate, s^2, given by the mean square deviation from the fit

$$s^2 = \frac{\sum (y_i - mx_i)^2}{n-1}.$$ (8.4.10)

Quite often the line to be fitted to the data need not be constrained to pass through the origin and the equation of the line is then of the form

$$y = mx + c.$$ (8.4.11)

In this case a least squares analysis shows that χ^2 is a minimum when

$$m = \frac{\sum w \sum wxy - \sum wx \sum wy}{D},$$ (8.4.12)

$$c = \frac{\sum wy \sum wx^2 - \sum wxy \sum wx}{D},$$ (8.4.13)

where

$$D = \sum w \sum wx^2 - \left(\sum wx\right)^2.$$ (8.4.14)

Here the i subscripts have been omitted but the summations are understood to take place over all the measurements. The standard errors of m and c are given by

$$\sigma_m^2 = \sum w/D,$$ (8.4.15)

$$\sigma_c^2 = \sum wx^2/D.$$ (8.4.16)

If all the measurements have the same precision, σ, then these results simplify to

$$m = \frac{n \sum xy - \sum x \sum y}{D},$$ (8.4.17)

$$c = \frac{\sum y \sum x^2 - \sum xy \sum x}{D},$$ (8.4.18)

$$D = n \sum x^2 - \left(\sum x\right)^2,$$ (8.4.19)

$$\sigma_m^2 = \frac{n\sigma^2}{D},$$ (8.4.20)

$$\sigma_c^2 = \frac{\sigma^2 \sum x^2}{D}.$$ (8.4.21)

If σ^2 is not known it may be estimated as before using the mean square deviation from the fit

$$s^2 = \frac{\sum (y - mx - c)^2}{n - 2}.$$ (8.4.22)

Although these equations may look very formidable, their form is well suited to computer calculation and indeed several modern pocket calculators have these functions built into them.

8.4.4 Least squares fit to an exponential curve

Even data which do not inherently follow a linear relationship may often be put into a form suitable for a linear least squares fit by the use of a suitable transformation such as taking the logarithm of the data, the square of the data or some other suitable function.

A common application of this technique is to carry out a fit to data which falls exponentially [see IV, §2.11] with time. If we have measurements of a variable Y at various times t we are looking for a fit of the form

$$Y = Ae^{-\lambda t}.$$ (8.4.23)

If we take the logarithm of this equation we have

$$\log_e Y = \log_e A - \lambda t,$$ (8.4.24)

so we can perform a normal linear least squares fit, (8.4.11), by putting

$$y = \log_e Y,$$ (8.4.25)

$$x = t,$$ (8.4.26)

$$m = -\lambda,$$ (8.4.27)

$$c = \log_e A.$$ (8.4.28)

Using the theory of propagation of errors [see VI, §2.7.1] the errors σ_λ, σ_A and σ_Y are related to σ_m, σ_c and σ_y by

$$\sigma_\lambda = \sigma_m,$$ (8.4.29)

$$\sigma_A = A\sigma_c \text{ (approx.)},$$ (8.4.30)

$$\sigma_Y = Y\sigma_y \text{ (approx.)}.$$ (8.4.31)

Thus by carrying out a linear fit to the logarithm of the data we can find m and c and hence λ and A using the above relationships. If all the measurements have the same precision we can, of course, use the equations for equal weights, (8.4.17) to (8.4.22), rather than equations (8.4.12) to (8.4.16).

An interesting special case arises if the variable Y represents a measurement of counts obtained in a given time from some radioactive tracer samples. In this case the standard error of Y is given by (Section 8.3.1)

$$\sigma_Y = \sqrt{Y} \text{ (approx.)}, \tag{8.4.32}$$

but the weighting factor is related to the standard error of y so, from (8.4.6), (8.4.31) and (8.4.32),

$$w = \frac{1}{\sigma_y^2} = \frac{Y^2}{\sigma_Y^2} = Y. \tag{8.4.33}$$

Thus, in this particular case the weighting factors are equal to the counts themselves. If the counts do not change very much then one might be justified in using the simplified equations for equal weights. In using an exponential, however, the counts may fall by orders of magnitude over a series of measurements and then the weighting factors of (8.4.33) are important since they discriminate against the low counts, which have relatively greater statistical error.

8.4.5 Exponential stripping

A common form of curve encountered in tracer studies is the multiexponential— a sum of several decaying exponentials with different time constants. For example, with three exponentials we have

$$Y(t) = A_1 e^{-\lambda_1 t} + A_2 e^{-\lambda_2 t} + A_3 e^{-\lambda_3 t}. \tag{8.4.34}$$

It is convenient to assume that the terms are arranged in order of decreasing time constants so that

$$\lambda_1 > \lambda_2 > \lambda_3. \tag{8.4.35}$$

When trying to fit data of this form we make use of the fact that as t increases all the terms decrease but the last one (with the smallest λ) will fall most slowly. For sufficiently large t this term will dominate and Y will fall like a simple exponential,

$$Y(\text{large } t) \approx A_3 e^{-\lambda_3 t}. \tag{8.4.36}$$

Therefore if Y is plotted on a logarithmic scale, for large t it will fall linearly (Figure 8.4.1). A straight line can be fitted to this portion of the curve either using the least squares method or by eye, and thus A_3 and λ_3 are determined. If this fit is extrapolated back to smaller times the fit value may be subtracted from all previous points to give a new set of values which contains only two exponentials,

$$Y'(t) = A_1 e^{-\lambda_1 t} + A_2 e^{-\lambda_2 t}. \tag{8.4.37}$$

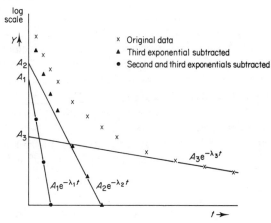

Figure 8.4.1 Exponential curve stripping.

If these points are replotted on the logarithmic scale the last few points will again appear linear because they are dominated by the second term. A fit to this linear portion will yield values of A_2 and λ_2. This fit is subtracted from the remaining points and a fit to the single exponential remaining gives A_1 and λ_1.

At each stage, when a fit has been made to the last few points of the curve it is only necessary to consider previous data points when subtracting the extrapolated fit and proceeding to the next stage. Indeed, if the fit is subtracted from the data over the range to which it was fitted, some negative values will result since some points are bound to lie below the fit due to statistical variations.

The advantage of this method of successively stripping off exponentials is that one does not need to know in advance how many exponentials there will be; one can continue stripping untill all the data points are accounted for. The technique does have some limitations, however. It will not distinguish components that have similar time constants and it will not determine the slowest time constant adequately unless measurements are continued long enough for this term to dominate over the others. At the other extreme, fast components will not be seen unless sufficient measurements are made at early times. In practice it is rarely necessary, or possible, to separate data into more than three separate components by this technique. The accuracy attainable will depend strongly on the precision with which measurements are made. An example of the application of exponential stripping is given in Section 8.5.5.

8.4.6 Curve-smoothing

When the measurement of a constant quantity is subject to random errors it is possible to improve the precision of the result by repeating the measurement several times and taking an average. When the quantity is known to be changing with time, however, this technique has to be modified. A series of measurements taken at regular intervals forms a curve showing the variation of the quantity with time [see VI, Chapter 18]. Each individual measurement is subject to random error but the precision with which the value of the quantity at any time is determined can be improved by taking a weighted average of the measurement and those immediately before and after it. A weighted average is used because neighbouring measurements are more accurately representative of the value to be determined than are more distant ones.

If we have a curve consisting of measurements (x_i, y_i) for $i = 1, 2, 3, \ldots$ at equally spaced values of x_i, then the smoothed values of y are defined by

$$y_i' = \frac{\sum_{j=-m}^{m} w_j y_{i+j}}{\sum_{j=-m}^{m} w_j}. \tag{8.4.38}$$

There are $2m + 1$ different weights in the smoothing function w_j and these must be symmetric so that

$$w_j = w_{-j}. \tag{8.4.39}$$

It is often convenient to normalize the weights so that their sum which appears in the denominator of (8.4.38) is 1.

To take a specific example, a five-point smooth ($m = 2$) with weights in the ratio 1:2:4:2:1 would put

$$y_3' = 0.1y_1 + 0.2y_2 + 0.4y_3 + 0.2y_4 + 0.1y_5$$
$$y_4' = 0.1y_2 + 0.2y_3 + 0.4y_4 + 0.2y_5 + 0.1y_6$$
$$\vdots \tag{8.4.40}$$

Notice that it is not possible to smooth the first m points or the last m points in the curve by this method.

The effect of smoothing is to filter out high frequencies (i.e. rapid changes) in the data. The smoothed curve will therefore not show such large random fluctuations as the unsmoothed curve, but any genuine rapid changes will also be reduced. The choice of suitable smoothing weights is therefore governed by the degree of noise (i.e. random statistical fluctuations) and the speed of genuine changes that might exist in the data. A high degree of smoothing (large m or nearly equal weights) will reduce random noise but will also tend to mask genuine changes in the data.

If the weights are all equal then the smooth is equivalent to carrying out a linear least squares fit to a point and its immediate neighbours and then taking the value of the fit at that point for the smoothed curve. This idea can be extended to polynomial least squares fits [see III, §6.1.3] for each group of points, and tables of corresponding weights have been compiled by Savitzky and Golay (1964). The same paper also gives sets of weights that can be used to calculate the derivatives of the data at the same time as smoothing.

Spline-fitting [see III, §6.5] is an alternative method of curve-smoothing (Reinsch, 1967). It has the advantage that even the end-points of a curve can be smoothed but it involves rather a lot of computation and this is not widely used. Another technique for reducing random fluctuations in curves is data-bounding (Diffey and Corfield, 1976). This method has the advantage that the degree of filtering applied automatically changes according to the precision of the individual data points.

8.4.7 Deconvolution

The observed response of any system to a stimulus depends not only on the properties of the system itself but also on the form of the input applied to the system. As a result of this the response $R(t)$ at time t is a particular kind of weighted average of the values taken by the input function $I(\tau)$ at times τ between 0 and t inclusive, the weights in question depending on the nature of the system. This is expressed mathematically as follows:

$$R(t) = \int_0^t I(\tau)H(t-\tau)\,d\tau \qquad (8.4.41)$$

The weight function H is called the *impulse response function* of the system. An integral of the particular form shown is called a *convolution*. The expression (8.4.41) states that the response at any time t is simply the cumulated effect of the input at all previous times, τ, modified by its passage through the system during the intervening time interval [see IV, §4.2]. This will be true provided that the system is linear (responses are additive) and stationary (does not change with time). The function $H(t)$ which describes the system behaviour is called the *impulse response function* because if the input is a true impulse or delta function, i.e.

$$I(\tau) = 0 \qquad \text{except when } \tau = 0, \qquad (8.4.42)$$

then the equation (8.4.41) reduces to

$$R(t) = H(t). \qquad (8.4.43)$$

Thus the response is obtained as the convolution of the input function and impulse response function. The converse problem, that of determining the impulse response from a knowledge of the input and the response, is the problem of *deconvolution* (see also Section 5.A.2).

The physical basis behind convolution and the reverse process of deconvolution has been described in simple terms by O'Reilly, Shields and Testa (1979). They show that if the functions are only measured at discrete times the integral in (8.4.41) is replaced with a sum [see IV, §4.1]:

$$R_i = \sum_{j=1}^{i} I_j H_{i-j+1} \Delta t \qquad (i = 1, 2, 3, \ldots), \qquad (8.4.44)$$

where I_j = system input measured at time $j\Delta t$,
         R_i = system response measured at time $i\Delta t$ and
         H_{i-j+1} = impulse response function (to be inferred from input and
         response measurements) at time $(i - j + 1)\Delta t$;

or

$$R_1 = I_1 H_1 \Delta t,$$
$$R_2 = (I_1 H_2 + I_2 H_1)\Delta t,$$
$$R_3 = (I_1 H_3 + I_2 H_2 + I_3 H_1)\Delta t$$ (8.4.45)
$$\vdots$$

Provided $I_1 \neq 0$ these can be rearranged to give

$$H_1 = \frac{1}{I_1} \frac{R_1}{\Delta t},$$

$$H_2 = \frac{1}{I_1}\left[\frac{R_2}{\Delta t} - I_2 H_1\right],$$

$$H_3 = \frac{1}{I_1}\left[\frac{R_3}{\Delta t} - (I_3 H_1 + I_2 H_2)\right]$$ (8.4.46)

$$\vdots$$

or, in general,

$$H_i = \frac{1}{I_1}\left[\frac{R_i}{\Delta t} - \sum_{j=1}^{i-1} I_{i-j+1} H_j\right] \qquad (i = 1, 2, 3, \ldots).$$ (8.4.47)

Thus if the input function and the corresponding response function are known the impulse response function can be calculated. This is the process of deconvolution. Using (8.4.46) the calculation must be done a term at a time because the value of H_1 is needed to calculate H_2, and so on. Because each value of H depends on the previous ones, any errors will propagate through the whole calculation. The technique is therefore very susceptible to random noise in the data and invariably this has to be reduced by smoothing (Section 8.4.6) before deconvolution can be applied.

The technique of discrete deconvolution using (8.4.47) is often called the matrix algorithm (Valentinuzzi and Volachec, 1975). Other deconvolution techniques using the Fourier transform [see IV, §13.2] (Niemi, 1976) or Laplace transform [see IV, §13.4] (Fleming and Goddard, 1974) are based on the continuous form of the convolution equation but they are also susceptible to noise in the data. Gamel et al. (1973) has compared the behaviour of several deconvolution methods with noisy data.

The concept of a system response in tracer studies can have two separate interpretations. If we consider the kidney, for example, the input function will be the rate of uptake of tracer from the blood, but the response can be measured either as the rate of out-flow of tracer in urine or as the amount of tracer remaining in the kidney. In renography it is the kidney contents which are considered to be the system response but in a urine sampling study the outflow rate might be a more convenient response to use.

If we consider the system contents, then (8.4.43) tells us that $H(t)$ would be the amount of tracer remaining in the kidney at a time t after a perfect bolus injection into the renal artery (if recirculation were also eliminated) and so we call this the *impulse retention function*. If we consider the outflow rate as the response, then the impulse response would correspond to the amount of tracer that takes a time t to pass through the kidney. We therefore call this the *transit time spectrum* and denote it by $h(t)$. The relationship between the two impulse response functions is simple because the rate of change of system contents is the difference between input and output rates

$$\dot{C}(t) = I(t) - O(t), \tag{8.4.48}$$

and so for the impulse input (8.4.42), when by definition the contents are $H(t)$ and the output rate is $h(t)$,

$$\dot{H}(t) = -h(t) \quad \text{except when } t = 0, \tag{8.4.49}$$

Since either content or outflow rate are valid measures of system response, (8.4.41) to (8.4.47) can be applied to either situation. If $R(t)$ represents contents then $H(t)$ is the impulse retention function. If $R(t)$ represents outflow then $H(t)$ should be replaced by $h(t)$, the transit time spectrum, in the above equations.

Figure 8.4.2 shows the shape of a typical impulse response for a system which exhibits a well-defined range of transit times between t_{min} and t_{max}. At $t = 0$ a bolus input causes $H(t)$ to rise, but then it remains constant until t_{min} as tracer traverses the system. Tracer leaves between t_{min} and t_{max} at a variable rate shown by the slope of $H(t)$ or equivalently by the magnitude of $h(t)$.

The *mean transit time* is defined by

$$\bar{t} = \frac{\int_0^\infty t h(t)\,\mathrm{d}t}{\int_0^\infty h(t)\,\mathrm{d}t} = \frac{\int_0^\infty H(t)\,\mathrm{d}t}{H(t=0)}, \tag{8.4.50}$$

and similarly the mean square transit time is calculated as

$$\overline{t^2} = \frac{\int_0^\infty t^2 h(t)\,\mathrm{d}t}{\int_0^\infty h(t)\,\mathrm{d}t} = \frac{2\int_0^\infty t H(t)\,\mathrm{d}t}{H(t=0)}, \tag{8.4.51}$$

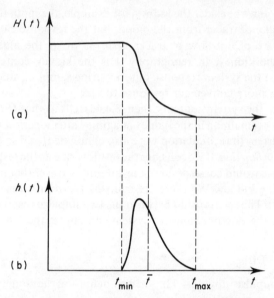

Figure 8.4.2 (a) Impulse retention function and
(b) transit time spectrum of a typical system.

using the method of integration by parts [see IV, §4.3].

A convenient measure of the range of transit times is the width of the transit time spectrum which can be quantified by σ, the root mean square deviation [see II, §9.2] from the mean transit time

$$\sigma^2 = t^2 - (\bar{t})^2. \tag{8.4.52}$$

The shape of the impulse response functions can easily be interpreted and quantified in terms of the behaviour of the system, whereas the observed response to a general input, which is a convolution of this input with the impulse response, is much harder to interpret since it depends on the input. Deconvolution of an observed response to unfold the underlying system behaviour is therefore an important technique in tracer studies whenever the input is variable or the results are to be quantified. The technique has been applied, for example, in renography (Britton and Brown, 1971; Diffey, Hall and Corfield, 1976) and in brain blood flow (Britton *et al.*, 1979).

8.4.8 Principal components analysis

If one measures a continuous variable $x(t)$ at n discrete instants, one obtains a data set $(x_1,...,x_n)$. This data set can be represented as a column vector $\mathbf{v}$ in an n-dimensional space. If one collects N such data sets, $\mathbf{x}_j(1 \leq j \leq N)$, it is possible to identify certain principal components in these [see VI, §16.3]. Section 2.2.2 gives a general introduction to this topic.

One starts with a 'training set' $\mathbf{x}_j^0$, collected under defined conditions. The derived mean set vector $\boldsymbol{\mu}$ for the training set is defined by $\boldsymbol{\mu}^0 = E(\mathbf{x}_j^0)$ the expectation value of the training set.

Next one defines the difference vectors $\mathbf{g}_j^0$ where

$$\mathbf{g}_j^0 = \mathbf{x}_j^0 - \boldsymbol{\mu}^0. \tag{8.4.53}$$

The covariance matrix [see II, §13.3.1] is then:

$$\mathbf{C}^0 = E(\mathbf{g}_j^0 \mathbf{g}_j^0) \tag{8.4.54}$$

i.e. the expectation value of the product matrix of the difference vector with its transpose (The product matrix $\mathbf{C} = \mathbf{ab}'$ of the two column vectors $\mathbf{a}$ and $\mathbf{b}$ has terms $C_{ij} = a_i b_j$). The matrix $\mathbf{C}^0$ is a symmetrical matrix with $n \times n$ elements [see I, §6.7]. It is now possible to find a transform $\mathbf{R}^0$ which diagonalizes $\mathbf{C}^0$ such that [see I, §7.4]

$$\mathbf{R}^{0'} \mathbf{C}^0 \mathbf{R}^0 = \mathrm{diag}(\lambda_1, \ldots, \lambda_n), \tag{8.4.55}$$

where $\quad \lambda_1 \geq \lambda_2 \geq \ldots \lambda_n$.

The eigenvectors of $\mathbf{C}$ constitute a new coordinate system in the n-dimensional vector space of the data sets $\mathbf{x}$. They define the principal components [see I, §7.8]. Any further data set $\mathbf{x}$ can now be decomposed into principal components of the training set by the transformation:

$$\mathbf{y} = \mathbf{R}^0(\mathbf{x} - \boldsymbol{\mu}^0). \tag{8.4.56}$$

The components of $\mathbf{y}$ indicate the content of the principal components in the new data set $\mathbf{x}$. Principal components analysis has been applied to gastric emptying curves (Barber *et al.*, 1974) and to renal studies (Schmidlin *et al.*, 1976). The same techniques can also be used to analyse static images in nuclear medicine.

It is first necessary to acquire a large set of data which contains examples of all the types of curves likely to be encountered. These curves are used as the 'training' set to calculate the eigenfunctions and then any further curves acquired can be analysed into their principal components. Sometimes it is possible to separate curves due to different clinical conditions on the basis of the values of their principal components and so the method can provide a basis for the classification of curves into clinical groups.

Although the technique of principal components analysis is quite sophisticated and necessitates a lot of computer calculation, in essence it does no more than replicate what an experienced human observer would do. Based on experience of many other similar curves (the training set) an observer extracts the features that can be recognized in a curve (principal components) and associates them with conditions that are known to normally show these features (classification). The advantage of the computer analysis is that it is reproducible and that it quantifies the result. However, it has the disadvantage that it can easily be confused by an unusual type of curve that it has not experienced in its training set, whereas a human observer is more flexible.

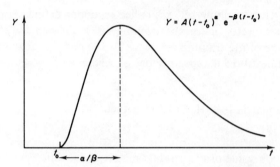

Figure 8.4.3 A function of the same form as the gamma distribution in probability theory used in fitting concentration data from tracer flow studies.

8.4.9 Gamma fit

It is common in several tracer techniques involving the rapid inflow of tracer into an organ followed by its more gradual washout to find a curve of tracer concentration against time which has the form shown in Figure 8.4.3. It is sometimes desirable to be able to fit data of this type and a function based on the form of the gamma distribution [see II, §11.3.1, IV, §10.2] can be used. This is of the form

$$Y = A(t - t_0)^\alpha e^{-\beta(t - t_0)} \qquad \text{for } t \geqq t_0. \tag{8.4.57}$$

If $\alpha > 0$ the function rises rapidly from $t = t_0$, reaching a maximum at $t = t_0 + \alpha/\beta$, and then falls asymptotically towards zero. Since t_0 is the time at which the curve first rises above zero this parameter can usually be determined by inspection of the data. The three remaining parameters α, β and A are determined by a least squares analysis.

If we take the natural logarithm of equation (8.4.57) and put

$$
\begin{aligned}
y &= \log_e Y, \\
c &= \log_e A, \\
x_1 &= \log_e(t - t_0), \\
x_2 &= t - t_0,
\end{aligned}
\tag{8.4.58}
$$

we have

$$y = c + \alpha x_1 - \beta x_2. \tag{8.4.59}$$

A fit can now be carried out using a multiple linear regression [see IV, §3.5.2] of y on the two new variables x_1 and x_2. The details are rather tedious but are readily performed by a small computer.

This procedure is sometimes known as a 'gamma-variate fit', but the measured concentration itself does not in fact have the gamma distribution as this name might seem to imply. Equally, although we are fitting a mathematical function to the concentration-time data, the term 'gamma function fit' may also mislead since the gamma function has another and rather specific connotation in mathematical analysis. A gamma fit is sometimes used in blood flow tracer studies in order to extrapolate the washout phase of the curve. This is necessary to allow for the effects of recirculation which obscure the later parts of the washout (see Figure 8.6.2). It can be shown (Davenport, 1983) that if the organ concerned behaves like a series of mixing chambers then the washout curve will indeed be of the gamma type (8.4.57). However, if the organ behaves like a single mixing chamber then compartmental analysis predicts that the washout curve will be a single exponential (see equation 8.5.6) which is the same as (8.4.57) with $\alpha = 0$.

In Section 8.6.2 an exponential fit to the downslope of the curve is used rather than a gamma fit. Unless several points on the downslope are included, the gamma fit curve will be well constrained on the upslope, but may deviate significantly from the data on the downslope. The extrapolation will thus be unreliable. If, on the other hand, there are sufficient points on the downslope to give a reliable fit in this region, then an exponential fit may be performed just as reliably.

8.5 COMPARTMENTAL ANALYSIS

The observable quantity in any tracer study in medicine is the time variation of the concentration of tracer in different organs and, in particular, biological pools such as blood or urine. However, the purpose of the study is to determine something about the transport of the tracee in the body, which is related to the particular physiological parameter under investigation, such as blood volume or renal plasma flow. Often the observable quantities can only be related to the parameters to be determined by using a suitable model of the system, and compartmental models are widely used for this purpose.

In a compartmental model the tracee is considered to be distributed through several *pools*, or *compartments*, in the body. These compartments might correspond to particular organs in the body or to some definite fluid volume distributed throughout the body, such as extracellular space, or even to a particular chemical state of the tracee, such as iodine bound in thyroid hormone. The identification of a compartment with a definable anatomical, physiological or chemical state is not always possible but this does not necessarily invalidate the model. The only essential requirement for a compartment is that it must be a space within which the tracer and tracee are perfectly mixed, so that the concentration of tracer is uniform throughout the compartment.

Flow of tracee between connected compartments is usually assumed to take place at a fixed *transport rate*, but new tracee enters in such a way that a steady state exists in which the total amount of tracee in a compartment remains constant. If tracer is initially introduced into one or more of the compartments the quantity of tracer in any compartment will change with time as it is carried around with the tracee. The number of compartments and the ways in which they are interconnected are chosen to model the system that they represent. Some examples are shown in Figure 8.5.1. A *closed system* is one that is self-contained, having only *exchange* between compartments (e.g. Figure 8.5.1b). An *open system* (e.g. Figure 8.5.1c) has *turnover* represented by '*washin*' from and *washout* to the outside world. An open system can always be thought of as an equivalent closed system, by the addition of one extra very large compartment representing the outside world (e.g. Figure 8.5.1d). If the size of this extra compartment is sufficiently large the tracer concentration in it remains negligibly low and it will act as a sink for tracer without allowing any significant quantities of tracer back into the system.

The two most important classes of compartmental systems are *catenary*, where compartments are connected in a linear array (Figure 8.5.1e), and *mamillary*,

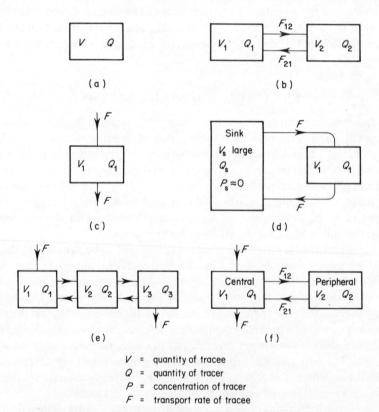

V = quantity of tracee
Q = quantity of tracer
P = concentration of tracer
F = transport rate of tracee

Figure 8.5.1 Examples of compartmental models: (a) closed single-compartment system, (b) closed two-compartment system—exchange only, (c) open single-compartment system—turnover only, (d) closed two-compartment system equivalent to (c), (e) open three-compartment catenary system and (f) open two-compartment mamillary system.

where a central compartment exchanges with one or more peripheral compartments (Figure 8.5.1f).

In this chapter we use Q to represent a quantity of tracer irrespective of whether this is measured as an activity of radioisotope, the mass of a chemical label or the optical density of a dye. We use V to represent the quantity of tracee (i.e. the size of the compartment) which, depending on the system concerned, may be measured as a volume, a mass or a number of molecules. We will refer to the ratio of tracer to tracee,

$$P = Q/V, \tag{8.5.1}$$

as the *tracer concentration*.

The theory of compartmental analysis has been analysed by Matthews (1957) and details of the use of the technique in a variety of medical applications have been given by Belcher and Vetter (1971) and Godfrey (1983). The following sections of this chapter will deal with the most commonly encountered systems and some typical applications.

8.5.1 Closed single-compartment system

The simplest of all compartmental models is a closed single compartment (Figure 8.5.1a). It is an essential requirement of any compartment that tracer concentration is uniform throughout, and in this model, since there is no outlet, the concentration also remains constant with time if no further tracer is added. If the size of the compartment (amount of tracee) is V and a quantity of tracer Q_0 is added, then the equilibrium concentration P is simply

$$P = \frac{Q_0}{V}, \tag{8.5.2}$$

whence

$$V = \frac{Q_0}{P}. \tag{8.5.3}$$

Thus the amount of tracee, V, may be found by measuring the equilibrium concentration of tracer, P, after a known amount, Q_0, is introduced into the system.

This technique is known as *dilution analysis* and is the basis of many methods for determining the size of body compartments (Haxhe, 1971). However, there are very few situations in which the compartment is truly closed (no turnover) and the method is often extended to an open system.

8.5.2 Open single-compartment system

In an open single-compartment system (Figure 8.5.1c) turnover of tracee is represented by washin of fresh tracee at a rate F with washout at the same rate, so that the total amount of tracee in the compartment, V_1, remains constant. The quantity of tracer, Q_1, and the tracer concentration, P_1, will, however, change with time. The system is equivalent to the closed two-compartment system of Figure 8.5.1(d) where the size of the sink compartment, V_s, is very large so that $P_s(=Q_s/V_s)$ is negligibly small. If a quantity of tracer Q_0 is introduced into compartment 1 the amount $Q_1(t)$ remaining after a time t will fall because it is being washed out at a rate given by

$$\dot{Q}_1 = -FP_1(t) = \frac{-FQ_1(t)}{V_1} = -k_1 Q_1(t), \tag{8.5.4}$$

where

$$k_1 = \frac{F}{V_1}. \tag{8.5.5}$$

Thus k_1 is the *fractional rate constant* for turnover, i.e. the fraction of tracee from compartment 1 that is turned over in unit time.

Equation (8.5.4) is a first-order differential equation which has the solution [see IV, §7.1]

$$Q_1(t) = Q_0 e^{-k_1 t}, \tag{8.5.6}$$

so

$$P_1(t) = \frac{Q_1(t)}{V_1} = \frac{Q_0}{V_1} e^{-k_1 t}. \tag{8.5.7}$$

Thus the concentration of tracer in compartment 1 falls exponentially with a *biological half-time*

$$t_{1/2} = \frac{0.693}{k_1}. \tag{8.5.8}$$

Clearly any tracer leaving compartment 1 ends up in the sink compartment so, since the total amount of tracer is conserved,

$$Q_1(t) + Q_s(t) = Q_0. \tag{8.5.9}$$

Using (8.5.7) and (8.5.9) we can find the compartment size V_1 where

$$V_1 = \frac{Q_1(t)}{P_1(t)} = \frac{Q_0 - Q_s(t)}{P_1(t)}, \tag{8.5.10}$$

or, in the special case when $t=0$ and all the tracer is in compartment 1,

$$V_1 = \frac{Q_0}{P_1(0)}. \tag{8.5.11}$$

The turnover rate can be found from (8.5.5) and (8.5.11):

$$F = k_1 V_1 = \frac{k_1 Q_0}{P_1(0)}. \tag{8.5.12}$$

These equations have many applications to dilution analysis as well as to turnover studies. Turnover rate is determined by taking sequential measurements of tracer concentration $P_1(t)$ and plotting these against time on log-linear graph paper. The exponential fall in $P_1(t)$ then appears as a straight line from which k_1 and $P_1(0)$ can be determined (see Section 8.4.4). This technique is the basis of most methods for the measurement of the metabolism of biologically important compounds; e.g. total water exchange (Roberts, Fisher and Allen, 1958) and iron turnover (Huff *et al.*, 1950). It can also be applied to organ blood flow measurement, such as liver blood flow, determined by the disappearance rate of colloid from blood (Vetter, 1971) and to organ function such as the glomerular filtration rate measured by clearance of EDTA (Chantler *et al.*, 1969).

In dilution analysis, (8.5.10) is often used instead of (8.5.3) for tracers which do not remain entirely in the body (see the example in Section 8.5.3).

8.5.3 Example—Exchangeable sodium determination

A single-compartment model can be used to measure the body's total exchangeable sodium pool using ^{24}Na as a tracer (Miller and Wilson, 1953). The following example is based on this method.

A dose of 2 ml and a standard of 1 ml are prepared from a stock containing approximately 0.75 MBq/ml ^{24}Na. A background blood sample is taken from the patient and then the dose is administered orally. All urine passed during the next 23 hours is collected together—this is the 'pooled urine'. At 24 hours a 'spot urine' collection is made and another heparinized blood sample is taken. Both blood samples are centrifuged and 1 ml of plasma is drawn off. Samples of 1 ml of the pooled urine and the spot urine are also drawn up. The ^{24}Na standard is diluted to 500 ml and a 1 ml sample is drawn off. All these samples are counted in a well-type scintillation counter with the electronics set to count the 1,369 keV gamma rays of ^{24}Na. A biochemical analysis of the 24-hour plasma sample and the spot urine is carried out to determine their sodium concentration.

Some sample results are as follows:

Dose/standard ratio	= 2
Standard dilution volume	= 500 ml
Pooled urine volume	= 1,625 ml
Spot urine volume	= 140 ml
Urine Na concentration	= 170 mmol/litre
Plasma Na concentration	= 143 mmol/litre
Patient's weight	= 50 kg

Sample	Counting time, sec	Counts	Count rate, count/sec	Background corrected, count/sec
1 ml sample from diluted standard	34.2	10,000	292.4	290.8
1 ml plasma sample at 24 h	418.4	10,000	23.9	22.2
1 ml of 24 h spot urine	363.6	10,000	27.5	25.9
1 ml of 0–23 h pooled urine	600.0	6,547	10.9	9.3
1 ml background plasma sample	600.0	1,016	1.7	
Room background	600.0	958	1.6	

These counts were obtained on an automatic sample counter set to terminate each measurement at 10 min or 10,000 counts, whichever occurred first. Section 8.3.1 shows that 10,000 counts gives a precision of 1 per cent and we do not wish to waste time improving on this since other errors in the test will be greater than 1 per cent anyway. Equation (8.3.6) shows that in fact we need not have counted the background samples for as long as the others, but in this situation the time saved is not worth the effort of changing the counter settings. Each measurement has been converted to a count rate and the background plasma sample rate has been subtracted from the 24-hour plasma sample rate and the room background rate subtracted from all other rates (Section 8.4.2).

We are going to use (8.5.10) for an open single-compartment model to calculate our results. Since the tracer quantities can be measured in arbitrary units, it is convenient to measure Q_0 and Q_s in units of counts per second, P_1 will then be in units of counts per second per millimole, which will give us V in millimole.

We know that the dose to standard ratio was 2 and that the standard sample was diluted by a factor of 500 before counting, so we have for the quantity of tracer administered

$$Q_0 = 290.8 \times 2 \times 500 = 291 \times 10^3 \text{ count/sec.}$$

The volume of the 0 to 23-hour pooled urine was 1,625 ml and the 23 to 24-hour spot urine was 140 ml so the quantify of tracer in the sink compartment (urine) at 24 hours is

$$Q_s(24\,h) = (9.3 \times 1,625) + (25.9 \times 140) = 19 \times 10^3 \text{ count/sec.}$$

We have two ways of measuring the tracer concentration P (ratio of tracer to tracee) because after 24 hours the ratio of ^{24}Na to stable sodium has had time to equilibrate, so both the concentration in the plasma and in the urine should be representative of the concentration within the compartment. In each case the tracer concentration is calculated by dividing the tracer count rate per litre by the sodium concentration in millimoles per litre. From the plasma sample,

$$P_1(24\,h) = 22.2 \times 1,000/143 = 155 \text{ count/(sec mmol).}$$

From the spot urine sample,

$P_1(24\,h) = 25.9 \times 1,000/170 = 152\,count/(sec\,mmol)$.

Using the mean of these two results for P_1 in (8.5.10) we have, for the exchangeable sodium space,

$$V = \frac{(291 - 19) \times 10^3}{153} = 1,780\,mmol.$$

Since the patient's weight was 50 kg,

Exchangeable sodium $= 36\,mmol/kg$.

We are careful to quote the results as exchangeable sodium because it is known that approximately 30 per cent of sodium is locked up in non-exchangeable forms (Forbes and Lewis, 1956) and hence will not contribute to the sodium space measured by this technique.

If instead of the open single-compartment model we had assumed a closed single-compartment model for this calculation we would have ignored the correction for excreted sodium and used (8.5.3) instead of (8.5.10). This would have given

$$V = \frac{291 \times 10^3}{153} = 1,900\,mmol,$$

an overestimate of 7 per cent.

Note that at no point in the calculation did we need to know the absolute tracer activity in meqabecquerels. This is because we made use of the diluted standard sample which was counted in the same apparatus and in the same arbitrary units as the other samples. Because the dose to standard ratio and the standard sample dilution factor are known the administered dose can be related to these same units.

8.5.4 Open two-compartment mamillary system

An open two-compartment mamillary system is shown in Figure 8.5.1(f). Turnover of tracee takes place through compartment 1 at a rate F and exchange between compartments 1 and 2 occurs at rates F_{12} and F_{21} as shown. The sizes of the compartments are V_1 and V_2. The quantities of the tracer in each compartment are Q_1 and Q_2 and initially all the tracer is assumed to be in the central compartment, so

$$Q_1(0) = Q_0 \qquad (8.5.13)$$

and

$$Q_2(0) = 0.$$

Now Q_1 will start to fall as tracer is washed out at a rate FP_1 and transferred to the peripheral compartment at a rate $F_{12}P_1$. However, as Q_2 begins to rise tracer begins to return to the central compartment at a rate $F_{21}P_2$. We can therefore write the rate of loss of tracer from each compartment as

$$\dot{Q}_1 = -FP_1(t) - F_{12}P_1(t) + F_{21}P_2(t),$$
$$\dot{Q}_2 = F_{12}P_1(t) - F_{21}P_2(t). \tag{8.5.14}$$

If we now define rate constants

$$k = F/V_1,$$
$$k_{12} = F_{12}/V_1, \tag{8.5.15}$$
$$k_{21} = F_{21}/V_2,$$

we can rewrite equations (8.5.14) as

$$\dot{Q}_1 = -(k + k_{12})Q_1(t) + k_{21}Q_2(t),$$
$$\dot{Q}_2 = k_{12}Q_1(t) - k_{21}Q_2(t). \tag{8.5.16}$$

This description follows exactly the same form as that for the modelling of intravenous bolus injection of drug considered in Section 7.2.2. The emphasis here is on the use of the two-compartment model to describe clearance of injected tracer substances and obtain indirect measurements of physiological function, as in the example in the next section.

The most general form of the solution to these simultaneous differential equations which is consistent with the initial conditions (8.5.13) is of the form (see Section 7.2 of Chapter 7):

$$Q_1(t) = \frac{Q_0}{A_1 + A_2}(A_1 e^{-\lambda_1 t} + A_2 e^{-\lambda_2 t}),$$

$$Q_2(t) = \frac{Q_0}{A_1 + A_2}(A_3 e^{-\lambda_1 t} - A_3 e^{-\lambda_2 t}), \tag{8.5.17}$$

[see IV, §7.9], so

$$P_1(t) = \frac{Q_0}{V_1(A_1 + A_2)}(A_1 e^{-\lambda_1 t} + A_2 e^{-\lambda_2 t}). \tag{8.5.18}$$

It is interesting to compare this bi-exponential solution of the two-compartment model with the single exponential of the single-compartment model (8.5.7) and the constant solution for the closed single compartment (8.5.2).

When $t = 0$ we have, from (8.5.18),

$$V_1 = \frac{Q_0}{P_1(0)}. \tag{8.5.19}$$

By substituting (8.5.17) into (8.5.16) we can show that

$$k = \frac{\lambda_1 \lambda_2 (A_1 + A_2)}{A_1 \lambda_2 + A_2 \lambda_1}, \tag{8.5.20}$$

$$k_{12} = \frac{A_1 A_2 (\lambda_1 - \lambda_2)^2}{(A_1 \lambda_2 + A_2 \lambda_1)(A_1 + A_2)},$$ (8.5.21)

$$k_{21} = \frac{A_1 \lambda_2 + A_2 \lambda_1}{A_1 + A_2},$$ (8.5.22)

so all three rate constants are determined if A_1, A_2, λ_1 and λ_2 are measured. These can be found by measuring P_1 as a function of time and fitting the data to a bi-exponential, as illustrated in the following example.

8.5.5 Example—Effective renal plasma flow (ERPF) determination

An open two-compartment mamillary system is the basis of a method for measuring effective renal plasma flow (ERPF) by the clearance of ^{131}I-labelled hippuran (Tauxe, Burbank and Maher, 1964). The following example is based on this method.

A dose and a standard, each of approximately 1 MBq of ^{131}I hippuran, are prepared from the same stock solution. The dose to standard ratio is determined by weighing. A background blood sample is taken from the patient and then the dose is injected intravenously. Blood samples are taken after 5, 15, 25, 35, 45 and 55 minutes. All blood samples are centrifuged and 2 ml samples of plasma are drawn off. The ^{131}I standard is diluted to 1 litre and a 2 ml sample is drawn off. All these samples are counted in a well-type scintillation counter set to count the 364 keV gamma rays of [131]I.

Some sample results are as follows:

Weight of dose	= 0.570 g
Weight of standard	= 0.629 g
Dose to standard ratio	= 0.91
Standard dilution volume	= 1,000 ml

Sample	Counting time, sec	Counts	Count Rate, count/sec	Background corrected, count/sec
2 ml sample from diluted standard	9.9	10,000	1,010	1,009
2 ml plasma sample at 5 min	128.2	10,000	78.0	77.1
2 ml plasma sample at 15 min	223.5	10,000	44.7	43.8
2 ml plasma sample at 25 min	315.8	10,000	31.7	30.8
2 ml plasma sample at 35 min	411.2	10,000	24.3	23.4
2 ml plasma sample at 45 min	502.6	10,000	19.9	19.0
2 ml plasma sample at 55 min	600.0	9,869	16.4	15.5
2 ml background plasma sample	600.0	556	0.9	
Room background	600.0	561	0.9	

The background corrected count rates from the 5 to 55 minute plasma samples are plotted on a logarithmic scale as a function of time and fitted to a sum of two exponentials by stripping (Section 8.4.5). Figure 8.5.2 shows the data with a straight line drawn through the last three points by eye. The value of A_2 is read off as the intercept of this line and λ_2 calculated from its logarithmic slope:

$$\lambda = \frac{\log_e Y_A - \log_e Y_B}{t_B - t_A}, \tag{8.5.23}$$

where (t_A, Y_A) and (t_B, Y_B) are any two convenient points on the line. The corresponding values of the fitted line are subtracted from the first three points and the result replotted. A fit to these new points gives A_1 and λ_1.

The results of the fit are

$$A_1 = 66 \text{ count/sec}, \qquad \lambda_1 = 0.14 \text{ per min},$$
$$A_2 = 48 \text{ count/sec}, \qquad \lambda_2 = 0.021 \text{ per min}.$$

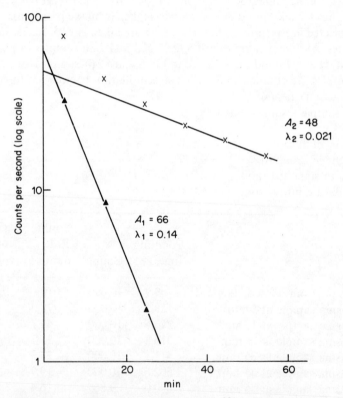

Figure 8.5.2 ERPF determination using ^{131}I hippuran. Count rate from 2 ml plasma sample versus time since injection.

Using (8.5.20) this gives a turnover rate constant of

$$k = 0.041 \text{ per min.}$$

Using the same approach as in Example 8.5.3 we measure Q_0 in units of counts per second and P_1 in units of counts per second per millilitre, which will give us V in millilitres:

$$Q_0 = 1,009 \times 0.91 \times 1,000/2 = 459 \times 10^3 \text{ count/sec.}$$

If the fits to the data are extrapolated to time zero we see that a 2 ml plasma sample would have given $(A_1 + A_2)$ counts per second so

$$P_1(0) = \frac{66 + 48}{2} = 57 \text{ count/(sec ml).}$$

The volume of the hippuran space is given by (8.5.19)

$$V_1 = 459 \times 10^3/57 = 8.05 \times 10^3 \text{ ml,}$$

so from (8.5.15)

$$\text{ERPF} = kV_1 = 330 \text{ ml/min.}$$

8.6 BLOOD FLOW

8.6.1 Mean transit time

In general, when blood flows through an organ there are many possible circulatory pathways from input to output and so individual blood cells will exhibit a range of transit times. However, the *mean transit time* of a system has already been defined by (8.4.50) in terms of the impulse response function. We can use this definition to measure mean transit time.

If we inject a bolus of tracer to the arterial input of an organ then the concentration appearing at the venous output, $P_V(t)$, will reflect the spectrum of transit times and so the mean transit time through the organ is given by

$$\bar{t} = \frac{\displaystyle\int_0^\infty t P_V(t)\,dt}{\displaystyle\int_0^\infty P_V(t)\,dt}. \tag{8.6.1}$$

This result assumes that there is no recirculation of tracer from output back to input, although in practice recirculation will usually occur. In the absence of recirculation the curve of $P_V(t)$ will follow the shape of $h(t)$ shown in Figure 8.4.2(b), but the effect of recirculation will be to prevent the downslope of the curve from falling to zero. The curve can therefore be corrected for recirculation effects by extrapolating the initial downslope on the assumption that it is falling

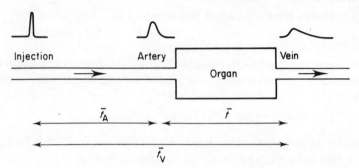

Figure 8.6.1 Mean transit time through an organ may be determined
as the difference in mean transit times to vein and artery.

exponentially (see the example in Section 8.6.3). After making this correction
(8.6.1) is simple to apply because $P_V(t)$ appears in both the numerator and
denominator and so can be measured in any convenient units since these will
cancel out. If a radioactive tracer is used, the count rate from blood leaving the
organ can be used instead of P_V and in some cases it is possible to measure this
non-invasively with an external detector.

An important property of mean transit times is that they are additive for
systems connected in series. For example, in Figure 8.6.1, if blood flows from the
injection site to the arterial input of an organ with a mean transit time $\bar{t}_A$ and from
the injection site to the venous output with a mean transit time $\bar{t}_V$ then the mean
transit time through the organ will be

$$\bar{t} = \bar{t}_V - \bar{t}_A. \tag{8.6.2}$$

This relationship obviates the necessity for a direct intra-arterial injection when
measuring mean transit time. In fact, when a difference of mean transit times is
calculated in this way, any error introduced due to not having a perfect bolus at
the injection site cancels out. It is easier to make the measurements if the injection
is made as rapidly as possible, however, due to the need to correct for
recirculation. An injection into a peripheral vein can be used and $\bar{t}_A$ and $\bar{t}_V$
measured by monitoring the arterial and venous count rates and applying (8.6.1)
to each. Then (8.6.2) gives the mean transit time through the organ.

An alternative method of determining the mean transit time is to measure the
tracer remaining in the organ, $Q(t)$. Following an intra-arterial bolus input this
would give the impulse retention function and so, from (8.4.50),

$$\bar{t} = \frac{\displaystyle\int_0^\infty Q(t)\,dt}{Q_0}. \tag{8.6.3}$$

It turns out that this result remains true even if the input is not a bolus,
provided that Q_0 is the total tracer entering the organ. This may be less than the

total injected if an intravenous injection is used. For a radioactive tracer a count rate proportional to $Q(t)$ is easily measured with an external counter or a gamma camera, but it is not always easy to determine Q_0 accurately in the same units. If the duration of the input is short enough for it to be over before any tracer has had time to leave the organ, then the peak value of $Q(t)$ will be a measure of Q_0. However, this condition cannot always be relied on when an intravenous injection is used.

The impulse retention function can, in principle, be calculated even if an intravenous injection is used by performing a deconvolution of the observed $Q(t)$ with the input function (Section 8.4.7). This requires that the input activity be monitored. It is sometimes possible to do this with a gamma camera and computer system by taking a region of interest over the aorta or the major artery supplying the organ. However, it is not easy to obtain data of sufficient quality to carry out deconvolution reliably.

It can be shown (Meier and Zierler, 1954) that the mean transit time through a system is related to the flow rate of the tracee by

$$F = \frac{V}{\bar{t}}, \tag{8.6.4}$$

where V is the volume of distribution of the tracer within the system. This fundamental relationship is very important in blood flow studies because it is not dependent on any preconceived model of the system. In fact, the reciprocal of the mean transit time of an intravascular tracer through an organ is a measure of the flow per unit vascular volume because, from (8.6.4),

$$\frac{1}{\bar{t}} = \frac{F}{V}. \tag{8.6.5}$$

The usefulness of mean transit time as an index of flow depends on the constancy of V. In comparing different patients, and even between repeat studies on one patient, there is no guarantee that the vascular volume will remain constant. An increase in mean transit time can be due either to a decrease in flow or an increase in volume or some combination of both. Nevertheless, mean transit time is a widely used parameter because it is easier to measure non-invasively than absolute flow since it requires no volume determination.

8.6.2 Cardiac output

Cardiac output can be determined by the intravenous injection of a non-diffusable (intravascular) tracer and measurements of the appearance of the tracer at some part of the circulatory system after passage through the heart. If measurements are made at a site which receives a fraction α of the cardiac output, CO, and in a short time, δt, an amount of tracer, δQ, passes in a volume δV, then

$$\delta Q = P(t)\delta V = \alpha CO\, P(t)\delta t, \tag{8.6.6}$$

where $P(t)$ is the tracer concentration. If we add up all such amounts of tracer we expect the total to be αQ_0, where Q_0 is the injected dose. Thus,

$$\alpha Q_0 = \alpha \text{CO} \int_0^\infty P(t)\,dt \qquad (8.6.7)$$

or

$$\text{CO} = \frac{Q_0}{\displaystyle\int_0^\infty P(t)\,dt}. \qquad (8.6.8)$$

This is the *Stewart–Hamilton equation* (Stewart, 1897). The only requirements that must be satisfied for it to be applicable to cardiac output measurement are that the tracer should be well mixed in the heart so that it is distributed to all organs in proportion to their blood flow, that no tracer is lost from the circulation and that there is no recirculation of tracer. In practice recirculation will occur but it can be allowed for in the same manner as already described for mean transit time measurements.

Use of (8.6.8) would require continuous blood sampling in order to determine the tracer concentration $P(t)$. However, if we use a radioactive tracer we can instead measure count rate $C(t)$ which remains proportional to $P(t)$ at all times. Since we are using an intravascular tracer it will eventually reach equilibrium and we have

$$\frac{C(t)}{P(t)} = \frac{C(\text{Eq})}{P(\text{Eq})}, \qquad (8.6.9)$$

and therefore

$$\text{CO} = \frac{Q_0}{P(\text{Eq})} \times \frac{C(\text{Eq})}{\displaystyle\int_0^\infty C(t)\,dt}. \qquad (8.6.10)$$

Here $P(\text{Eq})$ is the equilibrium tracer concentration determined from a single blood sample and $C(t)$ and $C(\text{Eq})$ are count rates determined with an external scintillation probe or a gamma camera. Now, from (8.5.3) we can identify the factor $Q_0/P(\text{Eq})$ in (8.6.10) with the volume of distribution of the tracer, in this case total blood volume. The remaining factor is sometimes referred to as the *circulation index*. It represents the fraction of the blood volume pumped through the heart in unit time. We therefore write

$$\text{Circulation index} = \frac{C(\text{Eq})}{\displaystyle\int_0^\infty C(t)\,dt}, \qquad (8.6.11)$$

$$\text{Cardiac output} = \text{total blood volume} \times \text{circulation index}. \qquad (8.6.12)$$

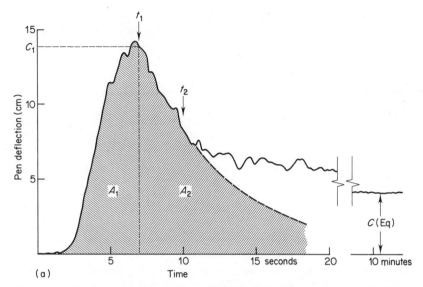

Figure 8.6.2(a) Chest recorder tracing of a first circulation curve from the head: vertical scale, $1\,cm = 100$ count/sec; horizontal scale, $1\,cm = 1$ sec.

The integral in the denominator of (8.6.11) is just the area under the first circulation part of the count rate curve [see IV, §4.1]. This is determined as the sum of two areas A_1 and A_2 (Figure 8.6.2a). A_1 is measured as the area under the curve up to time t_1 when the downslope starts. A_2 is the area under the exponential which may be shown to be

$$A_2 = 1.44C_1t_{1/2} \qquad (8.6.13)$$

[see IV, §§2.11 and 4.2], where $t_{1/2}$ is the half-time of the exponential obtained by fitting the downslope of the curve between t_1 and t_2.

The measurements can be taken over any part of the body with a good vascular supply, not necessarily the heart itself, and the head is often used for this purpose. Because all the injected tracer passes first through the heart it is the total cardiac output that is determined, not just blood flow to the measurement site.

8.6.3 Example—Blood volume and cardiac output measurement

Blood volume and cardiac output can both be measured using a single injection of ^{99m}Tc-labelled human serum albumin (HSA). A dose and a standard each of approximately 20 MBq are prepared and calibrated by weighing. A scintillation counter connected to a ratemeter and chart recorder is placed against the patient's head and the dose is injected intravenously as a bolus. Figure 8.6.2(a) shows the tracing obtained from a patient in chronic renal failure and with an arterio-venous fistula created for dialysis. The ratemeter time constant was 0.3 sec

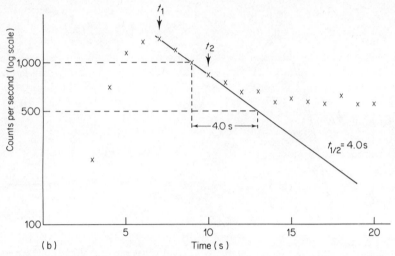

Figure 8.6.2(b) Data of Figure 8.6.2(a) replotted on a logarithmic scale with an
exponential fit to the downslope.

and the chart speed 1 cm/sec. After the first circulation had passed the time
constant was increased to 10 sec and the chart speed slowed down, but the
recording was continued until, after about 10 min, an equilibrium count rate was
reached. At this time a blood sample was taken and a 2 ml sample of plasma
prepared. The standard of ^{99m}Tc was diluted to 1 litre and a 2 ml sample was
drawn off. This standard sample and the plasma sample were then kept for 24
hours so that the activity had decayed to a low enough value to be counted in a
well-type scintillation counter without errors due to dead-time. Results obtained
were as follows:

Weight of dose injected   = 0.568 g
Weight of standard used = 0.647 g
Therefore,
Dose to standard ratio   = 0.88.

Standard diluted in 1000 ml
2 ml standard sample count rate = 1,554.8 count/sec
2 ml plasma sample count rate   = 456.6 count/sec

The standard sample represents 1/500 of the total standard and the dose to
standard ratio was 0.88, so if all the dose had been counted we would have

$$Q_0 = 0.88 \times 1,554.8 \times 500$$

$$= 6.84 \times 10^5 \text{ count/sec.}$$

The plasma concentration of the tracer is measured as the count rate per millilitre:

$$P = 456.6/2 = 228.3 \,\text{count}/(\text{sec ml}).$$

The volume of distribution of the tracer is calculated by dilution analysis using (8.5.3). Since the tracer is HSA we assume that its volume of distribution is equivalent to plasma volume. Therefore,

$$\text{Plasma volume} = \frac{6.84 \times 10^5}{228.3} = 3,000 \,\text{ml}.$$

The patient's haematocrit was determined as 34 per cent, so the total blood volume is

$$\text{Blood volume} = 3,000 \times \frac{100}{100 - 13.4} = 3,460 \,\text{ml}.$$

The circulation index is calculated from the head curve using (8.6.11). It is convenient to measure C in centimetres directly from the chart recorder tracing so

$$C(\text{Eq}) = 4.1 \,\text{cm}.$$

The area under the curve up to 7 sec is determined by counting squares and, noting that on the horizontal axis $1 \,\text{cm} = 1 \,\text{sec}$,

$$A_1 = 41.4 \,\text{cm sec}.$$

When the curve is replotted on a logarithmic scale (Figure 8.6.2b) the downslope between 7 and 10 sec is seen to be falling exponentially and is easily fitted by drawing a straight line on this graph. The half-time of the exponential is read directly from the graph as 4.0 sec because the line falls from 1,000 to 500 count/sec in this time. The height of the curve at 7 sec is 13.8 cm and the area under the exponential is found, using (8.6.13), to be

$$A_2 = 1.44 \times 13.8 \times 4.0 = 79.5 \,\text{cm sec}.$$

From (8.6.11) and (8.6.12),

$$\text{Circulation index} = \frac{4.1}{41.4 + 79.5} = 0.034/\text{sec} = 2.04/\text{min}$$

$$\text{Cardiac output} = 3,460 \times 2.04 = 7,060 \,\text{ml}/\text{min}.$$

8.6.4 Organ blood flow

The blood flow to an individual organ can be determined by a tracer dilution technique in a similar manner to cardiac output. If a non-diffusable tracer is injected into the arterial blood supply to the organ and its concentration, $P_V(t)$, is measured in the venous return from the organ, the blood flow, F, is given by the

Stewart–Hamilton equation (8.6.8) as

$$F = \frac{Q_0}{\displaystyle\int_0^\infty P_V(t)\,dt}.$$

(8.6.14)

The venous concentration–time curve must be corrected for recirculating tracer as for the cardiac output method. Although the equation used is the same as that applied to cardiac output it yields organ blood flow because all the injected tracer must pass through the organ. This necessitates catheterization for direct intra-arterial injection. Venous catheterization is also necessary to measure P_V.

A more convenient way to determine organ blood flow is to utilize a tracer which accumulates in the organ. The rate of clearance of tracer from the blood and the rate of uptake in the organ can then be used to measure blood flow.

The classic equation for determining blood flow is based on the *Fick principle*, which states that the rate of accumulation of tracer in an organ is the difference between its input and output rate. If the tracer enters and leaves only via the blood then its input rate is FP_A and its output rate is FP_V, where P_A and P_V are tracer concentrations in the artery and vein respectively. Therefore, if $Q(\tau)$ is the quantity of tracer in the organ at a time τ,

$$\dot{Q}(\tau) = FP_A(\tau) - FP_V(\tau).$$

(8.6.15)

If there is no tracer in the organ initially, we can integrate this equation for all times up to some time t [see IV, §7.2], giving

$$F = \frac{Q(t)}{\displaystyle\int_0^t [P_A(\tau) - P_V(\tau)]\,d\tau}.$$

(8.6.16)

The Fick principle can be applied to blood flow measurement in several ways. For example, if an organ actively removes a particular tracer from the blood then we can define its *extraction ratio*, E, by

$$E = \frac{P_A - P_V}{P_A}$$

(8.6.17)

and rewrite (8.6.16) as

$$EF = \frac{Q(t)}{\displaystyle\int_0^t P_A(\tau)\,d\tau}.$$

(8.6.18)

The product of the extraction ratio and blood flow (EF) can be thought of as an effective flow and if E is close to unity tracer clearance rates calculated in this way are often quoted as being measurements of blood flow, although this is only strictly true if the extraction ratio remains constant. In a disease state the effective flow may fall either because of a reduction in blood flow or because of a decrease in the extraction ratio. However, effective flow is a useful clinical parameter and

(8.6.18) is the basis of several methods for the measurement of effective renal plasma flow and glomerular filtration rate (Cohen, 1974). $Q(t)$ can be determined from the amount of tracer appearing in the urine and P_A approximated by sampling from a peripheral vein.

Blood flow to an organ, such as the brain, which does not actively concentrate any particular tracer, can be determined using the passive equilibration of an inert tracer which will easily diffuse from blood to tissue. We define the *partition coefficient*, s, for such a tracer to be the ratio of the quantity of tracer per gram of tissue to the quantity per millilitre of blood when at equilibrium. Thus, if Q is the quantity of tracer in the organ tissue, M is the mass of the organ and P the tracer concentration in blood, then

$$s = \frac{Q}{MP} \qquad\qquad (8.6.19)$$

or

$$s = \frac{V}{M}, \qquad\qquad (8.6.20)$$

because Q/P gives the volume of distribution, V, of the tracer within the organ, (8.5.3). If we assume that the tracer diffuses rapidly enough to equilibrate between blood and tissue during its passage through the organ, we can apply (8.6.19) to venous blood and obtain

$$Q(t) = sMP_V(t). \qquad\qquad (8.6.21)$$

Substituting this into (8.6.16) gives

$$\frac{F}{M} = \frac{sP_V(t)}{\int_0^t [P_A(\tau) - P_V(\tau)]\,d\tau}. \qquad\qquad (8.6.22)$$

It is therefore possible to determine the average flow per unit mass of the organ if the arterial and venous concentrations of a freely diffusable tracer are measured. This equation was originally used by Kety and Schmidt (1948) to measure cerebral blood flow using nitrous oxide, but the same technique can be applied using radioactive isotopes of the inert gases such as ^{133}Xe or [85]Kr. The gas is simply administered by continuous breathing but the method is invasive because arterial and venous catheters must be used to withdraw blood samples. P_A and P_V are measured for several minutes until the tissues become saturated and the two concentrations become equal.

8.6.5 Regional blood flow

Blood flow methods based on the accumulation of tracer in an organ can be extended to give the blood flow to different regions of the organ. Radioactive tracers are particularly suitable for this purpose because the quantity of tracer in each region can be measured by external monitoring. On the assumption that every region of the organ is presented with the same concentration of tracer in the blood then, at any given time, the quantity taken up by the organ will be proportional to its regional blood flow. Unfortunately it is not easy to obtain absolute values of regional blood flow in this way, but the technique is very suitable for relative blood flow. It forms the basis of the use of macroaggregated albumin (MAA) for lung perfusion scanning and thallium for myocardial scanning.

An absolute value of regional blood flow can be obtained using the washout of an inert freely diffusable tracer following a bolus injection into the organ. For a perfect bolus input with no recirculation the arterial concentration will be

$$P_A(t) = 0 \qquad \text{except when } t = 0. \tag{8.6.23}$$

Using this in the Fick equation (8.6.15) gives

$$F = \frac{-\dot{Q}(t)}{P_V(t)}, \qquad t \neq 0. \tag{8.6.24}$$

Since we are using a freely diffusable tracer we can substitute for P_V from (8.6.21), giving

$$\frac{F}{M} = \frac{-s\dot{Q}(t)}{Q(t)}, \qquad t \neq 0. \tag{8.6.25}$$

This gives the flow per unit mass to any region of the organ simply by measuring the quantity of tracer remaining in that region. $Q(t)$ may be measured in any units, which makes the technique particularly suitable for radioactive tracers and external counting with probes or a gamma camera. A review of the technique applied to regional cerebral blood flow measurements has been given by Lassen and Ingvar (1972). An injection of ^{133}Xe in solution is made into the carotid artery and the subsequent washout of tracer from several regions of the brain is observed over the next few minutes. Since gas that is washed out is removed in the lungs the problem of recirculating tracer is avoided.

The washout curves of $Q(t)$ against time can be analysed in one of two ways. If we use a compartmental analysis approach then the ratio $\dot{Q}/Q$ only yields a constant result, independent of time, for a single-compartment model which has an exponential solution (Section 8.5.2). In this case $\dot{Q}/Q$ gives $-k_1$ (8.5.4), the rate constant of the exponential. This can be determined from the slope of the graph obtained by plotting $Q(t)$ on a logarithmic scale. If $Q(t)$ is found to follow a multiexponential decrease rather than a single exponential then this implies that there are several compartments each with different rate constants. In this case the flow per unit mass for each compartment can be found by exponential stripping of the curve (Section 8.4.5), although it should be borne in mind that the partition coefficient may be different for each compartment.

The alternative method of analysing the washout curve makes no model assumptions but utilizes the fact that, following a bolus input, $Q(t)$ is really a measure of the impulse retention function $H(t)$ (Section 8.4.7). Therefore (8.4.50) gives the mean washout time of the tracer

$$\bar{t} = \frac{\text{area under curve}}{\text{initial height of curve}}.$$ (8.6.26)

Now if we combine equations (8.6.5) and (8.6.20) we obtain

$$\frac{1}{\bar{t}} = \frac{F}{V} = \frac{F}{sM},$$ (8.6.27)

and thus

$$\frac{F}{M} = \frac{s}{\bar{t}} = s \times \frac{\text{initial height of curve}}{\text{area under curve}}.$$ (8.6.28)

This expression emphasizes the fact that determination of regional blood flow per unit mass is really a mean transit time measurement. However, the mean transit time in this case is that for a diffusable tracer through the tissues of the organ and so it does not suffer from the variability of blood volume, discussed in Section 8.6.1 in connection with non-diffusable tracers.

R.L.

REFERENCES

Barber, D. C., Duthrie, H. L., Howlett, P. J., and Ward, A. S. (1974). Principal components: a new approach to the analysis of gastric emptying, in *Dynamic Studies with Radioisotopes in Medicine* (Proc. Symp. Knoxville, 1974) Vol. 1, pp. 185–196, IAEA, Vienna.

Bayley, R. J., Bell, T. K., and Waters, A. (1971). A dual isotope modification of the Schilling test, In *Ergebnisse der Klinischen Nuklearmedizin* (Eds. W. Horst and H. W. Pabst), pp. 911–915, Schattauer, Stuttgart.

Belcher, E. H., and Vetter, H. (Eds) (1971). *Radioisotopes in Medical Diagnosis*, Butterworths, London.

Britton, K. E., and Brown, N. J. G. (1971). *Clinical Renography*, Lloyd Luke, London.

Britton, K. E., Granowska, M., Rutland, M., Lee, T. Y., Nimmon, C. C., Petrosino, I., and Lumley, J. S. P. (1979). Non invasive measurement of regional cerebral flow before and after microvascular surgery, in *Progress in Stroke Research : 1* (Eds R. M. Greenhalgh and F. C. Rose), pp. 307–318, Pitman Medical, London.

Chantler, C., Garnett, E. S., Parsons, V., and Veall, N. (1969). Glomerular filtration rate measured in man by the single injection method using ^{51}Cr EDTA, *Clinical Science*, **37**, 169–180.

Cohen, M. L. (1974). Radionuclide clearance techniques, *Seminars in Nuclear Medicine*, **4**, 23–38.

Davenport, R. (1983). The derivation of the gamma-variate relationship for tracer dilution curves, *J. Nucl. Med.*, **24**, 945–948.

Diffey, B. L., and Corfield, J. R. (1976). Data-bounding technique in discrete deconvolution, *Med. Biol. Eng.*, **14**, 478.

Diffey, B. L., Hall, F. M., and Corfield, J. R. (1976). The ^{99m}Tc DTPA dynamic renal scan with deconvolution analysis, *J. Nuc. Med.*, **17**, 352–355.

Fleming, J. S., and Goddard, B. A. (1974). A technique for the deconvolution of the renogram, *Phys. Med. Biol.*, **19**, 546–549.

Forbes, G. B., and Lewis, A. M. (1956). Total sodium potassium and chloride in adult man, *J. Clin. Invest.*, **35**, 596.

Gamel, J., Rousseau, W. F., Katholi, C. R., and Mesel, E. (1973). Pitfalls in digital computation of the impulse response of vascular beds from indicator-dilution curves, *Circ. Res.*, **32**, 516–523.

Godfrey, K. (1983). *Compartmental Models and their Application*, Academic Press, London.

Haxhe, J. J. (1971). Body composition and electrolyte studies, in *Radioisotopes in Medical Diagnosis* (Eds E. H. Belcher and H. Vetter), pp. 258–297, Butterworths, London.

Huff, R. L., Hennessy, T. G., Austin, R. E., Garcia, J. F., Roberts, B. M., and Lawrence, J. H. (1950). Plasma and red cell iron turnover in normal subjects and in patients having various hematopoietic disorders, *J. Clin. Invest.*, **29**, 1041.

Kety, S. S., and Schmidt, C. F. (1948). The nitrous oxide method for the quantitative determination of cerebral blood flow in man: theory, procedure and normal values, *J. Clin. Invest.*, **27**, 476.

Lassen, N. A., and Ingvar, D. H. (1972). Radioisotopic assessment of regional cerebral blood flow, in *progress in Nuclear Medicine*, (Eds E. Potchen and V. R. McCready), Vol. 1, pp. 376–409, S. Karger, Basel.

Matthews, C. M. E. (1957). The theory of tracer experiments with ^{131}I labelled plasma proteins, *Phys. Med. Biol.*, **2**, 36.

Meier, P., and Zierler, K. L. (1954). On the theory of the indicator dilution method for the measurement of blood flow and volume, *J. Appl. Physiol.*, **6**, 731–743.

Miller, H., and Wilson, G. M. (1953). The measurement of exchangeable sodium in man using the isotope ^{24}Na, *Clin. Sci.*, **12**, 97.

Niemi, A. J. (1976). On discrete deconvolution, *Med. Biol. Eng.*, **14**, 582.

O'Reilly, P. H., Shields, R. A., and Testa, H. J. (1979). *Nuclear Medicine in Urology and Nephrology*, Butterworths, London.

Reinsch, C. H. (1967). Smoothing by spline functions, *Numerische Mathematik*, **10**, 177–183.

Roberts, J. E., Fisher, K. D., and Allen, T. H. (1958). Tracer methods for estimating total water exchange in man, *Phys. Med. Biol.*, **3**, 7.

Savitzky, A., and Golay, M. J. E. (1964). Smoothing and differentiation of data by simplified least squares procedures, *Anal. Chem.*, **36**, 1627–1639.

Schmidlin, P., Clorius, J., Kubesch, R., and Dreikorn, K. (1976). Evaluation of dynamic studies by means of factor analysis, in *Medical Radionuclide Imaging* (Proc. Symp. Los Angeles, 1976), Vol. 1, pp. 397–408, IAEA, Vienna.

Stewart, G. N. (1897). Researches on the circulation time in organs and on the influence which affect it. IV. The output of the heart, *J. Physiol. Lond.*, **22**, 159.

Tauxe, W. N., Burbank, M. K., and Maher, F. T. (1964). Renal clearances of radioactive ortho-iodohippurate and diatrizoate, *Mayo Clin. Proc.*, **39**, 761–766.

Valentinuzzi, M. E., and Volachec, E. M. M. (1975). Discrete deconvolution, *Med. Biol. Eng.*, **13**, 123–125.

Vetter, H. (1971). Studies of hepatic circulation function and morphology, in *Radioisotopes in Medical Diagnosis* (Eds E. H. Belcher and H. Vetter), pp. 518–545, Butterworths, London.

BIBLIOGRAPHY

Belcher, E. H., and Vetter, H. (Eds), *Radioisotopes in Medical Diagnosis*, Butterworths, London, 1971.

Welch, T. J. C., Potchen, E. J., and Welch, M. J., *Fundamentals of the Tracer Method*, W. B. Saunders, 1972.

9

Control Techniques in Drug Administration

9.1 INTRODUCTION

The human body contains a large number of control mechanisms with complex behavioural characteristics and inter-connections. These are found at all levels within the hierarchy of cellular function, organ function and in organ systems. It is not surprising, therefore, that the techniques developed in the analysis of control systems in engineering have been applied to many aspects of biomedicine. In a *control loop*, measurement of a variable which it is desired to control is processed and applied ('looped' or fed back) as a perturbing input to the system to alter its state and bring the variable under consideration towards the desired level. An example of such a loop would be the measurement and use of processed values of blood pressure to control an infusion pump delivering a drug into the body which influences the interacting mechanisms which determine blood pressure.

The techniques of *systems identification* are being used to elucidate the dynamic characteristics of component parts of the human physiological system. The aim of this chapter, however, is not to cover this aspect of systems analysis in biomedicine (which is discussed in some detail in Part II of the Guidebook), but to describe current research into the use of external automatic controllers to regulate certain variables in the body. Thus, rather than describing the inherent homeostatic control mechanisms of the body, we shall consider the design and analysis of systems where the body is only a part (albeit the main part) of the overall control loop. External control systems become necessary, for example, as part of life support during illness or during and after general anaesthesia and in the following sections we shall consider as examples both the direct control of important physiological variables, such as blood pressure or blood glucose levels, and clinical assistance under operating theatre conditions involving control criteria such as the levels of unconsciousness or muscle relaxation. Although all the applications described involve a drug administration regime as the output of the automatic controller, it should be noted that any other physical quantity which would affect the controlled variable could be considered, e.g. an electrical impulse regime stimulating the heart.

The basic mathematical principles of feedback system analysis and design are described in a companion Guidebook in this series [see *Mathematical Methods in Engineering*, Chapter 14]. A brief glossary of the control systems terminology used here is included at the end of this chapter. For details of techniques mentioned, the references themselves should be consulted. In the examples which are described here, a wide range of control systems techniques is involved. These include classical *single-loop feedback* design, *system identification, self-adaptive control* and *state estimation*. These concepts are illustrated in Figure 9.1.1 which

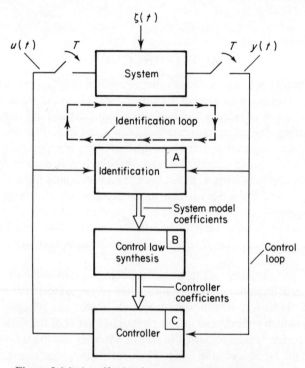

Figure 9.1.1 A self-adaptive control structure. In the identification loop, known inputs $u(t)$ are applied to the system and the measured responses $y(t)$, contaminated by noise about which assumptions must be made, are used to estimate parameters of a model of the dynamic characteristics or performance of the system (A). This information is then used in a process of control law synthesis (B) where the aim is to devise a suitable algorithm or procedure for controlling or regulating the system in normal operation. The controller (C) works by sampling the output signal $y(t)$ and varying system inputs in a feedback loop in order to achieve the desired objectives in regulating system behaviour.

shows the basic structure of a self-adaptive control scheme. The outer part of this structure comprises a feedback control loop, with $y(t)$ and $u(t)$ representing the output and input signals, respectively, of the process to be controlled. $\zeta(t)$ represents noise disturbances [see VI, §1.1] which enter the process and contaminate the output signal. If no identification is involved then the controller must be designed off-line from existing knowledge of the *system dynamics*. It must have a fixed structure, with parameters which can be 'tuned' on-line if necessary. Prior knowledge of the system dynamics can be gathered by using simple test input signals such as step functions or impulses, and calculating time delays and exponentials characterizing the system transfer function from the resulting measured system response. Alternatively, more complex input signals such as *pseudo-random binary sequences* (PRBS) [see II, §5.1] may be used and the response analysed using *correlation analysis* or *least squares identification* to determine the system model. Using simple inputs, the system dynamics are usually obtained in terms of time constants for a *continuous system model* and the controller design may be based on classical graphical techniques using *Nyquist* or *Bode diagrams*. More complex identification schemes require digital computation and necessitate sampling of the input and output data. These utilize a representation of the system dynamics in linear discrete form as shown in Figure 9.1.2 and described by

$$y_t = \frac{z^{-b}B(z^{-1})}{A(z^{-1})}u_t + \frac{C(z^{-1})}{A(z^{-1})}\zeta_t, \qquad (9.1.1)$$

where z is the *unit delay operator* and A, B and C are power series [see IV, §1.10] given by

$$A(z^{-1}) = 1 + a_1 z^{-1} + a_2 z^{-2} + \cdots,$$
$$B(z^{-1}) = b_0 z^{-1} + b_1 z^{-1} + \cdots,$$
$$C(z^{-1}) = 1 + c_1 z^{-1} + c_2 z^{-2} + \cdots,$$

where y_t, u_t and ζ_t are discrete values of the output and input signals and noise disturbance, as discussed above.

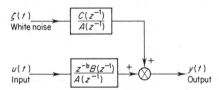

Figure 9.1.2 A linear discrete time model with additive noise at the output. A, B, and C, used in describing the system, are polynomial functions for which the coefficients have to be estimated from measurements using identification (parameter estimation) techniques.

Given the system dynamics in the form of (9.1.1), a fixed *sampled-data* feedback controller can be designed using *root-locus* techniques, which ignores the noise components. Alternatively, *optimal control theory* can be used for the design, incorporating knowledge of the additive output noise. Each of these approaches has a counterpart in adaptive schemes referred to as *self-tuning controllers*.

The most commonly used type of feedback controller is the so-called PID algorithm given by

$$u = K_p \left(e + \frac{1}{K_1} \int e \, dt + K_d \frac{de}{dt} \right),$$ (9.1.2)

where e is the error signal, usually the difference between a desired set level and the system output $y(t)$, K_p is a *proportional* gain constant, K_i is an *integral* term time constant and K_d is a *derivative* term component. Such controllers are used widely in the process industry because of their simplicity, robustness (in terms of feedback loop stability) and ease of tuning of parameters. PI regulators are the most commonly used since the derivative term, which is used to improve the closed-loop *transient performance* of the controller, is often too sensitive to noise in the system. PI controllers feature largely in the medical applications described below. The integral term is required to remove 'offset' (i.e a constant difference between actual and desired output levels under steady state conditions). Initial values of the K_p, K_i and K_d parameters are often obtained from recordings of the system output after a step change in input, using the so-called Ziegler–Nichols rules (Ziegler and Nichols, 1942).

Systems identification techniques are important both for the design of fixed controllers and as part of self-adaptive controllers as shown in Figure 9.1.1. A wide range of methods is available for estimation of parameters for system models, and some of these are described in detail by Eykhoff (1974). Commonly used techniques employ sequential least squares methods for updating parameter values [see VI, §12.3.5] using algorithms closely related to the *Kalman filter* [see VI, Chapter 20]. For example, to estimate the A and B polynomials in (9.1.1), the following parameter estimation [see VI, §3.1] equations can be used:

$$\hat{\theta}(t) = \hat{\theta}(t-1) + \mathbf{K}(t)[y(t) - \mathbf{x}'(t)\,\hat{\theta}(t-1)],$$ (9.1.3)

where θ is a parameter vector [see VI, §13.1] given by

$$\theta' = (a_1, a_2, \ldots, a_n, b_0, b_1, \ldots, b_n),$$

and $\mathbf{x}$ is a data vector given by

$$\mathbf{x}' = [-y(t-1), -y(t-2), \ldots, -y(t-n), u(t-b), \ldots, u(t-b-n)].$$

In (9.1.3) $\mathbf{K}(t)$ is the so-called 'Kalman gain' vector given by

$$\mathbf{K}(t) = \frac{\mathbf{P}(t-1)\mathbf{x}(t)}{\beta + \mathbf{x}'(t)\mathbf{P}(t-1)\mathbf{x}(t)},$$ (9.1.4)

where β is a 'forgetting factor', $0 < \beta \leq 1$, used to weight the past values of the output to allow for tracking of slowly-varying parameters. In (9.1.4), $\mathbf{P}(t)$ is the covariance matrix [see II, §13.3.1] which is also updated iteratively using

$$\mathbf{P}(t) = \frac{[\mathbf{I} - \mathbf{K}(t)\mathbf{x}'(t)]\mathbf{P}(t-1)}{\beta}. \tag{9.1.5}$$

The covariance matrix determines correlations [see VI, §2.1.2(d)] between elements of the estimated vector of parameters; in particular the variances of the parameter estimates are given by the main diagonal terms of the matrix [see II, Definition 9.6.3].

Only in the restricted case of white noise output contamination (i.e. $C/A = 1$ in equation 9.1.1) does the least squares algorithm defined by (9.1.3), (9.1.4) and (9.1.5) converge to give unbiased estimates [see VI, §3.3.2] of the polynomials A and B. In the presence of non-white noise [see VI, Chapter 18] the identification algorithms must be modified, two popular techniques being those of *generalized least squares* [see VI, §8.2.6] and *maximum likelihood* [see VI, Chapter 6] (Clarke, 1967; Eykhoff, 1974, p. 145).

In the adaptive scheme shown in Figure 9.1.1 the system identification is performed on-line and used to continually update the controller parameters. Adaptive schemes are of particular interest in biomedical feedback control because of the large patient-to-patient variability in system dynamics, and also because of changes over a period of time in parameters for an individual patient. In this situation, a fixed controller strategy is unlikely to give satisfactory closed-loop transient control for all patients. One form of adaptive control which is being exploited in industrial applications is that of the self-tuning controller. This and other forms of adaptive control are described in Billings and Harris (1981). In one form, the self-tuning control design is based on optimal control principles, and the identification stage comprises estimation of the controller parameters directly (Clarke and Gawthrop, 1975). By using different cost functions [see VI, §19.3.2] for the optimization [see III, Chapter II] other interpretations of this self-tuner relating to *model reference* adaptive control and *Smith predictor* control can be realized (Gawthrop, 1977). An alternative design of self-tuner referred to as *pole-assignment* is based on classical control system design techniques (Wellstead, Prager and Zanker, 1979). In this approach, the system model is identified first, followed by controller synthesis. The problem of biased estimates in the presence of non-white noise contamination has been tackled using an *extended least squares* identification algorithm (e.g. Wellstead and Sanoff, 1981).

Finally, in this introductory section we mention two other techniques relevant to the biomedical applications. These are the use of Kalman filtering and Smith predictor control. The Kalman filter equations, related to (9.1.3), (9.1.4) and (9.1.5), can be used for the purpose of filtering noisy data and also for the estimation and prediction of inaccessible states of the process using noise-contaminated measurements. For a long time it has been known that systems manifesting pure time delay in their dynamic response are difficult to control well. A component exhibiting pure time delay has no effect on the input signal other than to delay it by a specified time interval, Δt, where the output at time $t + \Delta t$ equals the input at time t. Such transport delays are commonplace in medical systems and the Smith predictor approach is of considerable interest. The principle of this is that, based on a knowledge of the system dynamics, a delay-free controller loop is designed, while in addition a predictor element is incorporated in the overall control strategy to offset the pure time delay in the process dynamics (Smith, 1957). When the dynamics are not known perfectly, the Smith predictor scheme is of questionable robustness. The performance, under conditions of a mismatch between the actual system dynamics and those assumed in the control strategy, and other aspects of Smith predictor schemes are discussed in detail by Marshall (1979).

In the following sections a series of examples is given which illustrate the use of all of the above techniques in clinical drug administration.

9.2 POST-OPERATIVE CONTROL OF BLOOD PRESSURE

This example is described first because of the large number of patients who have been treated post-operatively using automated feedback control of blood pressure. Over the past few years more than 10,000 hypertensive patients have been treated in this way by J. Kirklin, L. C. Sheppard and their coworkers at the University of Alabama Medical Centre, Birmingham, USA. Techniques involving simple classical control, systems identification and adaptive control strategies have all been applied to this situation, and clearly illustrate the way in which further knowledge of the dynamics of a physiological system and improved control can be achieved via an inter-disciplinary approach.

Before attempting closed-loop control, some knowledge of systems dynamics is essential, and this was obtained using PRBS excitation of the blood pressure control system (Sheppard and Sayers, 1977). In this work the mean arterial pressure (MAP) response to a number of hypotensive agents was determined. The later studies, involving computer control, have concentrated on the use of just one of these hypotensive drugs, sodium nitroprusside. Cross-correlation [see II, §13.3.3] between the MAP response and the PRBS drug input revealed information about the *impulse response* of the physiological system (i.e. the function which describes the output or response measured in the system over time after it is disturbed by an impulsive input). This indicated the presence of a time delay of about a single blood circulation time (30 to 40 sec) together with at least one time constant of decay. The impulse response typically showed a first minimum after one minute and a second after three minutes and a return to baseline within five minutes. Detailed modelling of these dynamic responses was performed later, by the initial information was sufficient for the design of a simple classical PI feedback controller.

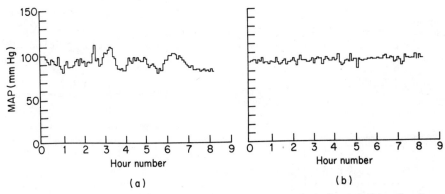

Figure 9.2.1 Blood pressure measured at 5 minute intervals during infusion of sodium nitroprusside under (a) manual control and (b) computer control (from Sheppard *et al.*, 1979).

Using typical impulse responses, simulation studies were used to select suitable parameters for a PID controller. It was found that these values required 'tuning' when closed-loop control was implemented (Sheppard *et al.*, 1979). Although this was partly due to simplications in the modelling, it was also due to patient-to-patient variability in system parameters. To give satisfactory response it was found to be necessary to include a 'decision table' in conjunction with the PI controller to keep the drug input consistent with a number of imposed clinical and physiological constraints. In this way, the control system became effectively non-linear in behaviour. An example of the improvement in the blood pressure variability caused by using automatic rather than manual control is shown in Figure 9.2.1. In a range of trials, significant improvement in the quality of control was achieved with the use of this constrained PI regulator.

More detailed modelling studies have revealed further dynamic features in the blood pressure response, including a recirculation effect and background activity containing both stochastic [see VI, Chapters 18 and 19] and sinusoidal (i.e. like a sine curve) components [see IV, §2.12] (Slate *et al.*, 1979). The detailed model obtained as a result of these studies is shown in Figure 9.2.2. The *transfer function* $G_d(s)$ contains two time delays T_i and T_c and one exponential time constant τ and is given by

$$G_d(s) = \frac{Ke^{-T_i s}(1 + \alpha e^{-T_c s})}{1 + \tau s}, \tag{9.2.1}$$

where T_i (30 seconds) represents the initial transport lag for the drug from the injection site and T_c (45 seconds) the recirculation time, α is the fraction of drug recirculating and τ is the time constant associated with drug metabolism. Using this model for a range of drug sensitivity factors, K, under the fixed controller strategy, previously mentioned, showed that such a structure could be unstable

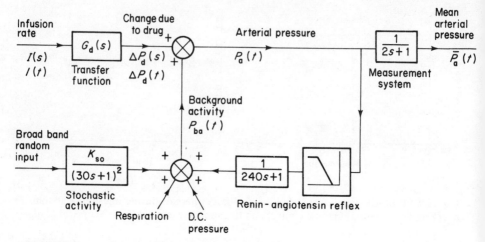

Figure 9.2.2 Arterial blood pressure model for vasoactive drug infusion control (from Slate *et al.*, 1979).

and this has been confirmed in clinical usage. Because of the non-robust nature of this method of control, an adaptive control structure was then investigated.

The adaptive control scheme studied by Slate (1980) is shown diagrammatically in Figure 9.2.3. This scheme incorporates a number of control modes and makes use of different sampling rates and filtering of the measured signals. Thus, blood pressure is sampled with a period of 1 second. This noisy signal is low-pass filtered (i.e. high frequency components are attenuated) and subsequently re-sampled at a 2-second period. This signal is used to form the closed-loop error signal (i.e. the difference between desired and actual MAP) which is further sampled at a 10-second period for processing by the controller algorithms. The derivative of this error signal is also required and is obtained from the 2-second sampled signal by passing it through a differentiator, followed by a low-pass filter, with subsequent sampling at the 10-second period. Based upon these error and derivative of error signals, a control coordinator selects either a transient control mode or a regulator mode to calculate the necessary change in control action required. In the transient control mode, the infusion rate increment is switched between two values by means of a controller that includes a Smith time delay compensator. Scheduling of the feedback loop gain is included in the transient controller to produce a fast speed of response to hypotensive pressure transients. In the regulator mode, the infusion rate increment is calculated from the error and its derivative. Adaptation to the patient drug gain (i.e. change in MAP caused by a unit change in drug input) is accomplished in an initial period after closed-loop control has begun.

A recursive least squares [see VI, §12.3.5] estimation algorithm is used to provide a measure of the drug gain parameter from data acquired at 2-second

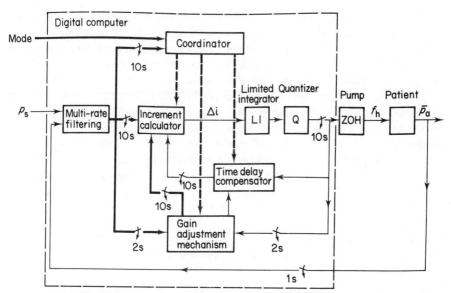

Figure 9.2.3 A self-adaptive control strategy for blood pressure control of hypertensive patients. $\bar{P}_a$ is the measured mean arterial blood pressure, $\bar{P}_q$ is the adjustable set point for the controller. (from Slate, 1980)

intervals. The estimated gain and the variance of this estimate are used to adjust (at 10-second intervals) the overall gain of the regulator, the relay output levels and the Smith compensator gains. These adjustments are based on decisions made by the coordinator.

The performance of this multi-rate adaptive scheme was initially assessed in simulation studies using the blood pressure described above (Slate, 1980). It has subsequently been implemented in microcomputer format and evaluated in dog trials and is currently undergoing clinical evaluation.

9.3 CONTROL OF ANAESTHESIA

Three major areas of responsibility for the anaesthetist are those of controlling general anaesthetics in the operating theatre, drug-induced muscle paralysis during operations and pain relief (analgaesia) during post-operative care. Each of these areas has been explored with respect to the use of feedback control as exemplified in the following sections. It should be noted that most of the work described is of very recent origin and is still undergoing considerable development.

9.3.1 Drug-induced unconsciousness

This is the most commonly recognized role of the anaesthetist and reveals the earliest attempts to produce automated feedback control in this discipline, under the title of the 'servo-anaesthetizer' (Bickford, 1949). As pointed out in a review article by Chilcoat (1980), the major problem with this, and subsequent attempts, was the dubious nature of the use of the EEG as a measurement for the depth of unconsciousness. A number of alternative approaches have been made to obtain a better quantitative measure of unconsciousness.

In the work of Coles, Brown and Lampard (1973) a multivariable system was proposed to control several inter-related variables in sheep, including arterial blood pressure as a measure of depth of anaesthesia (Figure 9.3.1). Their system maintained constant levels of end-expired PCO_2, inspired PO_2 and reservoir-bag volume in a closed anaesthetic breathing system. Oscillation of the controlled variable proved to be a problem in the blood pressure control loop, a point also noticed by Smith and Schwede (1972), illustrating the problems of good feedback control in the presence of time delays, as mentioned in the previous section.

The measurement of unconsciousness has also been approached using clinical signs such as pulse rate, arterial blood pressure, respiratory rate, tidal volume,

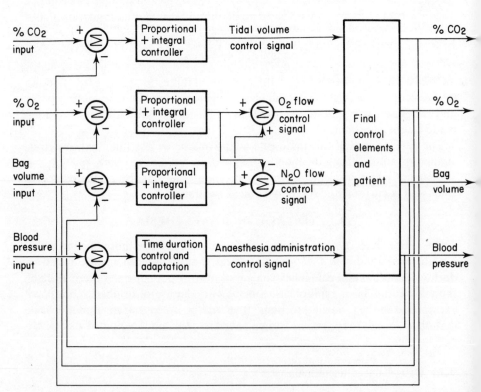

Figure 9.3.1 Block diagram of a multi-variable anasthesia control system (from Coles, Brown and Lampard, 1973).

sweating, movement, etc. In the work by Suppan (1972), one of these variables could be selected by the anaesthetist for control via a motor-driven vaporizer administering halothane. In recent work a 'clinical storing' approach has been used, whereby a number of clinical signs are summed together with selected weighting to give a single measure of depth of anaesthesia (Davies *et al.*, 1982). This has been used clinically with a microcomputer-based system which allows for entry of the scores via a keyboard, and provides control of a motor-driven syringe for the administration of drugs intravenously to mtaintain unconsciousness at a desired level.

The problems of designing adequate feedback controllers for biological systems, which often contain time delay components, is compounded by the large patient-to-patient variations in parameters for the dynamic models. This has prompted the investigation of adaptive control schemes for depth of anaesthesia. Beneken *et al.* (1974) showed, using a multicompartment model of the anaesthetic system, that a parameter-estimation adaptive control system could give superior performance to a conventional fixed-parameter controller. This type of approach has been followed by Tatnall and Morris (1977) for anaesthesia in neonates. Using a twelve-compartment body model, they showed via simulation that a fixed PI controller would not give acceptable control when allowances were made for differences in patient uptake characteristics. Their self-adaptive system is based on a simplified equation for halothane uptake in the lungs given by the differential equation [see IV, Chapter 7]

$$\frac{\mathrm{d}p_{\mathrm{alv}}}{\mathrm{d}t} = K_1(p_{\mathrm{v}} - p_{\mathrm{alv}}) + K_2(F_{\mathrm{i}} - p_{\mathrm{alv}}), \tag{9.3.1}$$

where p_{alv}, the alveolar halothane partial pressure, is regarded as the control variable; p_{v} is the mixed venous halothane partial pressure, F_{i} is the inspired halothane partial pressure, and K_1 and K_2 are patient parameters. K_1 and K_2 are identified during the first few breaths when p_{v} can be assumed to be almost zero. Under these conditions (9.3.1) reduces to

$$\frac{\mathrm{d}p_{\mathrm{alv}}}{\mathrm{d}t} = - K_1 p_{\mathrm{alv}} + K_2(F_{\mathrm{i}} - P_{\mathrm{alv}}) \tag{9.3.2}$$

and K_1 and K_2 can be estimated using on-line measurements of p_{alv} and F_{i} made with a rapid-response halothane meter. Identification is stopped and control initiated when p_{alv} reaches 95 per cent of the desired level p_{d} set by the anaesthetist. At this point the controller takes the form

$$F_{\mathrm{i}} = - \frac{K_1'}{K_2'} p_{\mathrm{v}}' + \frac{K_1' + K_2'}{K_2'} p_{\mathrm{d}}, \tag{9.3.3}$$

for which it has been shown that transient performance is significantly affected by any errors in the estimates K_1', K_2' and p_{v}'. Five minutes after the introduction of halothane, control is switched to a conventional PI regulator which is used to maintain p_{alv} at the desired level. Successful clinical trials have been undertaken using this structure of self-adaptive control (Tatnall, Morris and West, 1981). It should be noted that, in this work, depth of unconsciousness is being inferred solely from levels of gas concentration in the alveoli.

An alternative approach to the feedback methods described above is the use of open-loop control based on a known model of drug uptake. In this case the dynamic model is used to predict the time course of the drug level in brain tissue, which is presumed to determine the depth of anaesthesia. Purely open-loop control of this nature would be unworkable because of variations in patient dynamics, and hence a number of schemes have been attempted in which the model is updated using infrequent measurement of certain process variables. Thus, Mapleson, Allott and Steward (1974) reported trials on dogs in which they attempted to achieve an arterial halothane tension of 4 mm Hg within 5 minutes, and maintenance of this tension for a further 75 minutes. An extensive model was used, whose parameters were updated every 10 minutes, based on measurements of cardiac output and alveolar ventilation. A more extensive system has been reported by Mapleson et al. (1980) which automatically controls the set point of a vaporizer. It bases this on a computed brain tension of anaesthetic agent, obtained from a detailed model of uptake and distribution. The model is initially set up using average standard values based on body mass, and is subsequently updated every 10 minutes using measurements of cardiac output, alveolar ventilation and arterial blood tension. The anaesthetist is included in the loop by means of manual control of the N_2O/O_2 mixture which carries the volatile agent. He specifies the desired brain level of the volatile agent in terms which include the contribution of N_2O.

9.3.2 Drug-induced muscle relaxation

In certain operations, such as abdominal surgery, correct levels of patient muscle relaxation are necessary. A number of drugs exist for this purpose and the types referred to in this section are of the non-depolarizing form, such as pancuronium. To attain automatically controlled muscle relaxation, a suitable measurement variable must be defined. The level of muscle relaxation can be simply quantified either in terms of an evoked electromyograph (EMG) or an evoked muscle tension response. In the work reported here, the former method has been adopted using supramaximal stimulation at a frequency of 0.1 Hz at the ulnar nerve above the elbow. The resulting EMG is measured using surface electrodes taped to the hand. The EMG signals are amplified with a gain of 1,000 within a bandwidth of 8 Hz to 10 kHz, then rectified, integrated and finally stored in a sample-hold amplifier to produce the variable which is controlled.

Computer control of muscle relaxation using stimulation of the masseter muscle on the face of sheep has been described (Cass et al., 1976). In human trials using a simple proportional gain feedback controller (i.e. $K_d = 0$, $K_I = \infty$ in 9.1.2), satisfactory regulation was achieved with a mean level of 74 per cent paralysis for an 80 per cent set point (Brown *et al.*, 1980). This offset has been successfully removed using a PI controller whose parameters were set using the Ziegler–Nichols tuning method. Use of a fixed PI controller occasionally gives an oscillatory closed-loop response, as already noted in Section 9.2 on blood pressure control. This emphasizes the need to identify the dose-response model for muscle paralysis.

The model required here is a combination of the drug pharmacokinetics (i.e. relationship of drug dose to blood concentration) and pharmacodynamics (i.e. blood relationship of concentration to evoked EMG response). Instead of classical bolus injection methods for pharmacokinetics determination, the use of PRBS excitation has been made for model identification (Linkens *et al.*, 1981). Using bit intervals of 33.3 seconds or 100 seconds with a sequence length of 63, successful identification has been made in dog trials. Employing an off-line technique, identification of the data has been obtained using a generalized least squares package. This revealed the presence of a pure time delay with a mean value of 64 seconds and two exponential time constants with mean values of 2.7 and 20.1 minutes. These parameters had a range of about 4:1 in a small number of trials, illustrating once again the large variability in dynamics which is common in biological systems.

The feedback system described is currently being used in a range of microcomputer studies. These include attempts to quantify the effects of other drugs, such as tranquilizers, on relaxation levels (Asbury *et al.*, 1981), and the interacting effects of other anaesthetic agents such as halothane and ethrane in potentiating paralysis (Asbury, Linkens and Rimmer, 1982). Simulation studies have shown the desirability of using Smith predictor schemes to counteract the pure time delay, based on a *sensitivity analysis* using the parameter ranges identified previously (Linkens *et al.*, 1982a). Adaptive control schemes are also currently being investigated using a pole-assignment form of self-tuning controller, with simulation studies showing promising results (Linkens *et al.*, 1982b). On-line recursive identification algorithms have been implemented and tried successfully in dog studies under either open-loop or closed-loop conditions. The aim, therefore, is to use a form of adaptive control which will give simultaneous control and identification of drug dynamics. This latter aspect is of interest since some of the newer relaxant drugs, such as Organon NC 45, do not at present have any known assay method for determination of drug pharmacokinetics from classical bolus injection methods. Thus, it can be seen that, as well as automatic regulation of relaxation levels, studies of this nature can give more detailed quantification of interacting drug effects.

9.3.3 Post-operative pain relief

The control of pain following major surgery, such as total hip replacement, is an important clinical requirement. In conventional clinical practice the necessary feedback is provided by nursing staff who administer pain-relief drugs based on observation of the patient at about four-hourly intervals. Such slow sampling cannot give optimal relief from pain. In an automatic 'demand analgesia' system, feedback is provided by the patient who is equipped with a button and instructed to press it whenever he or she feels uncomfortable.

The use of a simple proportional gain controller in such a system, employing a microcomputer programmed in a special form of 'control' BASIC, is described by Jacobs *et al.* (1981). In this work pain is quantified as the rate of button-pushing by the patient. Proportional control in this case is non-optimal because it requires the patient to experience some pain before he can receive any pain-relieving drug. This non-optimality cannot be removed simply in this case by introducing integral control action because it would require the possibility of negative drug input. One commercial system attempts to overcome this severe output non-linearity by introducing what amounts to a positive non-zero desired value of pain, thus allowing integral action control (White, Pearce and Norman, 1979).

In work by Jacobs and his coworkers (Jacobs *et al.*, 1982; Reasbeck, 1982) the non-linear problem is overcome, with a claimed significant improvement in performance, by using a controller in which a non-linear state estimator is operated in series with a one-step-ahead control law. The non-linear estimator comprises a Bayes algorithm in series (cascaded) with an extended Kalman filter. The model used in this work is shown in Figure 9.3.2 where perceived pain y is assumed to depend on the difference between 'comfort', due to drug adminis-tration, and 'discomfort', due to surgery performed, n. The pharmacokinetic relationship between drug infusion rate u and brain tissue drug concentration is assumed to be represented by three exponentials having a transfer function of the form

$$\frac{X(s)}{U(s)} = \prod_{j=1}^{3} \frac{K_j}{1 + sT_j}. \tag{9.3.4}$$

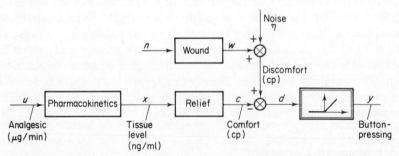

Figure 9.3.2 Structure of a mathematical model for control of postoperative pain (from Jacobs *et al.*, 1982).

Little is known about the relationship between comfort and tissue drug level and here a simple constant of proportionality is assumed, whose estimation is itself of importance and is included in the Kalman filter. The discomfort is modelled as the sum of an exponentially decaying stochastic term w, which represents a healing wound, plus a white noise term η. The term w starts from a positive initial value and is assumed to have a transfer function given by

$$\frac{W(s)}{N(s)} = \frac{1}{1 + sT_4}. \tag{9.3.5}$$

To define this model, five state variables are required as follows:

$x_1 \equiv x$ tissue drug concentration (ng/ml)

x_2, x_3 two further states for (9.3.4)

$x_4 \equiv w$ wound healing (cp) where p is a unit of pain defined as the amount of pain which produces button-pressing at the rate of one per second

$x_5 \equiv$ relief $(cp/(ng/ml))$

The corresponding dynamic equations are linear and can be written as

$$\mathbf{x}(i + 1) = \mathbf{A}\mathbf{x}(i) + \mathbf{b}u(i) + \boldsymbol{\xi}(i) \tag{9.3.6}$$

[see I, §5.7], where

$$\mathbf{A} = \begin{bmatrix} a_{11} & a_{12} & a_{13} & 0 & 0 \\ a_{21} & a_{22} & a_{23} & 0 & 0 \\ a_{31} & a_{32} & a_{33} & 0 & 0 \\ 0 & 0 & 0 & a_4 & 0 \\ 0 & 0 & 0 & 0 & 1 \end{bmatrix},$$

$$\mathbf{b} = [b_1 \quad b_2 \quad b_3 \quad 0 \quad 0]',$$

$$\boldsymbol{\xi}(i) = [0 \quad 0 \quad 0 \quad n(i) \quad 0]'. \tag{9.3.7}$$

and where $n(i)$ is given a value according to the surgical intervention.

Two non-linearities arise in the relationship between the states x and the output y. One is the estimation of nett pain d, given by

$$d = x_4 - x_1 x_5 + \eta. \tag{9.3.8}$$

The other is the severe demand non-linearity $y(d)$ shown in Figure 9.3.2.

The separated stochastic controller uses a novel non-linear estimation scheme which cascades (links in series) a Bayes algorithm with an extended Kalman filter. We describe below (a) how Bayes' theorem can be used to handle the severe non-linearity $y(d)$, (b) how the conditional mean and variance from Bayes' theorem [see II, §1.6.4] are weighted and then used to drive an extended Kalman filter (EKF) which handles the non-linearity of (9.3.8) and (c) how the control law is used.

The two non-linear estimators, Bayes' rule and EKF, are coupled by way of a new variable z defined by

$$z \equiv w - c = x_4 - x_1 x_5, \tag{9.3.9}$$

which is a rearrangement of the right-hand side of (9.3.8). Neither estimator is optimal. The non-optimality of each arises because it is assumed that probability distributions for the random variables can be approximated by Normal distributions [see II, §11.4]. This is the usual simplifying assumption made about non-linear states, x, estimated by an EKF; it is also applied here to the random variable z, estimated by Bayes' theorem, which could not really be Normal if the states x_i in (9.3.8) were Normal.

(a) Bayes' Theorem

Bayes' Theorem is the principal result in probability theory governing estimation of random variables observed through noise measurements. It gives an equation for a conditional distribution $p(z|y)$ [see VI, §15.2] in terms of a prior distribution $p_0(z)$ and a likelihood function $l(y|z)$:

$$p(z|y) = \frac{p_0(z)l(y|z)}{\displaystyle\int p_0(z)l(y|z)\,dz}, \tag{9.3.10}$$

which is directly applicable to estimating the variable z of (9.3.9). The assumed Normal prior distribution for z is written

$$p_0(z) = N(m_0, v_0), \tag{9.3.11}$$

where '$N(m, v)$' denotes 'Normal with expectation m, and variance v'. The white noise η is also assumed to be Normally distributed [see II, §11.4] according to

$$p_\eta(\eta) = N(0, v_\eta). \tag{9.3.12}$$

Whether or not the non-linearity of Figure 9.3.2 affects the output y depends on the sign of the sum d in (9.3.8), where

$$d = z + \eta.$$

When d is positive there is no non-linearity. A corresponding positive output y appears and the resulting conditional distribution for z is the well-known (Bayes' or Kalman) result

$$p(z|y) = N(m_1, v_1) \qquad \text{if} \quad y > 0, \tag{9.3.13}$$

where $\quad m_1 = \dfrac{m_0 v_\eta + y v_0}{v_0 + v_\eta}$

$$v_1 = \frac{v_0 v_\eta}{v_0 + v_\eta}.$$

When d is negative the demand non-linearity becomes effective and zero output y is observed. The likelihood function is then

$$l(0|z) = \text{Prob}\,(z + \eta < 0)$$
$$= \text{Prob}\,(\eta < -z)$$
$$= \Phi(-z/(v_\eta)^{1/2}) \tag{9.3.14}$$

where $\Phi(\cdot)$ is the standard integral of the normal distribution [see IV, §13.4.1, and III, §7.7.2]. The conditional distribution $p(z|0)$ can then be computed numerically using an algorithm obtained by substituting from (9.3.11) and (9.3.14) into (9.3.10). The sub-optimal approximation

$$p(z|0) \simeq N(m_2, v_2) \tag{9.3.15}$$

is reasonably valid when $p_0(z)$ is actually Normal. Values of the conditional mean m_2 and variance v_2, computed numerically, provide the coupling between Bayes' rule and the EKF, as discussed below.

(b) *Extended Kalman filter*

Whenever d and y are greater than zero, the estimation of states x_i, which satisfy dynamic equations (9.3.6) and have non-linear output $y(d)$ from equation (9.3.8), can be done using a standard extended Kalman filter (Eykhoff, 1974, p. 434). This EKF approximates the conditional distribution $p(\mathbf{x}|y)$ by a Normal distribution.

$$p(\mathbf{x}|y) = N(\hat{\mathbf{x}}, \boldsymbol{\Sigma}), \qquad \text{if} \quad y > 0, \tag{9.3.16}$$

updated from iteration $i - 1$ to i according to

$$\hat{\mathbf{x}}(i) = \tilde{\mathbf{x}}(i) + \mathbf{K}(i)[y(i) - \tilde{y}(i)],$$
$$\tilde{\mathbf{x}}(i) = \mathbf{A}\hat{\mathbf{x}}(i-1) + \mathbf{b}u(i-1),$$
$$\tilde{y}(i) = \tilde{x}_4(i) - [\tilde{x}_1(i)\tilde{x}_5(i) + \tilde{\sigma}_{15}(i)],$$
$$\boldsymbol{\Sigma}(i) = \tilde{\boldsymbol{\Sigma}}(i) - \mathbf{K}(i)\mathbf{f}(i)\tilde{\boldsymbol{\Sigma}}(i), \tag{9.3.17}$$
$$\tilde{\boldsymbol{\Sigma}}(i) = \mathbf{A}\boldsymbol{\Sigma}(i-1)\mathbf{A}' + \text{diag}\,[0 \quad 0 \quad 0 \quad v_\eta \quad 0],$$
$$\mathbf{f}(i) = [-\tilde{x}_5(i) \quad 0 \quad 0 \quad 1 - \tilde{x}_1(i)],$$
$$\mathbf{K}(i) = \tilde{\boldsymbol{\Sigma}}(i)\mathbf{f}'(i)[\mathbf{f}(i)\tilde{\boldsymbol{\Sigma}}(i)\mathbf{f}'(i) + v_\eta]^{-1}.$$

When d is negative the zero value of y produced by the demand non-linearity does not carry sufficient information to derive the EKF. The information is instead obtained from the conditional distribution $p(z|0)$ of (9.3.15) and is transmitted from Bayes' theorem to the EKF in the form of a synthetic output y' which is regarded as the sum of z and a synthetic noise η' having variance v'_η:

$$y' = z + \eta'. \tag{9.3.18}$$

Values of y' and v'_η, determined with reference to equation (9.3.13), are

$$y' = m_2 + \frac{(m_2 - m_0)}{v_0} v'_\eta,$$

$$v'_\eta = \frac{v_0 v_2}{v_0 - v_2}.$$

(9.3.19)

Their significance is in approximating the non-linear Bayes' theorem estimation by a linear output (9.3.18) which can be combined with (9.3.6) and (9.3.9) in an EKF to estimate x. This EKF, when y is zero, is specified by (9.3.16), but with y and v_η replaced by y' and v'_η of (9.3.19) using numerically computed values of m_2 and v_2 from Bayes' rule.

(c) Control law

The control law was designed to make the comfort c greater than the predictable component w of discomfort by an amount proportional to the magnitude of the unpredictable component η of discomfort. A suitable specification, in terms of one-step-ahead predictions, is

$$\tilde{c}(i + 1) - \tilde{w}(i + 1) \equiv - \tilde{z}(i + 1) = k \sqrt{v_\eta(i + 1)}, \tag{9.3.20}$$

where k is a positive constant of proportionality. The required value of $u(i)$, based on current estimates $\hat{x}(i)$ from the EKF and determined from the dynamic state equations (9.3.6), is

$$u = [k \sqrt{v_\eta(i + 1)} + a_4 \hat{x}_4 - a_{11}(\hat{x}_1 \hat{x}_5 + \sigma_{15})$$
$$- a_{12}(\hat{x}_2 \hat{x}_5 + \sigma_{25}) - a_{13}(\hat{x}_3 \hat{x}_5 + \sigma_{35})]/b_1 \hat{x}_5 \tag{9.3.21}$$

where the index (i) has, for greater clarity, been omitted from $u(i)$, $\hat{x}(i)$ and the elements $\sigma(i)$ of $\Sigma(i)$.

Simulation studies have been undertaken (Reasbeck, 1982) of the three systems referred to above, from which it was shown that the Kalman filter approach gave considerably fewer analgesia demands than the simple proportional or commercial controllers (23 demands against 166 or 122). This improvement is achieved, however, with a higher total drug consumption (674 μg against 332 or 473 μg). It is suggested that good estimates of the relief x_5 can be obtained using this method of stochastic control.

9.4 CONTROL OF BLOOD GLUCOSE LEVELS

The use of bolus subcutaneous injections of insulin in the control of blood glucose concentration in a diabetic patient is normal clinical practice. Better physiological response should be obtained if the glucose level is monitored regularly and insulin delivered in a regime more closely resembling the normal release mechanisms. In simple terms, the B-cell delivers insulin into the blood stream at two rates; a continuous, slow basal rate, which controls glucose output from the liver, and meal-time bursts which help dispose of the digested nutrients.

With the advent of continuous blood glucose monitoring and frequent sampling profiles it has become apparent that in most insulin-dependent diabetic patients it is difficult to sustain near normal blood glucose concentrations. The so-called 'artificial pancreas' is a closed-loop system, i.e. an extra-corporeal blood glucose sensor is coupled to a computer which controls the rate of infusion of insulin into a peripheral vein so as to maintain normoglycaemia (Albisser and Leibel, 1977). Although very successful in maintaining normoglycaemia in diabetic patients for up to a few days, it has major disadvantages for long-term use. Thus, it is limited by its bulk, complexity and cost, and its use of the intravenous route for insulin administration and blood sampling. Prolonged infusions carry the risk of thrombosis and infection.

The above considerations have prompted simpler portable infusion pumps without glucose sensing, and thus operate under open-loop conditions. In this approach, continuous subcutaneous insulin infusion (CSII) employs a portable electromechanical syringe pump capable of delivering insulin at two fixed rates. The lower level is continuous, while the higher rate is electrically engaged by the patient 30 minutes before each main meal (Pickup and Keen, 1980). A number of studies have now shown that near physiological blood glucose concentrations can be maintained by CSII for a number of days in ambulatory diabetics supervised in hospital. In terms of long-period outpatient treatment, a group of six diabetics treated at home via CSII for 2 to 4 months achieved overall mean blood glucose values varying from 4.8 to 7.7 m mol/1 (Pickup *et al.*, 1979). There are many intermediary metabolites and hormones which have abnormal concentrations in diabetics and may be contributory factors in the pathological processes. Treatment via CSII has been associated with a return to near-normal blood levels of lactate, pyruvate, 3-hydroxybutyrate, alanine, cholesterol, triglyceride and free fatty acids.

In spite of the success of CSII open-loop control in certain cases, there remain 'brittle' diabetics in whom large, fast and unpredictable swings in blood glucose concentration occur and for whom open-loop control cannot help. In such cases feedback control is the only way in which near-normal blood glucose levels could be achieved. Similarly, it has been observed that CSII does not allow for classical output disturbances caused by such things as severe stress or intermittent illness. The comment has been made that CSII should only be used, therefore, under close medical supervision—i.e. under closed-loop control! The situation begins to approximate to the combined open-loop/closed-loop system described above for drug-induced unconsciousness.

A number of control algorithms have been proposed for a closed-loop control 'artificial pancreas'. The simplest one was an on–off mechanism which activated syringe pumps containing insulin and glucagon, depending on threshold levels of

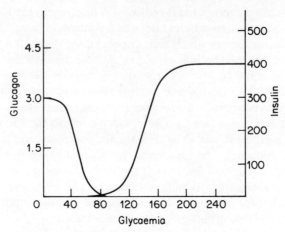

Figure 9.4.1 Graph from typical computer algorithms
for the artificial pancreas (from Albisser and Leibel, 1977).

blood glucose (Kadish, 1964). Kline *et al.* (1968) used a simple proportional
controller driven by the deviation from normal glucose levels. In the work by
Albisser and Leibel (1977), three relationships for controller synthesis were used,
as illustrated in Figure 9.4.1. Two of these are sigmoidal-shaped curves
relating insulin and glucagon delivery rates to the measured level of glycaemia,
while the third is a difference factor which depends on the rate of change of
blood glucose. These relationships are summarized by

Insulin delivery (mU/min) $= 200[1 + \tanh{(G_p - 140)/25}]$,

Glucagon delivery (μg/min) $= 1.5[1 - \tanh{(G\text{-}50/17)}]$, (9.4.1)

where $G_p = G + (A^3 + 10A)$,

$G =$ glycaemia (mg/dl),

$G_p =$ projected glycaemia (mg/dl),

$A =$ rate of change of glycaemia (mg/ml min).

An adaptive control scheme which allows for patient parameter variations and
selectable blood glucose profiles has been studied in dogs by Kondo *et al.* (1982).
Their adaptive scheme is outlined in Figure 9.4.2. The reference model used is a
linearized second-order model [see IV, §7.3] similar to that of Ackerman,
Rosevear and McGuckin (1964) and is given by

$\dot{y} = p_1(y - y_f) - p_2 x + p_3 v$,

$\dot{x} = - p_4 x_2 + p_5 y + u$, (9.4.2)

where y is blood glucose, y_f is its fasting value, x is the blood insulin level, u and v
are infusion rates of insulin and glucose respectively, and $p_1, ..., p_5$ are

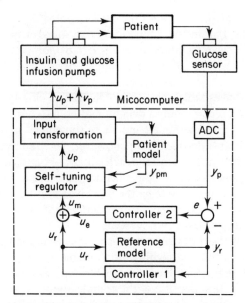

Figure 9.4.2 Schematic diagram of an adaptive and optimal blood glucose control system (from Kondo *et al.*, 1982).

parameters in the model. Controller 1 is designed to minimize the cost function

$$J_r = \Sigma[y_r^2(k) + \rho_r u_r^2(k)], \tag{9.4.3}$$

where y_r and u_r are reference values of blood glucose and insulin infusion respectively and proper choice of ρ_r gives the desired clinical profile. Controller 2 is designed from optimal principles to minimize the output error, $y_p - y_r$, which is caused by errors in initial estimates of parameters and disturbances due to meals. The self-tuning regulator is used to make the input/output relationship of the diabetic subject the same as that of the reference model. To do this requires recursive estimation of the patient parameters, together with updating of the controller law. The scheme has been successfully used in simulation studies including non-linear patient dynamics and in dog trials.

9.5 CONCLUDING REMARKS

The applications involving automated drug administration have demonstrated that a wide range of control techniques are currently being explored in biomedicine. These range from simple on–off control to complex adaptive control schemes. Classical PID, three-term controllers are commonly being used, but suffer from robustness problems when the system dynamics for a particular patient are either unknown or time-varying. Biomedical systems often include pure time delays, which encourages the use of controllers based on the Smith predictor principle. Parameter estimation is an integral part of many adaptive systems, and this may become an important component in the control scheme where knowledge of drug dynamics is a desirable byproduct of regulation.

Measurement of a suitable variable which reflects closely the physiological state to be controlled is commonly a difficult matter. As a result of this, open-loop control based on a predetermined model is sometimes mandatory. The inadequacies of such an approach must, however, be circumvented using techniques such as feedforward and infrequent feedback of sampled information. The majority of applications use linear controller designs, since this reflects the current field of major knowledge in systems theory. Since non-linearity is endemic in biological systems it is clearly desirable that attention should be given to improved design of controllers for such cases.

It is clear that the field of drug administration in biomedicine is fruitful for systems technologists and is stretching the available techniques for the design of adequate feedback regulators. Each control strategy will have to be tailored to the particular application because of the complexity of living dynamic systems. Such tailoring will require interdisciplinary knowledge of systems theory and physiological behaviour. The frontiers of knowledge in both areas should be advanced by such studies. In addition to examples described in this chapter, other areas of automated drug administration include the control of intracranial blood pressure during severe head injury using drugs such as Mannitol (Mason and Price, 1981) and the administration of anticoagulant drugs such as Warfarin (Sheiner, 1969).

D.L.

GLOSSARY OF TERMS

Bayes' estimators: methods of state or parameter estimation based on the well-known Bayes' rule in statistics [see VI, §15.2].

Bode diagram: a graphical plot, using logarithmic scales, of the response of a dynamic system to sinusoidal inputs.

classical feedback design: use of frequency response methods, such as Bode and Nyquist diagrams, to design controller algorithms.

closed-loop control: use of feedback information from a measured output to obtain satisfactory control.

continuous dynamic system: any time-dependent system which can be described by differential equations.

cost function: a function of system variables used to indicate optimal performance, either as a minimum or maximum value.

generalized least squares: a method of parameter estimation based on a least squares technique which does not require that the noise contamination be Gaussian [see VI, §8.2.6].

Kalman filter: a discrete-time algorithm for optimal estimation of parameters and/or states in noise-contaminated data.

maximum likelihood estimation: a technique of parameter estimation which maximizes a likelihood function involving *a posteriori* measurement values based on *a priori* probability density function knowledge of the data [see VI, Chapter 6].

Nyquist diagram: a graphical plot, using polar coordinates, of the frequency response of a dynamic system.

on-line control: application of parameter estimation and control techniques to a dynamic system in real-time ('as it happens').

open-loop control: maintenance of control of a dynamic system without the use of measured output information.

optimal control theory: design of controllers based on the minimization of some cost function.

pseudo-random binary sequence: a continuous signal having only two amplitudes and a random switching pattern between them. The times of switching are determined by the **bit interval** and the **sequence length** [see II, §5.1].

recursive estimators: methods of identification in which estimations are updated sequentially as new data become available.

robustness: the ability of a control algorithm to perform statisfactorily when there are changes in the system dynamics.

root-locus design: a method of classical feedback design based on the roots of a system transfer function.

sampled-data system: a dynamic system described and/or designed using discrete formulation based on difference equations.

self-adaptive control: feedback control in which the controller parameters are adjusted automatically depending on current estimates of the system dynamics.

self-tuning control: a particular form of self-adaptive control involving simultaneous parameter estimation and controller synthesis.

sensitivity analysis: investigation of system robustness by determining performance over a range of parameter values.

state(s): a set of variables whose values determine the behaviour of a dynamic system at any given instant in time.

system dynamics: a mathematical description of a system involving time-dependent behaviour.

system identification (parameter estimation): the determination of parameters and/or states of a dynamic system.

transfer function: definition of a dynamic system based on Laplace transforms and expressed as a ratio of output to input performance.

transient response: the response versus time of a system subjected to input changes such as step transitions.

unit delay operator: a difference equation operator usually related to sampling time which forms the basis of discrete system description and the concept of the z-transformation. If the difference equation uses a time interval Δt then $z(u(t)) = u(t + \Delta t)$, the value of u after a time delay Δt. Likewise $z^{-1}(u(t)) = u(t - \Delta t)$.

REFERENCES

Ackerman, E., Rosevear, J. W., and McGuckin, W. F. (1964). A mathematical model of the glucose-tolerance test, *Phys. in Med. & Biol.*, **9**, 203–213.

Albisser, A. M., and Leibel, B. S. (1977). The artificial pancreas, *Clin. Endocrin & Met.*, **6**, 457–479.

Asbury, A. J., Henderson, P. D., Brown, B. H., Turner, D. J., and Linkens, D. A. (1981). Effect of diazepam on pancuronium-induced neuromuscular blockade maintained by a feedback system, *Br. J. Anaesth.*, **53**, 859–863.

Asbury, A. J., Linkens, D. A., and Rimmer, S. J. (1982). Identification of interacting dynamic effects on muscle paralysis using Ethrane in the presence of pancuronium, *Br. J. Anaesth.*, **54**, 790.

Beneken, J. E. W., Sluijter, M. E., and Blom, J. A. (1974). Computer models of halothane anaesthesia, application leading to servo-anaesthesia, in *Measurement in Anaesthesia* (Eds. S. A. Feldman, J. M. Leigh, and J. Spierdijk), p. 183, Leiden University Press, Leiden.

Bickford, R. G. (1949). Neurophysiological applications of automatic anaesthetic regulator controlled by brain potentials, *Am. J. Physiol.*, **159**, 562.

Billings, S. A., and Harris, C. J. (1981). Self-Tuning and Adaptive Control: Theory and Applications, IEE Control Engineering Series 15, Peter Peregrinus, London.

Brown, B. H., Asbury, A. J., Linkens, D. A., Perks, R., and Anthony, M. (1980). Closed-loop control of muscle relaxation during surgery, *Clin. Phys. Physiol. Meas.*, **1**, 203–310.

Cass, N. M., Lampard, D. G., Brown, W. A., and Coles, J. R. (1976). Computer controlled muscle relaxation: a comparison of four muscle relaxants in sheep, *Anaesth. Intens. Care*, **4**, 16–22.

Chilcoat, R. T. (1980). A review of the control of depth of anaesthesia, *Trans. Inst. M.C.*, **2**, 38–45.

Clarke, D. W. (1967). Generalised least-squares estimation of the parameters of a dynamic model, in *Proceedings IFAC Symp. Identification in Automatic Control Systems*, Prague, paper 3.17.

Clarke, D. W., and Gawthrop, P. J. (1975). Self-tuning controller, *Proc. IEE*, **122** 929–934.

Coles, J. R., Brown, W. A., and Lampard, D. G. (1973). Computer control of respiration and anaesthesia. *Med. Biol. Eng.*, **11**, 262–267.

Davies, W. L., Evans, J. M., Fraser, A. C. L., and Barclay, M. (1982). Closed-loop control of anaesthesia. Inst. M.C. Symp. on *Control Systems Concepts and Approaches in Clinical Medicine*, pp. 87–90, *Inst. M.C.*, London.

Eykhoff, P. (1974). *System Identification: Parameter and State Estimation*, Chap. 6, 7, Wiley, New York.

Gawthrop, P. J. (1977). Some interpretations of the self-tuning controller. *Proc. IEE*, **124**, 889–894.

Jacobs, O. L. R., Bullingham, R. E. S., Davies, W. L., Reasbeck, M. P. (1981). Feedback control of post-operative pain. IEE Conf. Pub. 194 '*Control and its Applications*', pp. 52–56, IEE, London.

Jacobs, O. L. R., Bullingham, R. E. S., McQuay, H. J., and Reasbeck, M. P. (1982). On-line estimation in the control of post-operative pain, in Proceedings 6th IFAC Symp. on *Identification and System Parameter Estimation*, Washington.

Kadish, A. H. (1964). The regulation and control of blood sugar level. Physiological and cybernetic simulation, in *Technicon International Symposium*, New York, pp. 82–85.

Kline, N. S., Shimano, E., Stearns, H., McWilliams, L., Kohn, M., and Blair, J. H. (1968). Technique for automatic in-vivo regulation of blood sugar. *Med. Res. Eng.*, Second Quarter, 14–19.

Kondo, K., Sano, A., Kikuchi, M., Sakurai, Y. (1982). Adaptive and optimal blood glucose control system designed via state space approach, in Proceedings Inst. M.C. Symp. on *Control Systems Concepts and Approaches in Clinical Medicine*, pp. 103–106, Inst. M.C., London.

Linkens, D. A., Asbury, A. J., Brown, B. H., Rimmer, S. J. (1981). Identification of the model in the control of neuromuscular blockade using **PRBS** testing, *Br. J. Anaesth.*, **53**, 666.

Linkens, D. A., Asbury, A. J., Rimmer, S. J., and Menad, M. (1982a). Identification and control of muscle relaxant anaesthesia, *Proc. IEE*, **129**, 136–141.

Linkens, D. A., Asbury, A. J., Rimmer, S. J., and Menad, M. (1982b). Self-tuning control of muscle relaxation during anaesthesia, in Proceedings IEEE Conf. on *Applications of Adaptive and Multivariable Control*, Hull, 96–102.

Mapleson, W. W., Allott, P. R., and Steward, A. (1974). A non-feedback technique for programmed anaesthesia. *Br. J. Anaesth.*, **46**, 805.

Mapleson, W. W., Chilcoat, R. T., Lunn, J. N., Blewett, M. C., Khatib, M. T. and Willis, B. A. (1980). Computer assistance in the control of depth of anaesthesia. *Br. J. Anaesth.*, **52**, 234.

Marshall, J. E. (1979). *The Control of Time-Delay Systems*, Chap. 6, IEE Control Eng. Series, Peter Peregrinus, London, England.

Mason, J. and Price, D. J. (1981). The control of intracranial pressure, IEE Coloquium on *Control Techniques in Anaesthesia and Drug Administration*, Digest No. 1981/45, Itt, London.

Pickup, J. C., and Keen, H. (1980). Continuous subcutaneous insulin infusion: a developing tool in diabetes research. *Diabetologia*, **18**, 1–4.

Pickup, J. C., White, M. C., Keen, H., Kohner, E. M., Parsons, J. A. Albert, K. G. M. M. (1979). Long term continuous subcutaneous insulin infusion in diabetics at home. *Lancet*, **II**, 870–873.

Reasbeck, M. P. (1982). Modelling and control of post-operative pain. D. Phil. Thesis, Oxford University.

Sheiner, L. C. (1969). Computer-aided long term anticoagulation therapy. *Comput. Biomed. Res.*, **2**, 507–518.

Sheppard, L. C., and Sayers, B. McA. (1977). Dynamic analysis of the blood pressure response to hypotensive agents, studied in post-operative cardiac surgical patients. *Comput. Biomed. Res.*, **10**, 237–246.

Sheppard, L. C., Shotts, J. F., Roberson, N. F., Wallace, F. D., and Kouchoukos, N. T. (1979). Computer-controlled infusion of vasoactive drugs in post cardiac surgical patients, in Proc. First Ann. Conf. IEEE *Eng. in Medicine & Biology Society*, Denver Colorado, pp. 280–284.

Slate, J. B. (1980). Model-based design of a controller for infusing sodium nitroprusside during post surgical hypertension. Ph.D. thesis, University of Alabama, Birmingham.

Slate, J. B., Sheppard, L. C., Rideout, V. C., and Blackstone, E. H. (1979). A model for design of a blood pressure controller for hypertensive patients. *5th IFAC Symp. Ident. & Sys. Par. Est.*, Darmstadt, F. R. Germany, pp. 867–874.

Smith, O. J. M. (1957). Closer control of loops with dead-time. *Chem. Eng. Prog.*, **53**, 217–219.

Smith, N. T., and Schwede, H. O. (1972). The response of arterial pressure to halothane: a systems analysis. *Med. Biol. Eng.*, **10**, 207–221.

Suppan, P. (1972). Feedback monitoring in anaesthesia. II: pulse rate control of halothane administration. *Br. J. Anaesth.*, **44**, 1263–1271.

Tatnall, M. L., and Morris, P. (1977). Simulation of halothane anaesthesia in neonates, in *Biomedical Computing* (Ed. W. J. Perkins), Chap. 31, Pitman Medical, London.

Tatnall, M. L., Morris, P., and West, P. G. (1981). Controlled anaesthesia: an approach using patient characteristics identified during uptake. *Br. J. Anaesth.*, **53**, 1019–1026.

Wellstead, P. E., Prager, D., and Zanker, P. (1979). Pole-assignment self-tuning regulator. *Proc. IEE*, **126**, 781–787.

Wellstead, P. E., and Sanoff, S. P. (1981). Extended self-tuning algorithm. *Int. J. Contr.*, **34**, 434–455.

White, W. P., Pearce, D. J., and Norman, M. (1979). Post-operative analgesia. *B.M.J.*, **ii**, 166–167.

Ziegler, J. G., and Nichols, N. B. (1942). Optimum settings for automatic controllers. *Trans. Am. Soc. Mech. Eng.*, **64**, 759.

Mathematical Methods in Medicine
Edited by D. Ingram & R. F. Bloch
© 1984 John Wiley & Sons Ltd.

10

Linear Graphs: an Approach to the Solution of Systems of Linear Equations

10.1 INTRODUCTION

Living organisms are never static; change is the very essence of life. Mathematical models of living processes must therefore be able to represent and quantify rates of change. A major theme of Part II of this Guidebook is the formulation of mathematical models applicable to clinical measurements of various kinds. We therefore describe here an approach to linear systems analysis, based on graphical techniques, which has been found helpful by less mathematically versed medical researchers.

The temporal rate of change of a variable $x(t)$ is denoted by dx/dt [see IV, §3.1.1]. Many biological processes can be described or approximated by a first-order relationship of the form

$$\frac{dx}{dt} = ax + b(t), \tag{10.1.1}$$

where a is a constant, or is effectively constant within a certain range of values of x, and $b(t)$ is some function of time [see IV, §7.2].

Biological processes rarely occur as simple isolated systems and so we must often consider the dynamic interactions of multiple systems. As long as each variable and its interaction with others can be described by linear relationships then the process may be modelled by a set of first-order linear differential equations [see IV, §7.9] of the form

$$\frac{dx_1}{dt} = a_{11}x_1 + a_{12}x_2 + \cdots + a_{1n}x_n + b_1(t),$$

$$\frac{dx_2}{dt} = a_{21}x_1 + a_{22}x_2 + \cdots + a_{2n}x_n + b_2(t),$$

$$\vdots$$

$$\frac{dx_n}{dt} = a_{n1}x_1 + a_{n2}x_2 \cdots + a_{nn}x_n + b_n(t). \tag{10.1.2}$$

431

Linear systems of interest in biology and medicine tend to be somewhat simpler in form than (10.1.2) since commonly many of the elements of the matrix $[a_{ij}]$ are in fact zero. Use of the general algorithms for manipulating sparse matrices [see III, §4.12] is not efficient in calculation effort and may introduce unnecessary numerical errors. The method of linear graphs is particularly suitable for such sparse systems.

10.2 THE LAPLACE TRANSFORM

The Laplace transform [see IV, §13.4] of the continuous variable $x(t)$ is defined by

$$\bar{x}(s) = \int_0^\infty e^{-qs} x(t)\,dt. \tag{10.2.1}$$

This is often written in the notation

$$\bar{x}(s) = \mathcal{L}[x(t)]$$

and

$$x(t) = \mathcal{L}^{-1}[\bar{x}(s)].$$

Properties of the Laplace transform which make it particularly useful in solving linear systems are

$$\mathcal{L}\left[\frac{dx}{dt}\right] = s\bar{x}(s) - x(0), \tag{10.2.2}$$

where $x(0)$ is the value of $x(t)$ at time zero, and also

$$\mathcal{L}[ax(t) + by(t)] = a\mathcal{L}x(t) + b\mathcal{L}y(t), \tag{10.2.3}$$

which means that it is a linear operator for constant a and b. As discussed in Chapter 7, a set of linear ordinary differential equations in the time domain may be translated into a set of simultaneous algebraic equations in the Laplace domain. These are solved algebraically and the solution in the Laplace domain is then transformed back (inverted), if possible using standard tables of inverse transforms, to yield the solution in the time domain.

10.3 LINEAR GRAPHS: NOTATION AND RULES FOR GRAPH REDUCTION

We now develop a graphical notation (Mason, 1953, and Lorens, 1964), which may be used to express algebraic relationships among variables. Certain rules used in simplifying algebraic expressions will be analysed as graph operations. These tools will then enable us to set up a graph depicting a set of linear first-order differential equations in the Laplace domain and provide the basis of techniques for reducing the graph to solve for the particular variable or variables of interest.

The linear relationship between two variables x and y,

$y = Ax,$

can be described graphically in the form

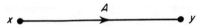

referred to as a *digraph*, where x and y are represented by two nodes and the factor A by an arrow connecting the two nodes [see V, Chapter 6]. The variables x, y and A are time-dependent. A is often referred to as a transfer function [see the Appendix to Chapter 5].

The expression

$z = Ax + By$

can be depicted graphically in the form

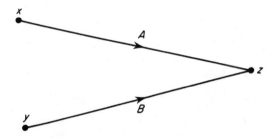

and this can easily be generalized for multiple digraphs incident at node z.

In solving or reducing linear graphs, we make use of algebraic relationships which have useful graphical correlates which help us to simplify or 'reduce' the graph and, by this process, arrive at a solution of the system.

There are four of these:

(a) *The serial-associative rule*
   Algebraically this rule tells us that

   if $y = Ax$
   and $z = By$
   then $z = BAx.$

   In graphical terms, the graph $x \xrightarrow{A} y \xrightarrow{B} z$ may be reduced

to the graph

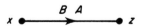

(b) *The parallel-associative rule*

This tells us algebraically that

$$Ax + Bx = (A + B)x.$$

In graphical terms, the graph

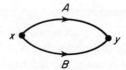

may be reduced to

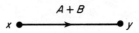

(c) *The distributive rule*

Algebraically,

if $z = Ax + By$

and $v = Cz$

then $v = CAx + CBy$.

In graphical terms,

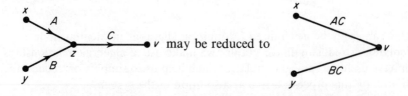

This may readily be generalized for any number of digraphs incident at a given node.

(d) *The feedback rule*

Algebraically, we may describe a feedback relationship in the form

$$z = Ax + Cz. \tag{10.3.1}$$

A proportion of the variable z feeds back as an input to the process determining the value of z. This may be visualized as a black box where z is an output and x and z are inputs.

The algebraic solution for z as a function of x is

$$z = A(1 - C)^{-1}x. \tag{10.3.2}$$

Graphically, we may depict the alternative algebraic expressions (10.3.1) and (10.3.2) as two equivalent graphs,

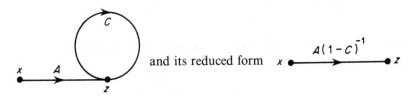

Once again we may generalize for multiple incident digraphs. In graphical terms, for two input variables x and y, the graph

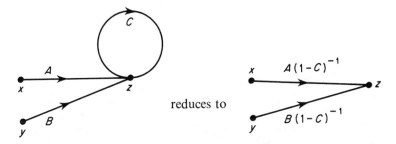

A system of linear equations such as (10.1.2) can be depicted as a graph where the nodes represent variables and the transfer functions are the coefficients. To show how the graphical formalism can be used in practice, we give a fully worked example of the three-compartment model.

10.4 SOLUTION OF A THREE-COMPARTMENT MODEL USING A LINEAR GRAPH

We consider here the solution of the system of linear differential equations arising in the mathematical description of a typical three-compartment model. Chapters 7 and 8 have given examples of the use of such models in pharmacokinetics and nuclear medicine. The treatment here is brief and aims only to demonstrate the application of the foregoing techniques of graph reduction to the solution of the equations.

In Figure 10.4.1 we depict the model. Drug concentrations are denoted by x, y and z. Rate constants determining flow of drug between compartments are depicted by a, b, c and d as shown. Input of drug is described by the function $g(t)$. Elimination of drug is determined by the rate constants e and f as shown.

Comparing the treatments in Section 7.2, the model gives rise to the set of linear

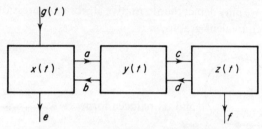

Figure 10.4.1 A three-compartment model with input $g(t)$. The flow between compartments is determined by rate constants a, b, c and d; the loss from the system by rate constants e and f.

differential equations:

$$\frac{dx}{dt} = -(a + e)x + by + g(t),$$

$$\frac{dy}{dt} = ax - (b + c)y + dz, \tag{10.4.1}$$

$$\frac{dz}{dt} = cy - (d + f)z.$$

Applying the Laplace transform to both sides of the equations and using (10.2.2), we have the following system of algebraic equations:

$$(a + e + s)\bar{x} = b\bar{y} + \bar{g} + x(0),$$
$$(b + c + s)\bar{y} = a\bar{x} + d\bar{z} + y(0), \tag{10.4.2}$$
$$(d + f + s)\bar{z} = c\bar{y} + z(0).$$

To simplify the graph notation, we substitute the variables

$$x^* = (a + e + s)\bar{x},$$
$$y^* = (b + c + s)\bar{y},$$
$$z^* = (d + f + s)\bar{z}. \tag{10.4.3}$$

Equations (10.4.2) can then be rewritten as

$$x^* = Ay^* + \bar{g} + x(0),$$
$$y^* = Bx^* + Cz^* + y(0), \tag{10.4.4}$$
$$z^* = Dy^* + z(0),$$

with $A = (b + c + s)^{-1}b,$

$B = (a + e + s)^{-1}a,$

$C = (d + f + s)^{-1}d,$

and $D = (b + c + s)^{-1}c.$

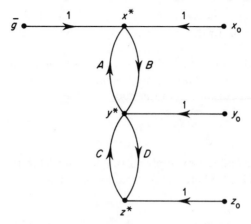

Figure 10.4.2 Representation of the three-compartment model as a linear graph.

We may now use linear graph techniques to solve this set of equations. We first set up a graph (Figure 10.4.2) depicting the system of equations (10.4.4).

Solutions of interest show the dependence of one or more of the unknown dependent variables (x^*, y^*, z^*) on the known independent variables $(\bar{g}, x(0), y(0), z(0))$ and the constants (a, b, c, d, e, f).

The linear system in the Laplace domain (10.4.4), represented by the above graph, can be solved by systematic graph reduction operations leading to a fully reduced graph (Figure 10.4.3) which relates the variable of interest, say x^*, to the independent variables via the transfer functions, Q^*, R^*, S^* and T^*. Algebraically this gives a solution of the form:

$$x^* = Q^*\bar{g} + R^*x(0) + S^*y(0) + T^*z(0) \tag{10.4.5}$$

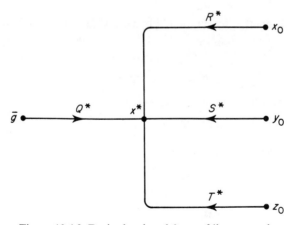

Figure 10.4.3 Desired reduced form of linear graph.

In many situations, one starts out with a system which is undisturbed, i.e. $x(0) = y(0) = z(0) = 0$. In this case it is only necessary to calculate the transfer function Q^*.

Having decided upon the variable for which we want to find the solution (e.g. x^*), we proceed in stages by progressively eliminating one node at a time, starting with the node most distant from the node of interest.

Stage 1

We first eliminate node z^* by applying rules (c) and (a) to the section of graph below node y^*. This leads to the first reduction (Figure 10.4.4).

Stage 2

We next eliminate the feedback loop at node y^* by applying rule (d). In doing so, we note that three digraphs (from x^*, $y(0)$ and $z(0)$) are incident on y^*. This results in a further reduced graph (Figure 10.4.5).

Stage 3

In a similar manner, we eliminate node y^* by application of rules (c) and (a). We substitute the variable

$$F = (1 - CD)^{-1}. \tag{10.4.6}$$

All three digraphs incident at y^* must be transferred to node x^* (Figure 10.4.6).

Stage 4

The feedback loop at x^* is eliminated by rule (d) (Figure 10.4.7), where we write

$$G = (1 - ABF)^{-1}. \tag{10.4.7}$$

Algebraically, this graph can be expressed as

$$x^* = G\bar{g} + Gx(0) + AFGy(0) + ACFGz(0).$$

We can now use (10.4.3) and obtain

$$\bar{x} = Q\bar{g} + Qx(0) + Ry(0) + Tz(0), \tag{10.4.8}$$

where $Q = (a + e + s)^{-1} G,$

$$R = (a + e + s)^{-1} AFG, \tag{10.4.9}$$

$$T = (a + e + s)^{-1} ACFG.$$

where A, B, C, D, F and G have been defined in (10.4.4), (10.4.6) and (10.4.7).

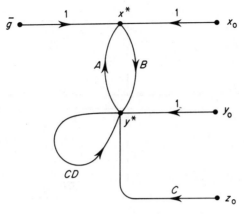

Figure 10.4.4 Linear graph after step 1.

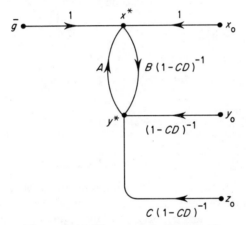

Figure 10.4.5 Linear graph after step 2.

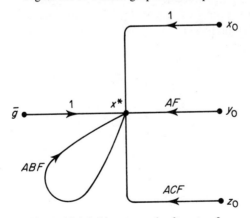

Figure 10.4.6 Linear graph after step 3.

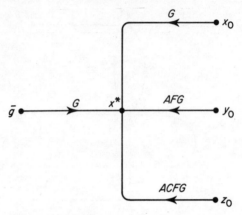

Figure 10.4.7 Linear graph after step 4 (final reduction).

Back-substitution results in

$$Q = \frac{(b + c + s)(d + f + s) - cd}{(a + e + s)[(b + c + s)(d + f + s) - cd] - ab(d + f + s)},$$

$$R = \frac{b(d + f + s)}{(a + e + s)[(b + c + s)(d + f + s) - cd] - ab(d + f + s)}, \qquad (10.4.10)$$

$$T = \frac{bd}{(a + e + s)[(b + c + s)(d + f + s) - cd] - ab(d + f + s)}.$$

The denominator in all three expressions is a polynomial of degree 3 in s. Except for special degenerate values of a, b, c, d, e and f, it will have three distinct zeros, which we designate α_1, α_2 and α_3. Because of the nature of the system these roots will be real and negative [see I, §§14.1 and 14.8]. The expressions represent proper rational functions [see I, §14.10]. They can therefore be expanded into partial fractions in the forms

$$Q = \sum_{i=1}^{3} \frac{q_i}{s - \alpha_i},$$

$$R = \sum_{i=1}^{3} \frac{r_i}{s - d_i}, \qquad (10.4.11)$$

$$T = \sum_{i=1}^{3} \frac{t_i}{s - \alpha_i},$$

where the q_i, r_i and t_i are constants.

We will examine the solution of equation (10.4.1) for two different driving function $g(t)$, representing continuous infusion (step function) and bolus input (delta function) respectively.

(a) *Step function input.* Here $g(t) = 1$ for $t > 0$. Then $\bar{g}(s) = \mathcal{L}[g(t)] = 1/s$ [see IV, §13.4]. The solution for $\bar{x}(s)$ is therefore, from (10.4.8),

$$\bar{x}(s) = \frac{1}{s}Q + Qx(0) + Ry(0) + Tz(0).$$

Since

$$\frac{1}{s(s-\alpha)} = \frac{1}{\alpha}\left[\frac{1}{s-\alpha} - \frac{1}{s}\right],$$

using (10.4.11) we have

$$\bar{x}(s) = \sum_{i=1}^{3}\left[\frac{q_i}{\alpha_i} + q_i x(0) + r_i y(0) + t_i z(0)\right]\frac{1}{s-\alpha_i} - \left(\frac{q_1}{\alpha_1} + \frac{q_2}{\alpha_2} + \frac{q_3}{\alpha_3}\right)\frac{1}{s}.$$

(10.4.12)

In the time domain, the solution is [see IV, §13.4]

$$x(t) = \sum_{i=1}^{3}\left[\frac{q_i}{\alpha_i} + q_i x(0) + r_i y(0) + t_i z(0)\right]e^{\alpha_i t} - \left(\frac{q_1}{\alpha_1} + \frac{q_2}{\alpha_2} + \frac{q_3}{\alpha_3}\right).$$

(10.4.13)

(b) *Bolus input.* Here $g(t)$ is an impulse function at time $t = 0$ with $\int_{0}^{\infty} g(t)dt = 1$ and using the definition of the Laplace transform [see IV, §13.4]:

$$\bar{g}(s) = \mathcal{L}[g(t)] = 1.$$

Therefore, (10.4.8) becomes

$$x(s) = \sum_{i=1}^{3}[q_i(1 + x(0)) + r_i y(0) + t_i z(0)]\frac{1}{s-\alpha_i},$$

(10.4.14)

which transforms back to

$$x(t) = \sum_{i=1}^{3}[q_i(1 + x(0)) + r_i y(0) + t_i z(0)]e^{\alpha_i t}.$$

(10.4.15)

For the degenerate case, where there are not three distinct roots, α_1, α_2 and α_3, the solution differ slightly [see IV, §13.4].

The reduction of linear systems by means of the graphical methods described in this chapter involves essentially the same manipulations as are traditionally performed algebraically. The major advantage of using the graphical method is that it gives a visual overview of the complex process and enables one to choose strategically those operations which most directly lead to the desired solution. A further application of the technique will be given in Chapter 8 of Part II of the Guidebook, where the modelling of uptake of inhaled anaesthetic agents is considered.

REFERENCES

Lorens, C. S. (1964). *Flowgraphs*, McGraw-Hill, New York.
Mason, S. J. (1953). Feedback theory: some properties of signal flow graphs, *Proc. IREEE*, **41**, 1144–1156.

R.F.B.
D.I.

Index

Absorption isotherm 322
Accuracy 275
Actuarial method 139
Adaptive control 409, 412
Admixture 183, 184
Adsorption isotherms 355
Affinity profile 337, 347
Albinism 173
ALGOL 105
Allele distribution 161, 179
Allele frequency 164–8, 175, 179, 180, 185, 187
Alternative hypothesis 33
Alveolar ventilation 416
Anaesthesia control 413–22
Analogue signals 227
Analogue-to-digital converter (ADC) 256–7
Analysis of covariance (ANCOVA) 75, 86–8
Analysis of covariance (ANCOVA) table 87
Analysis of variance (ANOVA) 69–73, 286
  Friedman two-way 75
  Kruskal–Wallis one-way 75–6
  many-way 76
  non-orthogonal missing values 79–81
  non-parametric 75
  one-way 71
  two-way 73–6, 79
Analysis of variance (ANOVA) table 71, 72, 74, 76, 77
Analytical method comparisons 293–4
Analytical techniques 283–4
1-Anilino-8-naphthalene sulphonate 352–5
Anorexics 36
APL 105

a posteriori probabilities 231
Arcsine transformation 91
Area-under-the-concentration-time curve 322
Arterial pressure waves 238–9
Artificial intelligence 149
Ascertainment 194, 205, 209
Ascertainment bias 196
Ascertainment probability 196, 205, 209
Assay 275
Assay bias 288
Assay imprecision 289–91, 301
Assay performance 291, 296
Assay run 275, 295–7
Association constants 350, 352, 355
Asymptotic relative efficiency (ARE) 53
Attributable risk 192
Attributes 42
Auto-covariance function 260, 262
Auto-regressive filters 263
Availability concept 328
Average 12
AZTEC algorithm 243

Back-stripping 323
Background corrections 370
Bahadur expansion 146
Bartlett's test 96, 97
BASIC 105, 418
Bayes' independence model 140, 143–6, 156
Bayes' theorem 25, 55, 140, 230–2, 419–21
Bayesian analysis 64
Bayesian inference 55
Bayesian methods 55
Becquerels 362

Berkson's bias 59
Between-subject variation 10
Between-treatment variation 10
Bias 22, 99, 210, 275, 288
Bias assessment 300
Binary data 11
Binomial distribution 17, 25, 45
Binomial theorem 17
Bio-assay data analysis 285–6
Bio-equivalence 329
Biological half-time 386
Biological rhythms 279–83
Biological samples 277–83
Biological signal processing 225–72
    stages of 226
Block design 75
Blood clotting factor X levels 208
Blood flow 393–403
    regional 401–3
    to individual organ 399–401
    traces studies 383
Blood glucose levels 422–5
Blood pressure, post-operative control of
    410–13
Blood pressure measurements 10
Blood volume measurement 397–9
Blunder index 302
BMDP (Biomedical Computer Package)
    106
BMDP3F computer program 92–3
BMDP7M computer program 99
Bode diagram 407
Bovine plasma albumin 352
Box and whisker plot 23
Branching ratio 362

Calibration factors 366
Canonical correlations 100
Cardiac output 395–7
    measurement of 397–9, 416
Case-control study 57, 58
Categorical data 91–4
Categories 11, 12
Catheterization laboratory 249–50
Cauchy distribution 54
Censored observations 102
Central limit theorem 20, 28, 45
Central tendency 13
Centroids 100
Chebyshev polynomials 268
Chebyshev transformation 268–9

Chi-square for trend 91
Chi-squared distribution 21, 177, 179
Chi-squared test 25, 27, 40–3, 46, 66, 68,
    91, 102, 144, 184, 192
Chondrodystrophy 173
Circadian rhythm 279–80
Circulation index 396, 399
Classical discriminant analysis 98
Classification rule 137
Clearance concept 329
Clinical algorithms 141
Clinical decision-making 119, 124–9, 149
Clinical decision problem 120–2
Clinical laboratory
    mathematics in 274
    role of 273–4
Clinical life table 102
Clinical trials 56
Closed-loop control 410, 423
Cluster analysis 101, 142
Clusters, 101, 252, 254
Cobalt-57 isotopes 367–8
Cobalt-58 isotopes 367–8
Coefficient of kinship 183
Coefficient of variation 275, 364, 365
Coherent averaging 266–7
Cohort studies 57, 58
Compartmental analysis 308–23, 383–93
    first-order absorption 314
    fundamental assumptions 308
    multiple dosing 320–1
    non-linear systems 321–3
    rapid intravenous injection 309
    theory of 385
    tracer studies 383–93
Compartmental models 307, 309
    catenary system 384
    closed single system 385
    closed system 383
    general input and output 317–20
    mamillary system 384
    open single system 385–7
    open system 383
    open two-compartment mamillary
        system 389–91
    solution using linear graph 435–42
    three-compartment 435–42
    two-compartment open 309, 314–17
Competing risks 103
Complex conjugate spectrum 262
Component mountains 148

Computation 103–10
Computer-assisted intensive care 251–4
Computer-assisted response curve
    regeneration 285
Computer-assisted systems 245
Computer programming languages 105
Computer programs 92, 94, 95, 99, 102,
    105–8, 149, 213, 344
Computers 108–10
    abuses of 109–10
    uses of 108–9
Concurrent processes 226
Conditional distribution 421
Conditional probability 25, 138, 207, 231
Confidence interval 43–5, 50
Confidence limits 30, 43–5, 49, 66, 67, 73,
    89, 286
    for the mean 43
    of a variance 45
Contingency tables 41–3, 89, 91, 92, 102,
    140, 141, 144, 145, 152, 177–9, 185
Continuity correction 46, 89
Continous data 18
Continous flow analysis 285
Continuous subcutaneous insulin infusion
    (CSII) 423
Continuous system model 407
Control chart 296, 297
Control law 422
Control loop 299, 405
Control systems 405–30
    glossary of terms 426–8
Controlled comparative trial 57
Controlled variables 58
Controls 57–9
Convolution 262, 377
Cook's distance 51
Coronary care 252–4
Corrected level of significance 178
Correcting for the mean 104
Correction factors 285
Correlation 52–3
Correlation analysis 407
Correlation coefficient 52–3, 68, 92, 293,
    295
Correlation matrix 96, 97
Counting measurements 364–5
Counting statistics 364
Covariance 260
Covariance function 260, 261
Covariance matrix 241, 381, 409

Covariates 86
Cox's method 102, 103
Cox's model 102, 103
Cross-correlation 234, 410
Cross-correlation matrix 241
Cross-covariance function 260
Cross-sectional studies 57, 58
Cross-spectrum 261
Cross-talk factors 368
Cross-validation 99
Çrossover designs 56
Crossover trials 58, 61–3
Comulative frequency distribution 24, 92
Cumulative sum techniques 297
Curies 362
Curvature index 286
Curvature significance 286
Curve-fitting 291, 295
Curve-fitting validity 286–8
Curve processing 369
Curve-smoothing 375–7

Data checking 109
Data exploration 109
Data reduction techniques 243
Data screening 108
Daughter atoms 362–3
Dead time zone 231
Decision analysis 127, 132
Decision comparisons 56
Decision-making 124, 128
Decision-making programs 324
Decision matrix 230
Decision problems 124, 128, 155
Decision space 54
Decision table 411
Decision theory 34, 54, 122, 124–36, 155
Decision tree 124, 130, 131, 133, 137
Deconvolution 377–80
Degrees of freedom 21, 35, 37, 42, 66, 70,
    73, 169
Descriptive statistics 12, 13, 15
Detection window 231
Deterministic signals 226
Diagnosis 122–3, 144, 145, 149–52, 246
    mathematical methods 136–49
Diagnostic nuclear medicine 361
Diagnostic rule 150–2, 156
Diagnostic systems, performance
    measurement 154–6
Diagnostic–therapeutic loop 225

Dichotomy 11
Dichrotic notch in arterial pressure
    waveform 238–9
Dicopac test 367
Digital filters 263–5
Digital signals 227
Digraphs 433, 435
Dilution analysis 385
Dirac delta function 318
Dirac impulse 227, 263, 264
Discordant pairs 47
Discrete data 11
Discrete deconvolution 378
Discrete distributions 16–18
Discrete scale 152
Discrete variables 12
Discriminant analysis 98–9, 123, 136–41
Discriminant function 98, 99
Discrimination level 241
Disease classes 122
Dispersion 255
Disposition coefficients 314
Distribution 15–27
    continuous variable 18
    see also under specific types
Distribution-free. *See* Non-parametric
    methods
Distribution function 317–19
Distributive rule 434
Dopamine β-hydroxylase activity 208
Dose-response curve 286, 288
Double blindness 59
Drift 180, 184, 291, 293
Drug absorption 307, 314–17, 323–4
Drug administration 418, 426
    control techniques 405–30
Drug availability 328–30
Drug binding 330
Drug clearance 328–30
Drug concentration 308, 318, 348, 435
Drug distribution 307, 348
Drug elimination 307, 310, 314
Drug-induced muscle relaxation 416–17
Drug-induced unconsciousness 413–16
Drug kinetics 308
Drug metabolism 328, 411
Drug–patient factors 328
Drug–protein binding 349–54
Drug–receptor interactions 307, 355
Drug sensitivity factors 411
Drug transport 328

Dual isotope counting 365–6
Dual isotope vitamin B12 absorption test
    367
Dummy values 80
Dummy variable 81
Dynamic function tests 280–3

Effective renal plasma flow (ERPF)
    determination 391–3
Eigenvalues 97
Eigenvectors 97, 381
Electrocardiogram analysis 249
Electrocardiogram segmentation 243–4
Electrocardiograms 240–3
Electroencephalogram analysis 250–1
Electroencephalogram histograms 253
Electroencephalogram segmentation 244–5
Electromyograph (BMG) 416
Elston model 209
Enzyme-catalysed reactions 355–6
Equality of variance 78
Ergodic signals 255, 256
Error combination 277–8, 283, 364–5
Errors 10, 150–4
    Type I 32–4
    Type II 32–4, 60, 89
    see also Random error; Standard error
Estimation 28–30, 40
Ethical problems 23, 59
Exchangeable sodium determination 387–9
Expected utility 131–2
Expected value 126
Expected weight of evidence 150
Explanatory variables 12
Exponential curve stripping 374–5
Exponential decay 362
Extended Kalman filter 418, 419, 421–2
Extended least squares 409
Extraction ratio 400

F distribution 22, 38, 70
F test 101
Factor analysis 99–100
Factorial experiments 77
False negative error rate 150
False positive error rate 150
Feathering 323
Feature likelihoods 146–8
Features 137
Feedback control 406–10, 413, 415
Feedback loop gain 412

Feedback rule 434
Feedback system analysis and design 406
Fick principle 400
Fisher's exact test 46
Fishing expeditions 109
Fitted sums of squares 71
Flog 91
Flowcharts 141
Foetal heart rate patterns 244
Folded log 91
Folded square root 91
Forgetting factor 409
FORTRAN 105, 106
Fourfold table 42
Fourier expansion 265
Fourier transform 258, 261, 262, 264, 378
Fractional rate constant 386
Frequency distribution 15, 28
Frequency of recombination 194, 210, 211, 214
Frequency of transmission 194
Frequency spectrum 240–1, 258, 259, 261, 263
Friedman two-way ANOVA 75
Froot 91
Full model 70
Full multinomial method 139
Function laboratories 246–51

Galactosaemia 174
Gametic association 185
Gamma distribution 382
Gamma-emitting nuclides 366
Gamma function fit 383
Gamma probability plots 97
Gamma-variate fit 382
Gauss–Newton programs 345
Gaussian distribution 20, 50, 98, 276
Gene counting 166, 185
Gene frequency 161, 163–5, 174–7, 180
Gene hypothesis 207–9
General linear models 86
Generalized control loop 299
Generalized least squares 409
Genetic analysis 161, 206
Genetic correlation 203
Genetic difference 184
Genetic disorders 193–4
Genetic distance 162, 179–84
Genetic drift 185
Genetic heterogeneity 206, 209

Genetic hypotheses 193–214
Genetic load 171
Genetic locus 177
Genetic markers 184, 189
Genetics 161–223
    glossary of terms 214
Genotype distribution 161, 165, 169, 170, 171, 177–80
Genotype frequency 161, 171, 174, 177, 184
Genotypes 161
GENSTAT 106
Geometric mean 44
GLIM (General Linear Interactive Modelling) 107
Glucose tolerance test 281
Goodness of fit 166–7, 204, 206, 209, 324, 371
Group matching 58

Half-life 362
Half-Normal plot 50
Haplotype frequency 187
Hardy–Weinberg equilibrium 165, 168, 170, 186
Hardy–Weinberg theorem 162–76
    application of 163–6
Hazard function 102, 103
Heart function 248
Heavy-tailed distribution 21
Height analysis 208
Hepatic clearance 329
Heritability 194, 201–5
Heteroscedasticity 346
Hill plot 343, 347
Histogram 19, 24, 290
Historical controls 58
Homoscedasticity 48
Hotelling's T^2 statistic 101
Hypercholesteraemia 208
Hypertriglyceridaemia 208
Hypothesis testing 30–2, 40, 46

Identification (parameter estimation) techniques 326, 407
Immuno-assay optimization 285
Immunology 161
Imprecision 275
Imprecision measurement 301
Impulse response 263, 264, 266, 410
Impulse response function 377, 378, 380

Impulse retention function 379, 394, 395, 402

Inaccuracy 275

Inbreeding coefficient 169, 172

Inbreeding effects 169–71

Independence 17–18, 92, 143–6

Independent variables 17

Indicants 137, 140, 142

Individual matching 58

Intensive care 251–4

Interactions 62, 79

Inter-quartile range (IQR) 14, 23

Inter-subject variability 10, 226

Interval estimation 43–5

Interval scale 11

Intra-assay 275

Intra-subject variability 10, 225

Intra-uterine pressure 252

Intrinsic error 275

Iodine-131 labelled hippuran 391

IQ inheritance 201

Iterative techniques 80, 345

Jack-knife 99

Joint probability 231

Kalman filter 245, 299, 408, 409, 419, 422
    extended 418, 419, 421–2

Kalman gain vector 408

Kappa statistic 153

Karhunen–Loeve expansion 267–8

Kendall's coefficient of correlation (tau) 53, 92

Kernel-based procedures 147–8

Kolmogorov–Smirnov statistic 24

Kolmogorov–Smirnov test 25, 39

Kruskal–Wallis one-way ANOVA 75–6

Kurtosis 21, 65, 109

Laboratory logistics 276–7

Laboratory medicine 273–306

Lancaster models 146

Langmuir binding isotherm 322

Laplace transform 264, 309, 312, 316, 317, 319, 320, 378, 432, 436

Latent class models 146

Latin squares 47, 75, 79, 80, 294, 369, 370–4

Least squares fit to exponential curve 373–4

Least squares identification 407

Least squares regression techniques 67, 280, 287, 345, 346

Least squares spectral analysis 280

Levey–Jennings control chart 296, 297

Life tables 102

Ligand binding. *See* Protein ligand binding

Ligand macromolecule interactions 352

Likelihood 25–6, 140, 146–8, 150, 196

Likelihood function 64, 421

Likelihood ratio 53, 200, 207, 210, 231

Linear analogue scales 136

Linear contrast 72

Linear discriminant function 98, 142

Linear effects 78

Linear equations 431–42

Linear graphs 431–42
    notation and rules for graph reduction 432–5
    solution of three-compartment model 435–42

Linear model 47

Linear regression 47, 284

Linear standard curves 284

Linear systems 431

Linearity 301

Linearity transformation 49

Linkage analysis 212

Linkage disequilibrium 162, 184–9

Linkage studies 194, 209–14

Location 19
    measures of 13

Lods score 210–3

Log likelihood 20, 206

Log–linear models 92, 146

Log-rank test 102

Logarithmic score 155

Logistic difference 90

Logistic discriminant 140, 143, 148–9

Logistic distribution 91

Logistic regression 86, 90

Logistic transform 90

Logit 90, 91

Logit transform 91

Lung perfusion scanning 402

M estimates 24

MACDOPE model 327

McNemar's test 47

Macroaggregated albumin (MAA) 402

Management decisions 121

Mann–Whitney U test 39
Mann–Whitney–Wilcoxon test 92
Many-way classification 76
Marginal distribution 95
Marginal tables 93
Matched filters 265–6
Mathematical models 139, 285, 325, 331–7, 431
Matrix algebra 82, 94
Maximization procedures 209
Maximum likelihood estimates 53, 90, 196, 200, 206, 213, 214, 409
Mean 12, 16, 20, 23, 28, 29, 30, 36, 44, 64, 296, 364
Mean absolute deviation (MAD) 14, 64
Mean arterial pressure 410
Mean inbreeding coefficient 169
Mean square 70
Mean square for treatments 70
Mean transit time 379, 393–5
Measurement error 10, 150–4
Measurement scales 137
Median 13, 23, 30, 39, 49, 50
Median polishing 76
Medical investigations, design of 55–64
Medical statistics, advanced techniques and computation 69–117
Mendelian segregation 207
Mendelian transmission 207
Michaelis–Menten coefficient 322, 356
Michaelis–Menten expression 327
Michaelis–Menten kinetics 324, 327
Michaelis–Menten mechanism 321, 322
Microcomputers 418
Mid-point 20
MINITAB 107
Missing values 80
Model building 69
Model parameters 139
Model reference adaptive control 409
Molar binding ratio 331, 332, 334, 342
Moving average filter 263
Multi-dimensional scaling 101
Multifactorial hypothesis 203, 204, 206, 208
Multifactorial phenotypes 201
Multiple comparisons 73
Multiple correlation 83
Multiple-dose function 320
Multiple-drug therapy 330
Multiple linear regression 81–6, 382

Multivariate analysis 48, 94–101
    introduction to 94–5
Multivariate analysis of variance (MANOVA) 100
Multivariate failure times 103
Multivariate Normal distribution 94–5, 143
Multiway contingency tables 92
Muscle relaxation, drug-induced 416–17
Mutation rate 172–3
MYCIN system 149
Myocardinal scanning 402

NAG library 105
Nearest neighbour models 142
Negatively skewed distribution 21
Newton–Raphson procedure 348
Noise 226, 244, 256–67, 407, 409, 421
Nominal data 11
Nominal scale 11
NONLIN computer program 345
Non-linear mapping 247
Non-linear models 284, 322, 327
Non-linear regression 49
Non-linear standard curves 284
Non-linear systems 321–3, 346
Non-orthogonal design 80
Non-parametric methods 38, 40
Non-stationary processes 226
Normal distribution 20–1, 23, 25, 29, 45, 52–4, 60, 420, 421
Normal plots 50
Normal probability graph paper 50
Normal range 276
Normal scores 50
Normality 24, 54
Nuclear decay 362
Nuclear families 196, 204, 208
Nuclear medicines 361–404
Null distribution 30, 32
Null hypothesis 30, 31, 34, 35, 43, 46, 52, 60, 63, 64, 97, 179, 186, 197
Numerical analysis 104
Numerical approximation 108
Nyquist diagram 407
Nyquist frequency 259

Observational studies 57
Observer error measurement 152–4
Observer variability 10
Odds ratio 89–92, 190

One-tailed test 30, 31
Open-loop control 416, 423
Operating characteristic curves 33
Operational research 277
Optimal control theory 408
Optimal filters 265–6
Optimization problems 285
Ordinal scale 11
Orthogonal design 71, 80
Orthogonal polynomial 104
Outliers 13, 21, 81, 287
Over-matching 58

P-values 109–10
P-waves detection 232–5, 243
    cross-correlation 234
    evaluation 235
    extrema 233–4
    filtering 232
    location of signal parts, windows 232
    threshold I 234
    threshold II 235
Pain levels 150
Pain relief, post-operative 417–22
Parallel-associative rule 434
Parameter estimation 426
Parameter identifiability 326, 407
Parameters 16
Parametric methods 102
Parent–daughter relationship 362–3
Parseval's theorem 262
Partial correlation 83
Partition coefficient 401
Path analysis 207
Pattern recognition 123, 226
Pedigree information 196
Pedigree studies 206
Performance assessment 154
Performance rankings 301
Peri-natal intensive care 251
Periodic components 260
Peri-operative intensive care 251
Pharmacokinetic parameters 323–7
    graphical technique 323–4
    numerical technique 324–5
Pharmacokinetics 307–30
    simulation 327–8
Phase angle 261
Phenotype distribution 178, 206
Phenotype frequency 166, 177–8, 184, 187

PI controller 408, 411, 415, 417
PID algorithm 408
PID controller 411, 425
Plotting 109
Point estimation 28–30
Point processes 103, 227
Poisson distribution 16, 17, 27, 289, 364
Pole-assignment 409
Polygenic hypothesis 200–5
Polygenic transmission 200–5
Polynomial least squares fits 376
Polynomial regression 84, 104
Population 15
Population distribution 15, 16
Population genetics 161–2
Population studies 193
Population survey 242
Positively skewed distribution 21
Power 32
Power curves 33
Power spectrum 261
Precision 99, 275
Precision profile 291, 293
Predictive procedures 141–3
Principal components analysis 95–7,
    380–1
Prior ignorance 55
Prior probability 54, 230, 231
Probabilistic models 149
Probability 15, 17, 33, 45, 46, 138–41,
    153–5
Probability density 147
Probability density function 228
Probability distribution 16, 55
Probability of ascertainment 195–6
Proband 195
Probit transformation 91
Proportional gain constant 408
Proportional hazards model 103
Proportions analysis 45–7, 88–91
Protein concentration 350
Protein–ligand binding 307, 330–56
    binding data analysis 337–47
    data analysis stratagem 346–7
    graphical techniques 337–43
    interpretation of binding coefficients
        347–8
    mathematical models 331–7
    numerical techniques 343–6
Pseudo-random binary sequences (PRBS)
    407, 410, 417

QRS typification 240–3
Quadratic effects 78
Quadratic score 155
Quality assessment, external techniques 300–2
Quality control 275, 283, 289, 294–302
    internal techniques 295–300
Quantization degree 256

Radioactive decay 362–4
    correction 369–70
Radioactive isotopes 361
Radioactive sample counting 364–9
Radioisotopes 361
Radionuclides 366
Random allocation rule 23
Random effects 77
Random errors 10, 18, 72, 83, 371, 375
Random numbers 22
Random sampling 22
Random variation 10, 50
Randomization 22–3, 59
Randomized block design 75
Range 13
Ranking 23, 27
Ranking indices 301
Rates, analysis of 88–91
Ratio scale 11
Recessive disorder 211
Recessive inheritance hypothesis 200
Recombination frequency 195, 210, 214
Recursive digital filters 263
Recursive least squares method 412
Reduced model 70
Reference range 276
Reference standards 287
Regression 47
Regression analysis 49, 294
Regression coefficient 49, 81, 103, 293
Regression technique 288, 291
Relative difference 192
Relative risk estimation 90, 162, 190–3
Reliability 15
Reliability assessment 155–6
Replicate analysis 290–1
Residual 14, 50–2, 79, 323
Residual mean square 70, 71
Residual mean squared error 67
Residual plots 51
Residual sum of squares 67, 70, 83, 343
Response–error relationship 291, 292

Response variables 12
Result assessment 294–302
Result derivation 283–94
Ridge regression 84
Ridit analysis 92
Risk factor 57, 102
Robust regression technique 346
Robustness 13, 23
Root-locus techniques 408
Runge–Kutta procedure 323

Sample 15
Sample size 59–61, 68
Sampled-data feedback 408
Sampling distribution 28
Sampling rate 258
Sampling theorem 258
SAS (Statistical Analysis System) 107
Satterthwaite's approximation 37
Scale 11
    measures of 14
Scatchard model 334, 336–8, 340, 347
Scatchard NIHH computer program 353
Scatchard plot 350–1
Scatter 19, 275
    diagram 47, 95
    measure of 13, 14
Scintillation 366
Segmentation 243–5
Segregation 206
Segregation analysis 198–200
Segregation frequency 194, 196, 197
Selection 180
Selection coefficient 172
Self-adaptive control structure 406
Self-tuning controller 406, 409
Sensitivity 301, 368
Sensitivity analysis 129, 417
Sequential designs 56
Sequential hypothesis testing 63
Sequential likelihood ratio 210
Sequential method 63–4
Sequential sign test 63
Serial-associative rule 433
Servo-anaesthetizer 414
Shape 19
Sheppard's corrections 257
Sickle cell anaemia 176
Sigmoid dose–response curve 287
Sign test 39
Signal classification 240

Signal processing systems 245–54
  biological 225–72
  mathematical definitions and techniques
    encountered 255–70
Signal sampling and quantization 256
Signal to noise ratio 230, 260, 266–7
Significance concept 30, 61
Significance level 30, 31, 34, 37, 38, 64
Significance test 30, 50, 102
Simple random sampling 22
Simpson's rule 281
Simulation 108
Simulation model 327
Simulation studies 422
Simulation techniques 277
Sinc function 259
Single-loop feedback design 406
SIR (Scientific Information Retrieval) 107
Site-binding coefficient 336, 338, 348
Site-binding model 333–7
Site equilibrium coefficient 333, 334
Skewness 21, 65
Slope factor 287
Smith predictor 409, 426
Smoothing function 376
Sodium concentration 387
Spearman's correlation coefficient (rho) 53,
  92
Spline-fitting 377
Spline functions 285
Spread, measures of 14
SPSS (Statistical Package for the Social
  Sciences) 106
Standard curve 283–6, 288, 291
Standard deviation (SD) 14, 20, 23, 28–30,
  36, 37, 44, 48, 60, 65, 275, 296, 364,
  371
Standard error 28–30, 37, 49, 50, 55, 65,
  66, 72, 73, 89, 102, 185, 187, 191,
  197, 204, 205, 374
Standard Normal distribution 20
Standard points 284, 285, 287
Standardization 88, 95
Standardized mortality ratio 89
State estimation 406
State vector 245
Statistical algorithms 105
Statistical calculations 104
Statistical inference 27–55
Statistical models 69–94
Statistical moments 255–6

Statistical significance 34
Stopwise regression 84
Stewart–Hamilton equation 396, 400
Stochastic signals 226–7, 259
Stoichiometric coefficients 335, 336, 345,
  348
Stoichiometric equilibrium coefficient 332
Stoichiometric (step-wise) model 332–7
Stopping rule 63
Stratified random sampling 22
Strongly stationary signals 256
Student's t test 286
Subjective probability 55
Sufficient statistics 25, 29
Sum of squares 70, 72, 74
Survival analysis 101–3
Symmetrical matrix 81
System dynamics 407, 409
System identification 405, 406, 408, 409
Systematic error 275

t distribution 22
t statistics 82
t tests 27, 39, 56, 59–61, 68, 101, 287
  one-sample 34–6, 65
  paired 38, 47, 66
  two-sample 36–8, 60, 66, 68, 75
  two-tailed 60
Technetium-99m generator 363–4
Technetium-99m labelled human serum
  albumin 397–9
Thyroliberin (TRH) test 280
Thyrotropin (TSH) measurement 280
Time series analysis 280
Tracer concentration 385
Tracer flow studies 382
Tracer techniques 361–404
Training set 98, 381
Transfer function 263, 264, 411, 418, 419,
  437
Transformations 26–7, 267–70
  arcsine 47
  monotonic 26
  normalizing 26
  to linearity 49
  variance stabilizing 27
Transient performance 408
Transit time spectrum 379, 380
Transmission frequencies 194
Transmission probability 207
Transport rate 383

Trapesium rule 281, 328
Trend detection 297
TRH (thyroliberin) test 280
Trigg's tracking signal 299
Trimmed means 13
TSH (thyrotropin) measurement 280
Tukey's test for non-additivity 79
Two-tailed test 31, 60
Two-way tables 93, 144
Type I error 32–4
Type II error 32–4, 60, 89
Typification 241, 243

Unbiasedness 28, 53
Unconditional probability 138
Unconsciousness, drug-induced 413–16
Unit delay operator 407
UNIVARIATE procedure 24
Utility 126
Utility assessment 134–6
Utility curves 135
Utility scales 136

Validity 23
Variables 11–12, 101
    non-numeric (or qualitative) 11
    numerical (or quantitative) 11
Variance 14, 20, 29, 37, 64
Variance components 194
Variance–covariance matrix 97, 241
Variance–covariance structure 143
Variance ratio 78
Variances, combination of 65
Variation in measurements 10
Variation sources 10
Vectorcardiogram 236, 248–9

Virtual flow 329
Visual analogue scales 91
V-shaped mask 298

Walsh functions 269
Walsh–Hadamard transformation 269–70
Washout curve 402
Washout time 403
Wave onsets and end points 235–8
    detection function 236
    training and templates 236
Waveforms 227, 229
Waveshape 227, 229
Weakly stationary signals 256
Weight analysis 208
Weighted regression 49, 85, 90
Weighting coefficients 264
Weighting factor 374
Weighting function 346, 377
White noise 409, 419
Wiener–Khintschin relation 261, 262
Wilcoxon matched pairs signed ranks test
    39
Wilcoxon rank sum test 39, 101
Wilks lambda 100–1
Winsorized means 13

X^2 statistic 40, 41

Yates' correction 46, 89

z-scores 95
z-transform 264, 265
Ziegler–Nichols rules 408
Ziegler–Nichols tuning method 417